Environmental Justice and the Rights of Unborn and Future Generations

Environmental Justice and the Rights of Unborn and Future Generations

Law, Environmental Harm and the Right to Health

Laura Westra

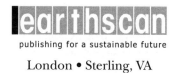

publishing for a sustainable future

London • Sterling, VA

First published in hardback by Earthscan in the UK and USA in 2006
Paperback edition first published in 2008

ISBN: 978-1-84407-550-8

Typeset by JS Typesetting Ltd, Porthcawl, Mid Glamorgan
Printed and bound in the UK by TJ International, Padstow
Cover design by Andrew Corbett

For a full list of publications please contact:

Earthscan
8–12 Camden High Street
London, NW1 0JH, UK
Tel: +44 (0)20 7387 8558
Fax: +44 (0)20 7387 8998
Email: earthinfo@earthscan.co.uk
Web: www.earthscan.co.uk

22883 Quicksilver Drive, Sterling, VA 20166-2012, USA

Earthscan publishes in association with the International Institute for Environment and
Development

A catalogue record for this book is available from the British Library

Library of Congress Cataloging-in-Publication Data

Westra, Laura.
  Environmental justice and the rights of unborn and future generations : law,
environmental harm, and the right to health / Laura Westra.
      p. cm.
  ISBN-13: 978-1-84407-366-5 (hardback)
  ISBN-10: 1-84407-366-1 (hardback)
  1. Unborn children (Law) 2. Right to life. 3. Environmental justice. I. Title.
  K642.W47 2006
  341.4'8572–dc22
                                    2006009673

The paper used for this book is FSC-certified and totally
chlorine-free. FSC (the Forest Stewardship Council) is an
international network to promote responsible management
of the world's forests.

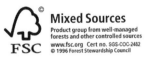

Mixed Sources
Product group from well-managed
forests and other controlled sources
www.fsc.org Cert no. SGS-COC-2482
© 1996 Forest Stewardship Council

FOR COLIN SOSKOLNE AND WILLIAM REES
THANK YOU FOR YOUR FRIENDSHIP, ENCOURAGEMENT AND SUPPORT –
THIS BOOK COULD NOT HAVE BEEN WRITTEN WITHOUT YOU

Contents

The globalization of human *rights* implies, too, the globalization of human *responsibilities*. For individual human rights holders, there is the responsibility to act in ways that show appropriate respect for the rights of fellow humans wherever they are located in the global community of rights. More significantly, for political and legal institutions – whether international, regional, national or sub-national – the responsibilities include promoting a culture of respect for human rights and exercising stewardship over those conditions that are essential for a flourishing community of rights.

In her latest book, Laura Westra proposes two important sets of responsibilities, one in relation to the next (and future) generations, the other in relation to the integrity of the environment. Yet, if the current generation of bearers of human rights have responsibilities only to one another, how can it be argued that their responsibilities extend to the unborn as well as to the environment? And, how can it be argued, as Westra suggests, that these are linked responsibilities?

First, if as fellow humans we must respect one another's rights, this means that we must not act in ways that threaten one another's freedom and well-being – or, at any rate, we must not so act without the authorization of the right-holder in question. If we take human rights seriously, so much is entirely straightforward.

Second, if (as surely is the case) the health of populations depends necessarily (if not sufficiently) on an adequate environmental infrastructure (clean air and water, and so on), then we threaten the well-being of human rights-holders if we damage that infrastructure. It follows that, even if the environment does not have rights, as fellow humans we owe it to one another to respect those environmental conditions that are essential for our well-being. In this sense, as members of a community of rights, we do have responsibilities in relation to the environment.

Third, even if (as the European Court of Human Rights has recently held in both *Vo v. France* and *Evans v. UK*) the unborn do not yet have human rights, it is arguable that once, as agents, we adopt reproductive purposes our responsibilities to embryonic rights holders are engaged. Even if we do no wrong by electing not to reproduce, it is arguable that the position changes once we elect to reproduce. Where we so elect, we must avoid damaging a future member of the community of rights.

Fourth, and quite simply, if we have responsibilities to future members of the community of rights and if we also have responsibilities to sustain the environment, then we must also owe those latter responsibilities to the former. In other words, our responsibilities in relation to the environment are ones that we owe to both existing and future members of a community of rights.

In a context of rapid technological innovation and change, it is crucial that communities of rights actively debate the nature and extent of their commitments – and, to this extent, it needs to be appreciated that the globalization of human rights is as much about process as about a finished product. Whether or not readers agree with the products of Laura Westra's arguments, it is a pleasure to introduce her book as a major contribution to the ongoing process of debate and discussion.

Roger Brownsword
Professor of Law, King's College London
and Honorary Professor in Law at the University of Sheffield

Acknowledgements

This book was inspired by the 2004 IV Ministerial Conference on Environment and Health, Budapest, Hungary, June 23–25, 2004, and by conversations with Dr Roberto Bertollini (WHO, Rome). This work extends the argument of my second doctoral thesis, *Ecoviolence and the Law* (2004a), to the most vulnerable in society, namely children, the unborn and future generations. Hence, I am grateful to Dr Marcus Stahlhofer and Dr Elizabeth Mason who allowed me to spend a month doing research in the Geneva Offices of the World Health Organization.

I am extremely grateful to Dr Colin L. Soskolne of the University of Alberta (Edmonton), for his constant help, collaboration and encouragement, as well as his recommendation to Dr Spady, which allowed me to participate in the important work of the Health Canada Health Policy Research Program Grant: 'Governance Instruments and Child Health: Informing Canadian Policy' (Spady, D. W., Soskolne, C. L., Buka, I., Ries, N., Nemer, L., Bertollini, R., and Osornio-Vargas, A. R. (August 1, 2004–January 31, 2006) (HC File #6795-15-2004/6450002).

The second half of the book was inspired by Dr William Rees, and his pioneering work on ecological footprint analysis, and supported by his grant from the Social Sciences and Humanities Research Council of Canada (SSHRC), 'Controlling Eco-Violence: Linking Consumption and the Loss of Ecological Integrity to Population Health, Eco-Justice and International Law'. Three year award from April 1, 2004 (File # 410=2004-0786);(PI: W. E. Rees, U.B.C., Co-applicant, C. L. Soskolne, Collaborator, L. Westra).

Thank are also due to Prof. Shelley Gavigan whose course on child law helped me to focus my research, and for her kindness and general encouragement.

Finally, special thanks to Osgoode Hall Librarian, Diane Rooke, who helped me throughout the writing of the book, and to Luc Quenneville of the University of Windsor for his outstanding technical support.

The somewhat radical views expressed in this work are entirely my own.

The traditional concept of social justice is challenged by a new philosophical vision of reality, characterized by interrelatedness and interdependence. It is only such a 'generality of outlook', to use A. N. Whitehead's own words to describe the vision of an interrelated and interdependent reality, that leads us to a 'morality of outlook' with its implied notion of social justice broadened to encompass the community of humankind as a whole, extending beyond present space and time.[1]

The most relevant point here is the question of 'broadened' social justice, that is, a notion to include 'the community of humankind'. It is undeniable that, thus far, future generations' rights have been linked to environmental regulations, at best, and cited primarily in aspirational and soft law documents, as well as making appearances in the preambular portions of general human rights conventions and environmental treaties, and we will look at those details in Chapters 5–7, below.

Most often, to speak of future generations, indicates, at best, a diffuse concern for the natural systems that are increasingly failing, because they are impoverished and depleted around the world. But, unless an immediate and forceful connection can be made with visible harms to nature or to human health, most view language about future generations to be the expression of a laudable but remote concern, not something that requires our immediate involvement, our efforts and energies.[2]

Their remoteness belies the interface between escalating ecological harms and humanity itself. Thus the erosion of global ecological integrity appears, at first glance, distant and even unrelated to social justice, in both its intragenerational and intergenerational aspects and, at times, it even appears to conflict with it. But both aspects of social justice, best captured in the concept of ecojustice, as I will argue below (Chapter 6), are neither distant nor remote, as they meet in the consideration of the rights of the first generation.

That generation is coming to be NOW, or it will come to be within our lifetime, without, however, losing its claim to be an integral part of the future of humanity as well. Perhaps then, from the point of 'ecological rights',[3] the presence of grave harms to this first generation, demonstrate precisely the connection between environment and humankind. That is where we can see exactly the havoc our current industrial practices are wreaking on the most vulnerable of humanity. The example of those harms force upon us a consideration of justice that is far more than the neo-liberal conception of freedom to embrace preferences. Such justice in fact, brings home the result of elevating the 'freedom' of natural and corporate persons to the status of ultimate goal in society.

This problem will become clear in the first four chapters, where the conflict between individual freedoms and rights, and the 'rights' of the first generation will be shown to come into conflict in most foundational legal instruments, both domestic and international, and – most violently perhaps – in the courts. These violent clashes and the circumstances that create them, will serve to diminish the importance of arguments stating that future generations don't exist now and that, even if they will come to be, we cannot be expected to modify law and morality on their behalf, as we don't know exactly who they are, and what their choices will be.

But the child born with flippers rather than hands or feet, because of pre-birth thalidomide exposure, or the baby with one eye because of dioxin exposure (as in the Seveso disaster, see Chapter 7), both clearly demonstrate without the need for complicated philosophical arguments, that (a) we do know what the first generation needs to be protected from, what they need for their security and what will harm them; and (b) we know that they will exist, and bear witness to our heedless pursuit of choice, to our tolerance of corporate, often criminal negligence and to what might be termed complicity on our part.[4]

No longer 'remote', or unreal, therefore morally unconsiderable and unfit to claim human rights like the rest of humanity, the first generation demonstrates the commonality of humankind, where neither time, nor age, nor geographical location should suffice to remove anyone from full consideration. At the same time as the plight of future generations comes 'alive' in the present and clear harms affecting the first generation, so too their own 'unreality', their lack of presence hence of considerability are no longer obvious. Their cause is linked with that of future generations who, paradoxically, appear to have more rights – at least in theory – than the first generation possesses.

Both future and first generations are far from being front and centre when human rights are at issue, even in the most prominent United Nations documents at present. I believe that viewing these two issues as one continuous aspect of justice for humanity, might help to shed light on both groups, so that neither will continue to remain invisible to either human conscience or international law. When both issues are studied side by side, we are struck by several points of similarity that are not considered as each issue is researched on its own.

The first point is that both are considered in law aside from their own intrinsic merits: as we shall see, for instance, future generations are considered in the context of environmental or trade issues, often against the background of conflicts arising between these two fields. When we turn to the child's rights to health, despite the presence of several international legal instruments devoted exclusively to child law, case law, for the most part views child law as derivative from family law. In the case of the preborn, this problem becomes acute, as the courts limit their consideration almost exclusively to the rights and the preferences of the pregnant woman: the situation is one where women's rights, based on proliferating instruments for their defence and protection, invariably trump whatever rights an unborn human might possess.

Thus we can observe that both issues are intrinsically hard to view objectively because they are significantly 'embedded', more or less literally, in other issues and concerns. Their underlying unity is thus disguised, although they are both issues of grave concern to humanity. But when considered in the way here proposed, that is as a unitary concern, they shed the limited perspective under which they were viewed and their common problems can best be appreciated and perhaps resolved.

Emmanuel Agius offers two other arguments in support of future generations' rights that, I believe, may apply equally to the first generations first, the argument from 'social justice and the weaker members of the human species',[5] and second, the argument for the development of human rights, after 'first' and 'second' generations' rights: the 'emergence of "solidarity rights" or "the third generation" of human rights in international environmental law'.[6]

These arguments will be defended below, in Chapter 8. For now, it may be sufficient to note that the description of both sets of circumstances, in support of evolving future generations' rights, fit as well the consideration of the first generation. The obligations generated by the acceptance of the former are equally significant for that of the latter:

> *In other words, social justice demands a sense of solidarity with the whole family of humankind. We have an obligation to regulate our current consumption: in order to share our resources with the poor and with unborn generations.*[7]

Thus, when we come to consider the best approaches in law to achieve this ideal of justice and solidarity, it is likely that whatever strategies we design for one issue, will ameliorate the situation for the other.

For now, we must start by showing clearly what is not there yet in the law: respect for either first or future generations is not embodied in the legal instruments that might be protective, either in domestic or international law. This fact needs to be demonstrated and in Part One we shall deal with the first generation in some detail, through the examination of both instruments and case law, before turning in Part Two, to future generations proper. We will then be in a better position to canvas existing regimes and jurisprudence, for the best available remedies presently existing, although perhaps not as well applied as they might be; but we will also consider all other possible options to bring about the necessary changes.

NOTES

1 Agius (1998), p4.
2 Westra (2000b), pp465–475.
3 Taylor, P. (1998).
4 Westra (2004a), Chapter 3.
5 Agius (1998), p9.
6 Agius (1998), p8.
7 Agius (1998), p10.

PART ONE

The Rights of the First Generation

The Child's Rights to Health and the Environment, and the Role of the World Health Organization

INTRODUCTION: CHILD PROTECTION AND FUTURE GENERATIONS' RIGHTS – THE ROAD TO ECOJUSTICE

This chapter starts with and is based on the foundational role played by the environment on these rights. The evidence amassed by the World Health Organization (WHO) is the starting point but, as we shall see, that evidence complements the findings of much of epidemiological, ecological and social literature on those issues. Hence all the evidence supports the expansion of human rights for which this work will argue. However, arguments based on science and moral principles are not enough to ensure that public policy will be consonant with our findings. We need to understand the full import of the harms perpetrated against children, now seen as the new 'canaries', by the present flawed and incomplete laws and regulations, both those that spell out their rights, and in general, the duty to protect children, and those which deal with environmental protection. These two forms of protection are inseparable, and their interface, we shall argue, forms the basis for 'ecojustice', that is justice that is both intragenerational and intergenerational at the same time (see Chapter 6).

The first of the future generations is at grave risk, as we shall see, right here and now. This must be the starting point, the basis of an understanding of the present situation, and of all present and future-oriented legal instruments. An example of a document that truly embraces all necessary requirements in its reach, is the *Earth Charter*.[1] The main point is that none of these issues can be fully appreciated when it is considered apart from others.

Environmental protection is insufficient if it does not include the consideration of all life, present and future; scientific uncertainty and the increasing use of the precautionary principle, make such an approach mandatory. Child protection, although it includes many important issues beyond the protection of life, health and normal function, *must* start with these 'basic rights', to paraphrase Henry Shue, as we shall see below. Protection of the child's right to religious freedom, to education, to a responsible and responsive family or substitute to nurture her growth and development, mean little if the child is born with serious mental, physical or emotional challenges, often irreversible, based on pre-birth or other early environmental exposure. Finally, future generations cannot be protected when the high-sounding rhetoric of the instruments designed for their protection does not generate immediate action, but is postponed indefinitely, while the first of those generations is negligently and carelessly harmed, often in ways that persist into the future.

To develop a just developmental ethic, we must seek to implement a form of global governance that includes the preconditions of human rights.[2] From that standpoint, the ecological basis for the developmental rights of infants and children, are also equally protected. As we will show, the foundations of children's rights to health must be built and respected long before the child sees light, or not at all. Thus '*developmental rights*' acquire a meaning analogous to the generally accepted meaning of the rights of peoples to development, when the referents are children.

No people or nation can truly achieve a successful development, now understood as including better social and economic conditions and the availability of education and personal freedom, unless each group member's rights are fully respected *from the start*, with the 'pre-conditions' of these rights,[3] as I will argue below. The rights of children to health and the environment[4] clearly demonstrate how early these 'preconditions' must be considered in this case, and these requirements must be factored into public policy and introduced in binding legal instruments, for the protection of all children.

The argument proposed below, however, is not that we ought to have as many children as possible, of course: 'responsible reproduction' means ensuring that reproductive choices include serious consideration of the rights of future generations and of those living now in the least developed countries, who have a strong right to their own resources and livelihood. It does mean instead, that the presence of a pregnancy imposes an immediate duty of respect for the health and the life of the embryo and the foetus. This responsibility accrues not only to the parents and their lifestyle choices: both national governments' and institutions', and multinational corporations' activities must reflect a similar duty in all their operations, from production, to the emphasis placed on consumption, to the so-called 'free trade' practices, to, ultimately, the problem of waste disposal.

This chapter will start with a consideration of the *Convention of the Right of the Child*, then continue to examine the foundation of child's rights, and the duty of institutional protection on the part of governments and individuals. The presence of an all-pervasive 'ecoviolence' against human life will be considered, before discussing the research of the WHO regarding harms to children. In conclusion, we will propose a stronger role for the WHO, and even the possibility of mandated interventions based on the 'international duty to protect'.

This chapter is intended as a survey of present circumstance, based on the WHO's research, and an initial discussion of obstacles and possible remedies for the child's health, before turning, in the next chapters, to a detailed examination of the status of the child in civil and in common law, through both instruments and cases, beyond the international approach here presented.

THE CONVENTION ON THE RIGHTS
OF THE CHILD AND ITS BACKGROUND

In Geneva the Fifth Assembly of the League of Nations (Records of the Fifth Assembly Supplement No. 23, League of Nations Official Journal, 1924), adopted the *Declaration of the Rights of the Child*. This declaration proposes five major principles to establish the duty of mankind regarding children:

a. *The child must be given the means requisite for its normal development, both materially and spiritually.*

b. *The child that is hungry must be fed; the child that is sick must be nursed; the child that is backward must be helped; the delinquent child must be reclaimed; and the orphan and the waif must be sheltered and succoured.*

c. *The child must be the first to receive relief in times of distress.*

d. *The child must be put in a position to earn a livelihood, and must be protected against every form of exploitation.*

e. *The child must be brought up in the consciousness that its talents must be devoted to the service of its fellow men.*

Nevertheless, unlike most modern human rights instruments, this document only 'invites States … to be guided' by these principles, yet does not even attempt to place binding obligations upon States.[5]

It is noteworthy that two of the major rights to be recognized at later dates are not specifically mentioned in this document: the right to life, and the right to nationality, hence, to protection. Both of these rights will be discussed below, as they represent core values and principles that support not only these principles (1924), and the recommendations of later documents, but also the findings of the WHO.[6]

Although the principles of the Geneva Declaration were non-binding, the instrument formed the basis of the Social Commission of the Economic and Social Council of the United Nations' instruments intended to form a *United Nations Charter of the Rights of the Child*. The Charter was eventually adopted by the General Assembly on 20 November 1959.[7] The Charter includes a 'Preamble' and ten Articles. Notably, according to Principle 3, a child is entitled to a name and nationality; and Principle 4 adds the right to 'adequate nutrition, housing, recreation and medical services'. Protection is explicitly mentioned in Principle 9 (the protection against neglect). This Charter will not be the main focus of attention here because it has been superseded by the *Convention on the Rights of the Child*[8] (1989), which is the instrument presently in force. But it is important to note with Geraldine Van Bueren, that:

By 1959, however, children are beginning to emerge no longer as passive recipients but as subjects of international law recognized as being able to enjoy the benefits of specific rights and freedoms.[9]

This emergent reality has a further effect:

> *the proposition that individuals can be subjects of international rights necessarily involves the corollary that they can be subjects of international duties; the cogency of the claim to the former gains by an admission of the latter.*[10]

Thus we must not lose sight of the fact that entrenching the right to life and that of protection (through 'nationality', see below), in international law, does far more that exhort states to ensure general human rights, and perhaps other special duties to children: it obligates both states and individuals (natural and legal) to fulfil these obligations.

As human rights instruments evolved and proliferated, it became increasingly clear that children require rights in addition to those enjoyed by adults, because of their 'social vulnerability and immaturity'.[11] Thus, even the same rights that are present in instruments intended for adult individuals, require different forms of interpretation when the focus intended is the child. For instance, there is far less controversy internationally on what defines an adult, within a certain age range being prevalent in domestic laws, than on the inception of childhood.[12]

This question is one of the major focuses of this work, given the ample evidence provided by the WHO and others on the violence that is environmentally caused prebirth,[13] and we will return to this topic. For now, it is sufficient to note that, for instance, although the general consensus is that states are allowed to establish the point where life begins, thus where the state is required to guarantee protection, the *American Convention on Human Rights* states:

> *Every person has the right to have his life respected. This right shall be protected by law and in general from the moment of conception.*[14]

The *Declaration of the Rights of the Child* of 1959, also provides:

> *Whereas the child by reason of his physical and mental immaturity needs special safeguards and care, including appropriate protection, before as well as after birth.*

But in 1924, no definition of the child was provided, thus leaving this critical issue undiscussed:

> *The issue, however, is critical, because if childhood begins from the moment of conception then the child's 'inherent right to life' contained in Article 6(1) of the Convention on the Rights of the Child and in other international treaties, applies from the moment of conception.*[15]

The *Convention on the Rights of the Child* (CRC) was adopted by the UN General Assembly on 20 November 1989[16] and it entered into force on 2 September 1990.

THE RIGHT TO NATIONALITY AND THE RIGHT OF THE DUTY OF PROTECTION IN LAW

Before venturing into the minefield of questions about the right to life and the defini-tion of the child, where the extent of the duty to protect those rights is the main con-cern, it might be best to establish the grounds upon which protection is based. Article 7 of the CRC states:

> *Article 7.1 The child shall be registered immediately after birth and shall have the right from birth to a name, the right to acquire a nationality and, as far as possible, the right to know and be cared for by his or her parents.*
>
> *2. States Parties shall ensure the implementation of these rights in accordance with their national law and their obligation under the relevant international instruments in this field, in particular where the child would otherwise be stateless.*

The language of this article follows upon that of Article 24(2)[17] of the *International Convention on Civil and Political Rights* (ICCPR). The question of nationality is particularly relevant, because a nationality is based on a state's responsibility to protect:

> *Nationality may be defined as the status of belonging to a state for certain purposes of international law. Each state regards itself as having certain rights and duties vis-à-vis other states and regarding its own nationals.*[18]

Nationality is present either 'by descent from parents who are nationals (*jus sanguinis*)', or 'by virtue of being born with the territory of the state (*jus soli*)' (ibid.) Nationality can also be acquired by marriage, adoption or naturalization. According to the *Universal Declaration of Human Rights* (UDHR)[19] Article 15, 'Everyone has the right to a nationality, and this declaration has now become customary international law'.[20] In addition, Article 24(3) of the ICCPR states that 'Every child has the right to acquire a nationality' as was already stated in the 1959 UN Declaration of the Rights of the Child. At Article 24(1), the ICCPR provides that:

> *1. Every child shall have without any discrimination as to race, colour, sex, language, religion, national or social origin, property or birth, the right to such measures of protection as are required by his status as a minor, on the part of his family, society and the State.*

State responsibility for the protection of its citizens is a given in international law, the existing case law focuses primarily on the relation between rights, and the citizens' duty of allegiance to the state, thus on the foundation of the right to nationality and protection.[21] These cases deal almost entirely with treason and with this allegiance due to one's state and one's nationality (even when abroad). Therefore these cases are far removed from the question of nationality, thus protection of the child.

Nevertheless, the discussion in the Joyce case shows most clearly the extent of the protection entailed by nationality. In this case, Lord Jowitt, L.C. discusses William Joyce, born in the US, one-time resident of Ireland, then for some years, a resident of England, who eventually, describing himself as a 'born British subject', applied for and received a British passport. Using this document he travelled to Germany, where he worked against the interest of his country of nationality (Britain), as an announcer for the German Radio, and a purveyor of German propaganda. In 1945 he was arrested and brought to trial for treason. His case is interesting because it analyses in detail the relation between the protection entailed by nationality and the duty of allegiance on the part of the citizen, based upon the acceptance of that protection.

Lord Jowitt L.C. appeals to feudal law as the origin of the relation between the citizen and 'the king':

> *Whether you look to the feudal law for the origin of this conception or find it in the elementary necessities of any political society, it is clear that fundamentally it recognizes the need of the man for protection and of the sovereign lord, for service.* Protectio trahit subjectionem et subjectio protectionem.

Thus the starting point is the inseparable connection between nationality and the *duty* to protect it engenders. The second step is the necessity for all natural born persons (as well as others, 'naturalized subjects') to remain nationals with all the responsibilities and duties that condition entails. This is vitally important because, as we saw above, nationality imposes duties but ensures protection:

> *The natural born subject cannot at common law any time cast it off. Nemo potest exurer patriam is a fundamental maxim of the law* ...[22]

But children cannot betray the 'sovereign', or be traitors, hence their nationality and the correlative right to protection is secure. Guaranteed by human rights instruments such as the ICCPR, as well as the CRC, their right to protection is absolute.

Glanville Williams argues that 'protection' must be understood to encompass two senses:

> *protection of the individual against the activities of others (whether such protection takes the form of force or persuasion), and respect for the individual by the sovereign in the course of his own activities.*[23]

Thus, in modern times, the state must (1) exert itself to protect each citizen against all harmful activities by others against the citizen; and (2) it must restrain its own activities (and decisions) to demonstrate the respect to which the citizen has a right. Williams views the state's or sovereign's duty of positive protection as including the provision of police protection, and in general of 'positive physical protection', as one which does not extend outside the state's territory. The additional occasional presence of diplomatic protection instead, is given 'as of grace', rather than by duty.[24]

On the other hand, the question of 'respect' is particularly important: the state must tailor its own activities and, I argue, the activities it permits all actors, natural and legal, to pursue, to be compatible with the respectful protection all citizens are entitled to have.

The second category, 'negative protection' as Williams terms it, includes both 'law abidingness of the sovereign', and 'abstention from interference'.[25]

Therefore a government that permits or provides licences for hazardous operations, acts in violation of the primary legal and moral maxim 'do no harm', a maxim that is routinely enforced in penal law. By permitting, perhaps even encouraging through tax cuts and other benefits, operations that may result in harm to life, the government may be interfering with the health of its citizens or be complicit in such interference on the part of other organizations, institutions or legal corporate persons.[26]

I have discussed citizens' responsibility in detail elsewhere.[27] I concluded that while such responsibility (for over consumption for instance) is a clear reality, it is modified by several mitigating factors that are absent from corporate and governmental responsibility instead. These factors include (a) the lack of clear scientific information about the harms inherent in present 'consumers' practices: not only does scientific uncertainty play a part, but it is deliberately emphasized and magnified by corporate marketing strategies, as they avail themselves of all possible legal protections as well (e.g. trades secrets acts); (b) the ongoing discourse that minimizes the harmful results through obscuring language,[28] and describes over consumption as normal, desirable and even patriotic (according to recent propaganda by the Bush administration); and (c) the psychological background of 'crimes of obedience' or as I have termed them, 'crimes of compliance',[29] as they are played out against the background of an increasingly amoral body politic, steeped in the neo-liberal economic agenda.

In addition, a large literature exists in philosophy and political theory on the inappropriateness of considering 'tacit consent' (of citizens) as a form of consent at all.[30] Finally we must realize that even in Western democracies, certain choices are not available even to an informed, altruistic and intelligent electorate (were it present): for instance, no election in Canada offers the choice of a party that would eliminate nuclear power.

Therefore, without denying the element of choice that is present for consumers in relation to various hazardous practices, such choice loses much of its meaning when it is manipulated by economic interests,[31] uniformed or even unavailable.

In contrast, corporate bodies have full information about their products and processes, a strong interest in the support and promotion of over consumption, and have the financial resources to produce the marketing strategies they need.

A final question is highly relevant: that is the 'physical' aspect of the basic protection to which all are entitled. This is the necessary protection as understood for instance by the European Court of Justice in its recent judgements, protection of the 'physical and biological integrity' of the citizens of two countries, Italy and Spain, over their respective governments' decisions to tolerate harmful industrial operations.[32]

In the next section we will discuss the interface between the duty of protection and the possibility of harm to the child.

THE POSITIVE DUTY OF PHYSICAL PROTECTION FROM HARM AND THE DEFINITION OF THE CHILD

There is no need to revisit the vast literature available on environmental hazards, many of which are fostered by current business practices, consumption patterns,[33] and climate change.[34] The most important issue from our standpoint is whether these hazards produce more significant harms when children are affected and if, so, what follows from this discovery.

The sequence appears to be: (1) a child has nationality from birth; (2) nationality entails physical protection; therefore (3) the latter is unequivocally due to the child who would have neither the motive nor the means to fail in their allegiance to the state. But a difficulty arises, in that modern science indicates that the child cannot simply be protected from birth, if the duty to protect is taken seriously.[35] If a child at birth, or thereafter, manifest the effects of exposure to a toxicant *in utero*, that harm to the present child and to the future adult denotes a failure on the part of the government in the duty to protect.

This duty could be discharged by controlling the production and distribution of the toxic substance, by insisting on mandatory disclosure of all possible effects of that substance, or even by disallowing the substance altogether. Such duty, of course, is not theirs alone. The industries and business corporations, including the pharmaceutical companies that may be producing these toxic substances, are also under the duty not to do harm, and to disclose fully what their R&D departments are discovering but first of all have the duty not to produce and distribute any substance that has not been fully tested.

The precautionary principle,[36] rather than economic necessities, should govern the decisions of when to release products that may not have been fully tested. According to the *Declaration of Helsinki on Human Testing*, individuals, let alone groups cannot be treated as guinea pigs to ultimately test these products at little or no cost to the producers, even if they would consider the costs of possible litigations arising from the resulting harms. An example of the dangers of these products is that of thalidomide: all drugs containing thalidomide were clearly not tested long enough to ensure that, once distributed, we should not confront the birth of children born with flippers instead of arms and legs, as well as many other malformations. These substances do not harm the mothers but they produce devastating effects because they affect embryos, thus the children that will be born. Any regulative instrument that limits its reach to what may affect born children misses the many ways embryos may be gravely affected, long before children are born.[37] Therefore, governments who are committed to the protection of human rights should be able to prioritize these rights, even when the resulting principles of justice may fly in the face of present day customs or political correctness, such as permitting normal day-to-day business practices without additional critical monitoring.

Indirect harms, perpetrated through the environment and through the ingestion or aspiration of toxicants must be taken in consideration when regulatory bodies enact laws. This need is particularly acute for children, as we shall see below, but it is vital for adults as well. For the issue of children's specific needs, the definition of the child in international law is a critical starting point:

> *Traditionally a child has been defined as a comparative negative: a child is an individual who is not yet an adult.*[38]

But the Preamble to the *Declaration of the Rights of the Child* (1959) is the first legal instrument to focus on the most debated point, that is, the start of the child's life:

Whereas the child by reason of his physical and mental immaturity needs special safe-
guards and care, including appropriate legal protection, before and after birth.

In addition, Article 4, *American Convention on Human Rights* provides that:

He shall be entitled to grow and develop in health; to this end, special care and protec-
tion shall be provided to him and his mother, including adequate pre-natal and post-
natal care.

These documents are clear, and correspond to the general popular belief in the
mother's right to prenatal care hence, to the pre-birth rights of the child, even though
the full extent to the effect of endocrine disruptors and other toxic substances on the
embryos was not fully known at the time. Only the *American Convention on Human Rights*
provides that, 'Every person has the right to have his life respected. This right shall
be protected by law and in general from the moment of conception'. The words 'in
general' allow states to intervene to save a mother's life, or in the case of rape. These
are also evident concerns of the European Commission, as it rejects the possibility of
guaranteeing an absolute right to life to the foetus, although it concedes that, 'certain
rights are attributable to the conceived but unborn child, in particular the right to
inherit'.[39]

Yet the right of the unborn not to be attacked through violence, directed also at the
mother, or through alcohol or drugs exists today. For instance, as early as 1987, Thomas
Murray in his paper 'Moral obligations to the not-yet born: the fetus as a patient',
argued that the age of the foetus is not relevant to the harms it may suffer in the womb.
If someone attacks a pregnant woman and beats her without killing either her or her
foetus, but the child is subsequently born paralysed the action is both morally wrong
and actionable.[40] Murray concluded that 'the timing of the harm is irrelevant', and his
position is supported by the US Congress, Office of Technology Assessment's document
Reproductive Health Hazards in the Workplace.[41]

In 1964 W.L.Prosser[42] argued that after 1946 began:

the most spectacular abrupt reversal of a well-settled rule in the whole history of the law
of torts. The child, provided that he is born alive, is permitted to maintain an action
for the consequences of prenatal injuries, and if he dies of such injuries after birth, an
action will lie for wrongful death.

All arguments proposing a role for viability in our consideration of foetal harms, are
not well taken, especially after the discovery of the effect a mother's exposure to endocrine disruptors and other environmental toxicants, as well as non-ionizing electromagnetic fields, alcohol consumption, tobacco smoke, pesticide residues and some
pharmaceuticals.[43] The effects of these exposures are particularly grave in the earlier
stages of embryonic life, not in the last trimester.

We will return to examine the clinical issues in more detail below, in 'World Health
Organization findings for policy guidance', after discussing why solid grounds for
human rights include general individual and institutional responsibility for the 'pre
conditions' of agency even for adults. The moral and logical basis for this position will
be the topic of the next section.

THE PRECONDITIONS OF AGENCY AND THE GROUNDS OF HUMAN RIGHTS

The connection between environmental degradation and human life, health and normal function rests upon the inviolability of human rights. Although a detailed analysis of all existing arguments in their support is beyond this scope of this work, we will revisit briefly some of those arguments in support of our own that these human rights extend beyond the right of the human person, to the generic right to life, including our habitat. The foundation arguments proposed by Alan Gewirth help to shed light on that basic connection between humans and their habitats. Gewirth argues that human rights are not based primarily on human dignity,[44] but this Kantian principle is only partially right. He prefers to base 'human rights on the necessary conditions of human action',[45] as morality is intended to give rise to moral action. Gewirth adds that 'human rights are the equivalent to "natural" right, in that they pertain to all humans by virtue of their nature as actual or prospective agents'.[46] He cites five reasons in support of his claim:

> *(1) 'the supreme importance, of the condition of human actions' (and we will return to this point below); (2) action is 'the common subject matter of all moralities'; (3) 'action' is more specific and less vague than 'dignity' or 'flourishing'; (4) thus 'action' ultimately secures 'fundamental moral status' for persons; (5) 'action's necessary conditions provide justification for human rights – as every agent must hold that he has a right to freedom and well-being as the necessary conditions of his actions'*[47]

Beyleveld and Brownsword argue that the 'basic' or 'generic needs' that represent the preconditions of all action including moral action are 'freedom or voluntariness' and 'well-being or purposiveness', where the former are procedural and latter 'substantive',[48] and they view freedom as instrumental to well-being. I want to propose inverting this order. Life, health and the mental ability to comprehend and choose precede the exercise of voluntariness and are not only necessary for it, but sufficient, when all these conditions are in fact present.

In essence 'basic rights',[49] represent the minimum all humans are entitled to, and they are prior to all other rights, both conceptually and temporally. For Gewirth as well, life and the capacities named can be 'threatened or interfered with'.[50] Thus to say we have a right to free agency is to say equally that the preconditions of these rights represents something we are entitled to have not only in morality but also in the law. In other worlds any legal instrument that supports the existence of human rights, *ipso facto* ought to proclaim the requirement that their preconditions be equally supported and respected.

Some argue that the dignity of human beings is only partially the ground of human rights and that dignity itself is based on agency, still the argument allows the introduction of at least a further point in favour of extending human rights to life and health. The introduction of 'preconditions' means the introduction of conditions that are not only conceptually but temporally prior to agency, hence the protection of these preconditions entails the acceptance of potential consequences in the protection of agency.

Arguments about potentiality have been discussed in a rather cavalier fashion in the extensive literature on abortion, only to re-emerge more recently because of the presence of the rights of the child (to be) while *in utero*. For instance, Deborah Mathiew says:

> *Thus even if the fetus is not considered a person in the moral or legal sense, there are still important interests of a person which must be weighted against those of the pregnant woman: the interest of the future child. A pregnant woman should act for the sake of the child that the fetus will become. Her obligations, in other words, are to her future child, not to her fetus.*[51]

Given that the potential for developing certain genetic conditions has been used to explain or justify abortion, is hard to see why the future should be viewed as suspect when it is used to proscribe it, instead, in cases where concern for the child's future health is not an issue.[52] Beyleveld and Brownsword argue that it is not necessary to support the presumed dignity of the embryo from conception:

> *it is the consideration of the possibility that the zygote might be an agent (and have dignity) even though there is little evidence of this.*[53]

The authors continue by citing the possible rights of the pregnant woman in this respect. To destroy the foetus by removing it from its first natural habitat, however, clearly violates the preconditions of its eventual agency, even if, with the authors, we accept the view that agency is the ground of human dignity.[54]

Moving instead to consider Singer's position, as foundational, thus grounding rights in sentience[55] or even that of David De Grazia on 'nociception',[56] we have more than dignity, or even dignity-as-agency, where the Gewirthian 'Principle of Proportionality' maintains that agents have 'duties to all living creatures (human or non-human) on a proportional basis'.[57]

A discussion of the detailed arguments for and against abortion or the use of embryos would take us too far afield. Yet even this brief analysis indicates that the presence of life ought to be the most important category to render beings worthy of respect and consideration, aside from their present or possible mental states.

Kant defends the infinite value of life, as someone whose generic capacities to be human, with all that it might entail, is not eliminated by a present adverse condition, such as regular drunkenness, for instance. Non-human animals have also been deemed to have purposiveness,[58] so that the same could be said of foetuses, according to the comparable development of their nervous system at various stages, and they certainly do have nociception as an indication of the capacities they will possess later in their development.[59] If at least duties are owed to all beings capable of sentience and agency in various proportions, then the duty is not specific, but it can be owed to all life, and to its preconditions, that is to the habitats whose 'fittingness' supports our own. That is to say, by extending the meaning of dignity from its modern sense of *dignitas*, to its classical Greek sense of being within the natural laws of the universe, one may be able to place Kant's imperatives within the more far-reaching imperatives of the 'principle of integrity'.[60] In this case, anything that conflicts with the 'dignity' of natural universal laws is prima facie suspect, hence – minimally – it requires serious justification, beyond 'preferences'[61] or economic advantages.

Although this philosophical discussion is peripheral to the main argument of this paper, some recent work by Michael Hauskeller also emphasizes not only the connection, but the possible identity of biological integrity and the dignity of human beings.[62]

In fact these extended rights, or the pre-conditions of the rights themselves are everyone's entitlement, and those who deliberately or negligently impose the harms described in the section entitled 'The positive duty of physical protection from harm and the definition of the child' should be considered to be guilty of crimes directly or indirectly, or of complicity in those crimes.

THE PRESENCE OF INSTITUTIONALIZED VIOLENCE: ECOCRIMES AND INTERNATIONAL LAW

In the preceding pages, the duty to protect from harm was located in the presence of nationality giving rise to state obligations. But many of the existing international legal instruments enshrine rights and obligations that – when violated – can be viewed as crimes committed in and through the environment, although children are not specifically mentioned in these documents.[63]

In addition, it is not only illegal activities that produce harmful and often lethal results, but also activities that are presently viewed as legal, because standards are not scientifically established, but negotiated. Christian Tomuschat says:

> *In a shrinking world, where any activity that modifies fragile ecological patterns tends to have repercussions beyond national borderlines, it becomes even more necessary to establish standards suited to save those natural cycles and thereby to ensure the foundations of human survival.*[64]

State responsibility arises both when an unlawful act has been committed and when there are harmful consequences from legal activities. In both cases *jus cogens* norms can be invoked to deal with environmental damage.[65] Two points must be clarified before proceeding. First, on the question of fault versus consequences, the hostages case in *United States v. Iran*, 1980 I.C.J.3, at 69, 70, shows that the duty of the Iranian government was to take 'every appropriate step' to bring 'the flagrant infringements' of international law to a speedy resolution. In fact, 'No such step was taken', although states have the duty to regulate private actors in their territory. In this cause it appears that the fault element makes this an even stronger case that 'Iran had violated ... its obligation toward the United States'.[66] Another point of clarification is that of moral implications of *jus cogens* norms, beyond their legal status.

In *Wiwa v. Royal Dutch Petroleum Co.*, for instance, it is clear that because no state was involved, one could not bring a case against Shell for the breach of a treaty obligation; Shell had to be charged with the breach of *erga omnes* obligations supported by *jus cogens* norms, because of the moral and legal principles they violated, in flagrant conflict with international law, especially 'crimes against humanity'. The second problem is the possibility that although the harm is visible and present, the act that generated the harmful consequences, was itself legal. The classic example is once again the Trail Smelter Arbitration.[67] As various forms of technology become more widespread and complex, the environmental harm that ensues, whether it is immediate or – as it is most often the case – delayed, it becomes precisely what this work suggests: a legal, institutionalized form of violence, producing harms that are often irreversible. `

The problem of transboundary harm was first considered in a study by a subcommittee of the International Law Commission in 1963 to deal with the 'conspicuous gap' left in international law by the exclusion of 'liability that derives from ... legal grounds'.[68] Several Rapporteurs and many iterations of that particular aspect of state responsibility uncovered several major points.

First, states are in a position to control specific activities. Hence, they should bear responsibility for the consequences arising from such activities. This appears unobjectionable. The second point, however, is more debatable, as it raises the question of transboundary liability for the 'global commons', as introduced by Rapporteur Barboza (1989 ILC Rep. 242, para. 348). The third point follows upon the other two: often negative effects are produced that reach well beyond the intended effects, thus producing a 'normative gap' that ought to be addressed by international law.[69] Fourth, modern scientific developments have indicated the immense scope of environmental problems such as climate change, global warming or biogenetic engineering, all of which are 'dangerous activities' and 'for whose consequences states must bear full responsibility'.[70]

Finally, whether the dangerous activities are undertaken by public or private sources, states must ensure that they assume full responsibility for all activities that place human rights in jeopardy. In addition, no private person or institution can ensure prevention, as a state can and must:

> *Experience has taught that more often than not damage to the environment cannot be made good after it has occurred. When a species of animals has disappeared it cannot be revived again. Soil that has been contaminated may have to rest for decades before it can be recultivated. Radioactive particles that have escaped a nuclear installation pose a threat to their environment as long as their radiation continues. The ozone layer, once destroyed may never build up again. Thus the primary goal must be to prevent harm from occurring. Second pollution caused by a major disaster, but also pollution caused by accumulation, may easily take on such huge dimensions that both in financial and in technological terms, reparation is simply impossible.[71]*

Against this background, we can consider now some specifics.

For instance, the 1996 ILC Report, chapter 4, defines the state obligation of 'due diligence'.[72] Germany and Switzerland disagreed on absolute liability for the pollution of the Rhine by Sandoz, but 'the Swiss government acknowledged responsibility for lack of "due diligence" in preventing the accident through adequate regulation of its pharmaceutical industries'.[73] The *Convention on the Protection of the Rhine* (1997), following the Rhine Action Programme adopted in 1987 (8th Ministerial Conference of the Rhine States, 1987), after the Sandoz accident,[74] adopts the ecosystem approach and is aimed at the sustainable development of the Rhine area, thus controlling not only the actions of the riparian states, but those of all states involved in industrial activities having an impact in the area (in the case of Sandoz, including Switzerland).

The UK defined due diligence as 'such care as government ordinarily employ in their domestic concerns'. A US definition can be found in the Alabama case (*United States v. Britain*):

> *[A] diligence proportional to the magnitude of the subject and the strength of the power which is to exercise it, a diligence which shall, by the use of active vigilance, and of all other means in the power of the neutral, through all stages of the transactions, prevents its soil from being violated; a diligence that shall, in like manner deter designing men from committing acts of war upon the soil of the neutral against its will.*

Returning to international law, the elements of the ILC convention's work on legal transboundary environmental harm were 'prevention, co-operation, and strict liability for harm', but they were considered 'too controversial'.[75] The 2001 amended draft of this convention,[76] divided the topic into two parts, 'prevention and liability' and the main concern remained the former, not the latter.[77] Although the latest draft prescribes 'all appropriate measures that must be taken to prevent or minimize the risk', it does nothing to prohibit the activites that give rise to transboundary harm.[78]

Risk itself is defined to encompass both 'a low probability of causing disastrous harm' and 'a high probability of causing significant harm.'[79] However, neither 'disastrous' nor 'significant' are defined, and neither international lawyers, nor judges nor even scientists can hope to express with any certainty what might constitute the desired 'clear and convincing' scientific proof of possible harm.

In addition, the standard of due care or due diligence must be proportional to 'the degree of risk of transboundary harm in the particular instance', and can be expected to change with time and must take into consideration 'location; special climate conditions; materials used in the activity;' and so on (at para. 12, 'Commentary' on Art. 3). Higgins, who analyses state responsibility, rather than liability, states that 'the only requirement is causality', which entails that 'responsibility is based on result, not fault'.[80] Special Rapporteur James Crawford explains:

> *In particular article [1] stated that every internationally wrongful act of a State entails its responsibility, and article [3] identified two and two only elements of an internationally wrongful act, (a) conduct attributable to a State which (b) is inconsistent with its international obligations. There was no distinct or separate requirement of fault or wrongful intent for an internationally wrongful act to be held to exist.[81]*

Hence, even in the latest iteration of the ILC, international law does not require intent for the commission of a 'crime' (although this language is no longer part of the ILC), and Higgins' point stands. Thus, the common argument of corporate or institutional wrong-doers, adducing lack of intent as exonerating or at least mitigating their responsibility, cannot be defended as even the due diligence defence is not allowed internationally.

The right to life is basic in law and, for instance, the *European Convention for the Protection of Human Rights and Fundamental Freedoms* (1950), has that right in its Article 2, and throughout the article by juridical extension, the right is coupled with that of 'physical integrity'.[82] Hence an activity that has even the potential to expose us to grave risks to life and our 'physical integrity' means that the state is allowing a corporate entity to use present and future generations as guinea pigs, effectively to test the result of their activities, and this practice should be eliminated.

In essence, presently existing international human rights instruments provide arguments to define as criminal the activities that result in harms to persons and especially to the most vulnerable among them – the children. These harms, I have argued, may be defined as 'ecocrimes', under several appropriate headings:

> 4.a   *Ecocrimes as a Form of Unprovoked Aggression;*[83]
> 4.b   *Ecocrimes as Attacks on the Human Person;*[84]
> 4.c   *Ecocrimes as a Form of Genocide;*[85]
> 4.d   *Ecocrimes as a Breach of Global Security;*[86]
> 4.e   *Ecocrimes as Attacks on the Human Environment;*[87]
> 4.f   *Ecocrimes as Breaches of Global Justice;*[88]

Hence this work stated at the outset the importance of the linkage between environment/ human rights and public health, and the need to ensure the presence of an international instrument such as the *Earth Charter*. Even if only considered to be 'soft law', or if it is viewed as a summary of customary principles accepted in international law, the *Earth Charter* would provide a basis from which to argue that even if domestic law does not provide sufficient protection at this time, international law's principles and the courts and ad hoc tribunals convened to defend these principles should do so.

In the next section we shall briefly sum up the findings of the WHO and others regarding the interface between the environment and children's health.

CHILDREN'S RIGHT TO HEALTH: OBSTACLES, CHALLENGES AND THE ROLE OF THE WHO

Before turning to the findings of the WHO, a true 'state of the art' summary of what science has demonstrated about the relations between an ecologically sound environment and human rights, specifically those of children, we need to start by defining public health and the role of the WHO in that regard. What is 'public health'? It can be defined as 'what we as a society do collectively to ensure the conditions in which people can be healthy'.[89]

Thus public health is understood to be more than disease control; it must involve society as a whole in both the activities required to achieve public health, and those that run counter to that ideal. The definition also emphasizes that it is *collective* responsibility, not exclusively a state responsibility as was argued above. The goal of Public Health requires consideration under three headings. David Fidler explains:

> Assessment *means collecting and analyzing data in order to identify and understand the major health problems facing a community.*
>
> Policy Development *establishes goals, sets of priorities, and develops strategies to address health problems.*
>
> Assurance of Services *involves the design, implementation and evolution of programs to address priority health problems in the community.*[90]

The largest and most authoritative body concerned with public health is the WHO, and their definition of health itself, in the 'Preamble' of the *Constitution of the World Health Organization*,[91] merits serious consideration:

> *Health is a state of complete physical, mental and social well-being and not merely the absence of disease or infirmity.*

In the same 'Preamble', the health of children is mentioned, and its relation to the environment is noted:

> *Healthy development of the child is of basic importance; the ability to live harmoniously in a changing total environment is essential to such development (see also chapter II, Article 2 (1)).*

The World Health Organization is an authoritative body, as part of the UN, thus it is not purely a medical/technical agency. The importance of their status was clearly demonstrated when the WHO requested an *opinio juris* from the UN General Assembly, after the International Court of Justice in the *Legality of the Use by a State of Nuclear Weapons in Armed Conflict*[92] determined that the WHO lacked the constitutional authority to ask the question posed.[93] The question posed was:

> *In view of the health and environmental effects, would the use of nuclear weapons by a State in war or other armed conflict be a breach of its obligations under international law including the WHO Constitution?*

The response of the Court, as indicated, was that although Article 65, para. 1 of the Court's Statute provides that, 'The Court may give an advisory opinion …' in this case, the Court refused because of the Court's lack of jurisdiction in this case, and because the question, as posed, was 'vague and abstract'. When the question was again posed by the General Assembly, 'the Court concluded that it has the authority to deliver an opinion on the question posed by the General Assembly, and that there exist no "compelling reasons" which would lead the Court to exercise its discretion not to do so'. This historic encounter between the International Court and the WHO ended with a debated and weak opinion; nevertheless it ended with an opinion being given after all. Kindred et al describe the event:

> *The Court held unanimously that there is in neither customary nor conventional international law any specific authorization of the threat or use of nuclear weapons; by 11 votes to 3, that there is in neither customary nor conventional international law any comprehensive and universal prohibition of the threat or use of nuclear weapons as such; unanimously, that threat or use of force by means of nuclear weapons that is contrary to Article 2, para. 4, of the U.N. Charter and that fails to meet all the requirements of Article 51, is unlawful;… As consequence, by the President casting his vote to break a 7to 7 tie, the Court held:*
>
> > *It follows from the above-mentioned requirements that the threat or use of nuclear weapons would generally be contrary to the rules of international law applicable in armed conflict, and in particular the principles and rules of humanitarian law;*

However, in view of the current state of international law, and of the elements of fact at its disposal, the Court cannot conclude definitively whether the threat or use of nuclear weapons would be lawful or unlawful in an extreme circumstance of self-defence, in which the very survival of a State would be at stake.[94]

The importance of this decision, incomplete and tentative though it is, has been emphasized in the work of Richard Falk[95] and many legal scholars, including the author.[96] Nevertheless, whatever its shortcomings, the 'opinion' places the WHO squarely in the realm of international players, with more than a research and advisory capacity. It is the argument of this work that capacity needs to be brought out fully once again in the services of humanity in general, and children in particular, in regard to the environmental threats we have noted. Although not immediately visible, as a mushroom cloud or other devastation arising from the use of nuclear power, nevertheless their insidious effects probably kill, harm and adversely affect many more than the Hiroshima disaster ever did.

The WHO's organizational ideology includes the formulation of broad goals and principles:

In 1977 the World Health Organization defined the broad goal of the organization as 'health for all by the year 2000'.[97]

Although (then) Director-General Halvdan Mahler laboured toward this goal, subsequent directors have taken a less idealistic and more managerial leadership style. Including placing more focus on specific issues and goals. With the appointment of Gro Bruntland, 'the WHO'S vision and political momentum' that had dissipated during the leadership of Makajima, were partially regained.[98]

Nevertheless, the increasing power of the World Trade Organization (WTO) and the World Bank posed a challenge to the role of the WHO. On global public health Kamran Abbassi says:

A WHO representative expressed a similar sentiment in arguing that 'the World Bank is the new 800 pound gorilla in world health care'.[99]

The *World Development Report 1993* introduced the concept of the 'disability-adjusted life year' (DALY).[100] Thus the World Bank introduced a regime intent on quantifying and rendering more cost-effective all health interventions, and Director Bruntland apparently also accepted this pragmatic approach.[101]

Nevertheless the traditional approach to the WHO sees health as a 'fundamental human right' that should be pursued for its own sake.[102] In order to ensure that this traditional vision prevails once again, the WHO needs to re-integrate its global public health mission into international law,[103] including trade law, environmental law and human rights law,[104] and, I add, the law concerning the rights of the child, as it did when it scrutinized South African policies in their area of competence during apartheid.

Hence it is vitally important to learn all that the WHO 2002 document (Tamburlini et al, 2002) can offer about children's health, perhaps recognizing in this document also a portent of the return to the vision and the traditional leadership of the WHO. This document is aware of the 1989 CRC, but it states that, contrary to the commitments on the part of that instrument and of several other international instruments, the situation does not show significant improvement.[105] The WHO concludes that:

> *Children are at risk of exposure to more than 15,000 synthetic chemicals, nearly all of them developed over the past 50 years and to a variety of physical agents. In addition, developing organisms are more vulnerable to environmental contaminants for several reasons, including greater and longer exposure and particular susceptibility windows. We are witnessing an unprecedented increase in the incidence of asthma; some childhood concerns also show an upward trend; injuries still represent a high burden for children and young adults; and there is increasing concern regarding the neurotoxicity, immunotoxicity and endocrine-disrupting properties of substances that are widely dispersed in the environment.*[106]

The magnitude of the problem demonstrates why the WHO should gain (or regain) world leadership and why it must have a significant role in the formulation of laws and the decisions about the appropriate punishment for non-compliance of either States or Juridical persons, whose interests and economic transactions give rise to most of the problems listed above. The role of the WHO ought not to be limited to responding to crises or proposing courses of treatment to various diseases. Following upon the 1997 *Declaration of the Environmental Leaders of the Eight*, the WHO is committed to:

> *(d) promote and encourage health measures into areas of emerging concern to children's health on the basis of the precautionary principles,*

and, in general 'to develop and implement' preventive measures in all areas of concern to children.[107] Given the global, transnational reach of the practices and products that put all children at risk, it is evident that the WHO must play a significant role in international law.

World Health Organization findings for policy guidance

> *Children are particularly vulnerable to many environmental threats, including contaminated and unsafe physical environment. This heightened susceptibility derives primarily from the unique biological features that characterize the various stages of development from conception to adolescence.*[108]

There are many examples of this heightened susceptibility. For instance, in the early years of a child's life, the brain and nervous system develop for the most part, so that cells destroyed by chemicals (e.g. lead or mercury) in this period, will not recover, and the resulting impairment will be 'permanent and irreversible'.[109] Another example is the greater exposure of children compared to adults 'per unit of body weight' to environmental toxins.[110] Because children eat, drink and even breathe air in larger quantities than adults, the effect of toxicants in these substances will be much more harmful to them than they might be to adults.[111] In addition, the child's life is mostly ahead of them, hence it is more likely that they will develop diseases engendered by environmental exposure.[112] For the same reason many chemicals will have long-term and even intergenerational effects through bioaccumulation.

Each period of a child's development, starting with preconception, has its own specific increased risks. Before conception, for example, ionizing radiation may affect the reproductive organs of either parent or may be stored in the mother's body to be reactivated during pregnancy, thus harming the foetus directly. The same is true of polychlorinated biphenyl (PCB) exposure or paternal exposure to occupational toxicants.[113]

During the embryonic and foetal period, many toxicants may reach the foetus directly or through the placenta, such as ionizing radiation, electromagnetic fields, environmental tobacco smoke.[114] Newborns have their own specific susceptibilities: exposure to parental occupational hazards, exposure to PVC plastics, and many substances that come in contact with their highly permeable skin, as well as receiving stronger, more severe effects from airborne pollutants, including tobacco smoke.[115] In the early years, not only diet and air, but harmful surroundings, from soil to carpets, can introduce harmful substances to the child, and environmental exposures are multiplied at the adolescent stages as exposure to the media becomes routine.[116]

These are some of the general findings addressing particular issues at various stages of a child's development. The next topic is a brief summary of some of the worse substances that harm children and some of the most serious effects that results, hence the gravest diseases and malfunctions to which children are exposed. Some of these are: (1) asthma and other respiratory problems, all on the rise in industrial countries;[117] (2) neuro-developmental disorders from chemical or pesticide exposure;[118] (3) cancers, as 'children are likely to be more prone than adults to events related to carcinogenesis', although cancer is and has been considered to be primarily a disease of adulthood and old age;[119] (4) birth defects, at a rate of about 5 per cent of live births; these also represent the 'leading cause of infant mortality in the developed world for more than 20 years, with a rate of 173.4 per 100,000 live births in 1994';[120] and (5) 'waterborne gastrointestinal disease due to biological contamination and acute and chronic poisoning by a variety of chemicals.'[121]

In addition, multiple health effects are the result of several environmental exposures, such as environmental tobacco smoke;[122] pesticides exposure;[123] ultraviolet radiation;[124] and the electromagnetic fields.[125] The weight of the evidence is so overwhelming that special policies need to be developed in order to protect children who surely have the right to that protection, as argued above. The WHO document we have briefly summarized proposes the following:

16.2 Rationale and guiding principles for Protective Policies for Children

- *Children cannot be regarded as little adults because their behaviour, physiology, metabolism and diet are different.*
- *Children have different susceptibilities from adults due to their dynamic growth and to their biological systems which are not yet fully developed.*
- *Children have very different exposure patterns from adults.*
- *For children the stage in their development when the exposure occurs is as important, if not more important, than the type and dose of exposure.*

- *Children are exposed to different types of toxicants in different combinations throughout their lives.*
- *Children can have very different health outcomes from adults exposed to the same toxicant; such health outcomes alter normal development and can be permanent.*
- *Children have more years during which they may be exposed to a variety of toxicants, which can lead to disease in later life.*
- *There is mounting evidence that certain types of childhood diseases may be related to environmental exposure, e.g. asthma and neuro-developmental effects.*[126]

CONCLUSIONS: THE RIGHTS OF THE CHILD AND THE DUTY TO INTERVENE (DOMESTIC), AND THE INTERNATIONAL RESPONSIBILITY TO PROTECT

Traditionally, the protection and the health of children have been the responsibility of the parents or family and community, in fact even the question of state intervention in hazardous situations has been debated. But, as the previous sections have indicated, most of the hazards to which the child is exposed are beyond the power of parents and families to control, without appropriate regulations to restrain industrial activities and the manufacture and distribution of unknown hazards. Even if complete transparency were a fact, globally, the lack of alternatives continues to militate against ascribing full responsibility to traditional family protectors.

Intervention, whether in a single case (as in social intervention in intolerable family situations), or general intervention aimed at a specific group (as in class action generating intervention that is eventually judicially decided), or the radical possibility of international intervention must be accepted. Clearly this is an ideal at this time, it does not exist explicitly in any legal instrument. Yet the two 1966 Covenants (ICCPR and the International Covenant on Economic, Social and Cultural Rights (ICESCR)) appear to support the legal foundation for such an intervention.

In his discussion of A.6 (ICCPR), Yoram Dinstein says:

> *Human rights aim at promoting and protecting the dignity and integrity of every individual human being. If there are any rights more fundamental than others for achieving that aim, surely they are the right to life, to physical integrity and liberty. On these all other human rights depend: without these, other rights have little or not meaning.*[127]

In addition, the rights defended in these Covenants (1966), when directed at specific groups, might trigger the forceful response of the UN, for instance against genocide, or other attacks against the human person;[128] they represent forms of aggression against the human person, in violation of the UN Charter (A.2). These rights include also the rights 'to an adequate standard of living and to health'

> *... which are recognized in Article 11 and 12 of The International Covenant on Economic, Social and Cultural Rights.*[129]

Deprivation of life by various means, that may include starvation, exposure to tempera-ture extremes or contamination by exposure to disease, means homicide.[130] Hence a solid ground for legal intervention appears to be present.

Only the European Court of Justice (ECJ), to my knowledge, has passed judgements that make such rights primary, that is, superior to economic considerations in general, and also to specific domestic laws in the respective countries where these cases originated in *Guerra v. Italy* and *Lopez-Ostra v. Spain*.[131]

The World Health Organization as we saw in the previous sections, has amassed a great deal of evidence about the causal connections between ecological degradation of various kinds and children's health.[132] This evidence may help to mitigate or even eliminate the concerns that have been expressed in regard to legal intervention on behalf of 'the best interest of the child'.[133] When the issue before the legal system is 'the best interest of children', in adoption debates, removal from family settings or educational choices, the 'prediction' and 'indeterminacy' problems emerge.[134]

Maximizing what is good for the child normally entails making very difficult choices. Mnookin says:

> *The judge would, for example, wish to compare the expected utility for the child of living with the mother, to that of living with the father. This requires considerable information as well as some source of values from which to measure utility for the child.*[135]

Some of the major problems with 'value conflicts' and 'prediction' are generally en-demic to utilitarianism; for instance, are the consequences that are decisive for choosing a moral action, to be viewed 'from a long-term or short-term perspective'? Or should one choose the conditions that will make the child happiest now, or 50 or 70 years from now?[136]

In contrast, the approach I have suggested, that is to consider at the outset the most 'basic rights'[137] as entrenched in the Covenants cited above, and as accepted globally today, eliminates most of the questions raised by legal interventions. The inherent right to life and to physical integrity is indisputably the foundation and the necessary and sufficient condition for the exercise of any right whatsoever. Thus that intervention remains justified and desirable, whatever one's predictive abilities or one's grasp of all the values involved.

Normatively and legally, therefore, at least in principle, intervention is both necessary and desirable if the most helpless and vulnerable of humanity are to be protected and defended. If a reasonably 'just war' could be waged against Germany for its terrible crimes against humanity, then force can and should be justly employed in defence of a much larger and most vulnerable group, that of children under environmental attacks.

The intervention in Germany's regime with its egregious human rights violations did not involve an international body as neither 'crime against humanity' nor 'genocide' were established as crimes at the time, nor was the United Nations in existence or their *Declaration of Human Rights*.

Although the argument above speaks of protection due to children because of their nationality, the international covenants of 1966 (ICCPR and ICESCR), also defend in general terms the right to life and imply the right to protection, although without the specificity I have argued for in the case of children. The international dimensions of the right to protection and thus the duty to intervene in case of 'state failure' are clearly present instead in the report of the *International Commission on Intervention and State Sovereignity*, appropriately titled 'The Responsibility to Protect'.[138]

With particular reference to children, I argued above that the duty to protect accrued inevitably to states. Yet the present pro-trade and economic-first climate, fosters a culture of neglect and disinterest toward environmental and public health concerns. This institutional or organizational 'culture' (as referred to for instance in Bill C-45, Canadian Criminal Law, in force 7 November 2003) renders institutions and organizations that enact, support or foster abuses and crimes such as those referred to in 'The presence of institutionalized violence: Ecocrimes and international law', as 'complicit' in the harmful consequences such as those demonstrated by the EEA Report No. 29 (Tamburlini et al, 2002) for instance. This complicity is analogous for peace-time consequences, to the complicity of individuals, organizations and institutions in the crimes committed in both war and peace by the Nazi regime in Germany, as clearly stated by the Nuremberg Charter.

But despite the *Declaration of Human Rights* (1948) and the presence of the two human rights covenants (1966), and even that of the *Convention of the Rights of the Child* (1989), the starting point of this work, most states have not advanced their protective practices and regulations. However, the supranational regime of the EU stands high above all others (with at least 150 human rights decisions by its human rights court by 1995). Jack Donnelly states:

> *In Western Europe there has been a significant transfer of authority from states to the regional community of states, which has redefined the limits of sovereignty. Human rights practices, which previously were an area of sovereign prerogative, are now subject to coercive regional enforcement.*[139]

The EU example, as indicated also in the two cases cited above *Guerra v. Italy* and *Lopez-Ostra v. Spain*, are not replicated in the Americas, Africa or Asia. Nevertheless it indicates the thrust and direction of today's international law approach to human rights, moving from state impunity to state responsibility, as indicated by the work of the Commission. A brief review of some of its principles will shed light on the right to protection for which I have argued.

The most important point to note is the terminology change the Commission emphasize[140] from 'the right to intervention', a confrontational expression that automatically places the onus of justification on the would-be-interveners, for their 'attack' on sovereignty, to the concept of 'responsibility to protect'. This concept indicates directly the moral strength of this position, and its basis both in domestic law, the 'duty to protect' because of nationality, and international principles and regimes, from natural law,[141] to the spirit of all human rights covenants.

Particularly relevant are (1) *Basic Principles*; (2) *Foundations*, as well as the 'Principles for Military Intervention': (1) *the just cause threshold*; and (2) *the precautionary principles* (ICISS, 2001: xi–xii), and the elaboration of the concept of 'Sovereignty as Responsibility'[142] The latter is most closely related to the changed conception of 'responsibility to protect'. The Commission's emphasis is on the change from 'Sovereignty as control' to 'Sovereignty as responsibility' (2.14).

The latter is the closest concept to the meaning of the changed conception of 'responsibility to protect'. This is an important move as it implies that (a) state authorities are responsible for the function of protection; (b) that this responsibility is both *internal* (to states), regarding their own citizens, and *international* (that is to the UN and its community of nations): and (c) it implies accountability 'for their acts of commission and omission' (2.15).

The most notable Basic Principles other than A, which states for the first time in the document the notion of state responsibility, is B, which spells out the reasons for possible international responsibility:

> *Where a population is suffering serious harm, as a result of internal war, insurgency, repression, or **state failure*** ... [emphasis added].

State failure, therefore, leads to the presence of 'just cause', or the justification for intervention, even for military force:

> *(1) A. large scale loss of life, actual or apprehended, **with genocidal intent or not**, which is the product either of deliberate state action, or **state neglect or inability to act*** ... [emphasis added].

It is important to note that intent is not an absolute requirement. As the lack of specific intent is one of the stumbling blocks to the criminalization of environmental attacks, this principle represents a significant improvement.[143]

The criterion upon which the international community will be impelled to intervene is not explicitly spelled out in the UN Charter. Some argue that it will be based upon a developed understanding that adheres quite closely to [the Charter's] 'spirit', if not to its letter.[144] It will not and cannot be the fruit of a 'customary' understanding, unless it is based on a *jus cogens* norm that is complementary to the Charter itself.[145] In addition, the criterion is based on the substance of human rights law, as it attempts to realize the ideal of 'universal justice', or 'justice without borders' (2.19). This ideal demonstrates the passage from a 'culture of sovereign impunity' to a 'culture of national and international accountability' (2.18).[146]

Finally, the 'precautionary Principles' enshrined in this document are nothing but a reiteration of 'just war' theory from Roman times, to Augustine, and finally to the work of St Thomas Aquinas, all of which spell out the conditions required for military intervention.[147] They are listed as:

> (2) A. *Right Intention* ...
> B. *Last Resort* ...
> C. *Proportional Means* ...
> D. *Reasonable Prospects* ...[148]

In addition, the requirement of a (3) Right Authority, completes the classical account of just war, as *jus ad bellum*. The appropriate authority may be found in the United Nations Security Council, when it chooses intervention as the proper response to a human rights crisis, or when the Secretary General brings a situation to the attention of the international community under Article 99 of the UN Charter.[149]

In sum, the argument here advanced starts with the established principle that children have a right to nationality. But nationality implies government protection of human rights, starting with the right to life, health and physical integrity. As was shown in the previous sections, effective protection implies, and requires, 'ecological rights',[150] or the consideration of the industrial activity right at the start against the environmental conditions it might engender, many of which may be hostile to health and normal function, particularly for children.

Since today's science increasingly demonstrates that 'protection' requires a specific sense in regard to children, this specificity must be reflected in the 'rights of the child' who, as the WHO has shown are not simply 'small adults' (see 'World Health Organization findings for policy guidance' above). In essence, since (a) the 'preconditions of human agency'[151] are established long before birth; (b) pre-birth and early infancy are the most vulnerable periods of human life, when the developing child requires the highest level of protection from various toxicants; and because (c) no difference can be made between different sorts of rights, some of which are accepted and entrenched in law, although based on potentiality, while others, although equally future-oriented, are not viewed as acceptable instead (as not politically correct), this distinction must be abandoned. The rights of the child must start with a healthy environment, capable of supporting and protecting her biological integrity, from the undisputable start of her individuated biological life.

Perhaps the most effective corrective would be to recognize the injustice inherent to the ecological footprint of affluent countries.[152] Thus although it can be argued that favourable socio-economic circumstances improve the health of the affluent populations in developed countries, there is no corresponding 'trickle down' effect on impoverished peoples for health, any more than there is for economics.

In fact, the favourable 'preconditions' of health, if understood in the sense of improved economic circumstances for some, often entail depriving those in developing countries of their resource base,[153] and future generations of theirs.

In contrast with the injustice of this approach, Ms Berglind Asglirdottir (Deputy Secretary General, OECD, Paris), argues that 'Health can be seen as a form of capital itself'. In this case, depriving some populations in the effort to improve our own health (in Western countries), is not only injust, but it should be viewed as criminal, given the effects produced by this form of appropriation, rather than being treated simply as a tort, like other property offences.[154]

All other rights, to education, to family life, non-discrimination, diminish in importance when compared to the basic, foundational right of health. It is our collective responsibility to ensure that these rights are fully researched in all their implications and that the duties they impose be fully embraced, if the Right of the Child is to be accepted as more than simply an incomplete, misunderstood extension of the present, limited, human rights instruments. In the following chapters, I will expand on many of the themes touched upon in this chapter. The connection between health and environment will be emphasized, as will the various ways of understanding the child and the environmental impacts on her health and safety. In the next chapter I will start with a consideration of child protection in countries governed by civil law regimes.

NOTES

1   Rockefeller (2002), ppx–xiv. See also www.earthcharter.org.
2   Taylor, P. (1998), p309.
3   Gewirth (1982).
4   Tamburlini et al (2002).
5   Van Bueren (1995), p7.
6   Tamburlini et al (2002).
7   *United Nations Charter of The Rights of the Child*, GA Res. 1386 XIV.
8   *Convention on the Rights of the Child*, U.N.Doc E/CN.4/1989/29; in force 20 November 1990
    (henceforth CRC).
9   Van Bueren (1995), p12.
10 Lauterpacht (1968).
11 Tamburlini et al (2002).
12 Van Bueren (1995), pp32–38; Detricks (1999), p5.
13 Tamburlini et al (2002); see also Soskolne and Bertollini (1999); Colborn et al (1996).
14 *American Convention on Human Rights*, (1969) OAS Tr.Ser./No. 36; 1144 U.N.T.S. 123.
15 Van Bueren (1995), p33; see Art, 6(1) *International Covenant on Civil and Political Rights*; Art.
    2.2 *European Convention on Human Rights and Fundamental Freedoms*; Art. 4 *American Convention
    on Human Rights*.
16 UN DOC.E/CN.4/1989/29/Rev.1, followed the *UN Declaration on the Rights of the Child,
    November 20, 1959.*
17 (1996) 999 U.N.T.S.171; and Article 18 of the ACHR (*American Convention on Human Rights*
    (1969) AS Tr.Ser/.No.36; 1144U.N.T.S. 123).
18 Detricks (1999), pp146–147.
19 (1948) Res. 217A(III) U.N.Doc.A/810.
20 Detricks (1999), p149.
21 *Joyce v. Director of Public Prosecution* [1946] A.C. 347 (H.L.); *In re Urios*, France's court of
    Cassation (criminal Chamber), 15 January, 192, (1919–1922), I Annual Digest 107; *Rex v.
    Nuemann* (Special Criminal Court, Transvaal), 1949 (3) S.A. 1238.
22 Williams (1948), p57.
23 Williams (1948), p58.
24 Williams (1948), p59.
25 Williams (1948), p63.
26 Westra (2004a), chapter 3.
27 Westra (1998, 2000a,b, 2004a).
28 Arendt (1964).
29 Westra (2004a), chapter 3.
30 Westra (2004a).
31 Chomsky (2004).
32 *Guerra v. Italy* (1998) 26 EHRR, 357; *Lopez-Ostra v.Spain* (1995) 20 EHRR 277, (1994) ECHR
    16798/90.
33 Westra (1998); Rees and Westra (2003).
34 McMichael (1995a, 2000).
35 Colborn et al (1996); Tamburlini et al (2002).
36 Raffensperger and Tickner (1999).
37 Tamburlini et al (2002).
38 Van Bueren (1995), p33.
39 Van Bueren (1995), p35.

40   Murray (1996), pp464–473.
41   *Reproductive Health Hazards in the Workplace,* Office of Technology Assessment's document, US Congress, US Government Printing Office, Washington, DC, 1985.
42   Prosser (1964).
43   Colborn et al (1996); Tamburlini et al (2002), pp104–110.
44   Gewirth (1982).
45   Gewirth (1982), p5.
46   Gewirth (1982), p7.
47   Gewirth (1982), p5.
48   Beyleveld and Brownsword (2001), p71
49   Shue, H. (1996a).
50   Beyleveld and Brownsword (2001), p70; Gewirth (1982) p54.
51   Mathiew (1996).
52   Marquis (1989) pp183–202.
53   Beyleveld and Brownsword (2001), p158.
54   Beyleveld and Brownsword (2001), p112.
55   Singer (1976).
56   De Grazia (1995).
57   Gewirth (1982), p112.
58   Regan (1983).
59   De Grazia (1995).
60   Westra (1994), pp96–97.
61   Westra (2000a).
62   Hauskeller (2002).
63   Westra (2004a).
64   Tomuschat (1991), p58.
65   Ago(1988), p237; Tanzi (1987), pp293–305.
66   Kindred et al (2000).
67   *Trail Smelter Arbitration (US v. Canada* 1931–1941-3 R.I.A.A. 1905).
68   Tomuschat (1991), p38.
69   Tomuschat (1991), p42.
70   Tomuschat (1991), p43.
71   Tomuschat (1991), p46.
72   The *ILC Convention on Transboundary Harm, Special Rapporteur Rao's 1st Report* (1988) UN Doc.A/CN 487/Add. 1; *2nd Report* (1999) UN Doc.A/Cn.4/501; *3rd Report* (2000) UN Doc. A/CN 4/510; ILC Report of the Working Group on International Liability for Injurious Consequences Arising Out of Acts not Prohibited by International Law, in Rpt. Of the ILC (1996) GAOR A/51/10, Annex 1.
73   Kiss (1989), pp719–727.
74   Birnie and Boyle (2002), p325; Kindred et al (2000), p1180; see also pp363–367.
75   Birnie and Boyle (2002), p105.
76   Rpt. of the ILC (2001) GAOR A/56/10.
77   Birnie and Boyle (2002), p106.
78   Birnie and Boyle (2002), p107.
79   Birnie and Boyle (2002), p115.
80   Higgins (1994), p161.
81   Crawford (2002), p12.
82   *Guerra v. Italy* 4 EHRC 63 (case 116/1996/735/932).
83   Barash (2000), p106.
84   Soskolne and Bertollini (1999); McMichael (1995a, 2000).
85   Schabas (2000).

86   Homer-Dixon and Gizewski (1996); Homer-Dixon (1999).
87   Noss and Cooperrider (1994); Karr and Chu (1999); Karr (2000); Westra (1998).
88   Rees (2000), p139; Brown (2000); Westra and Lawson (2001); D'Amato (1990), p190; Brown-Weiss (1990), p198; see also Westra (2004a).
89   Institute of Medicine 1988, US; as cited in Fidler (2000), p3.
90   Fidler (2000), p5.
91   EB101.R.2, January 1998.
92   [1996] I.C.J. Rep. 66.
93   Kindred et al (2000), p1180; see also pp363–367.
94   Kindred et al (2000), p367.
95   Falk (1998).
96   Westra (2004a).
97   Fidler (2000), p100.
98   Fidler (2000), p109; see also Gordenker (1994), pp167–191.
99   Abbassi (1999).
100   World Bank (1993).
101   Fidler (2000), p112.
102   Fidler (2000), p112.
103   Fidler (1998), pp1079–1126.
104   Fidler (2000), p119; see also Donnelly (1995), p131.
105   *Declaration of the UN Conference on Environment and Development,* UN Doc. A/CONF.151/26/ Rev.1, especially chapter 6; the *1997 Declaration of the Environmental Leader of the Eight on Children's Environmental Health* (Miami, FL, 5–6 May 1997; www.g7.utoronto.ca/g7/ environment/1997 Miami/children.html); *The State of the World's Children,* UNICEF, 1994, Oxford University Press, NY; the *UNECE Environment and Human Settlement Division,* 'Convention on access to information, public participating in decision-making and access to justice in environmental matters', Aarhus, Denmark, June 1998.
106   Tamburlini et al (2002), p12.
107   Tamburlini et al (2002), p14.
108   Tamburlini (2002), p18.
109   Rice and Barone (2002), pp511–533.
110   Tamburlini (2002), p19.
111   Snodgrass (1992), pp35–42; Bearer (1995), pp7–12.
112   Tamburlini (2002), p19.
113   Jacobson and Jacobson (1996), pp783–789; Ji et al (1997), pp238–244; Savitz (1989), pp1201–1210.
114   Tamburlini et al (2002), p20.
115   Plunkett, Turnbull and Rodricks (1992), pp79–94.
116   Tamburlini et al (2002), p22; Dyson (2000).
117   von Ehrenstein (2002), p44.
118   Grandjean and White (2002), p66.
119   Terracini (2002), p79.
120   Jensen (2002), p99.
121   Pond (2002), p113.
122   Courage (2002), p142.
123   Tirado (2002), p152.
124   Rehfuss and von Ehrenstein (2002), p161.
125   Ebi. (2002), p172.
126   Carlson and Tamburlini (2002), p207.
127   Dinstein (1981) p114.
128   Westra (2004a), chapter 7.

129   Dinstein (1981), p115; ICESCR, G.A. Res. 2000, 21 GAOR Supp. 16, UN *Doc.a/6316@49* (1996).
130   Dinstein (1981), p115.
131   See note 23.
132   Soskolne and Bertollini (1999); Tamburlini et al (2002).
133   Mnookin (1985), pp16–24.
134   Mnookin (1985), p17.
135   Mnookin (1985), p17.
136   Mnookin (1985), p18.
137   Shue (1996a).
138   ICISS, December 2001; www.iciss.gc.ca; see also Craig Scott (2001), pp333–369.
139   Donnelly (1995), p133.
140   ICISS (2001), pp11–12.
141   ICISS (2001), p16.
142   ICISS (2001), pp13; 2.14 and 2.15.
143   Westra (2004a), especially chapter 5.
144   Scott (2001), p337.
145   Scott (2001), p346.
146   ICISS (2001), p14.
147   Westra (2004a), Chapter 1.
148   ICISS (2001), pxii.
149   ICISS (2001), pxii
150   Taylor, P. (1998), p309.
151   Gewirth (1982).
152   Rees and Westra (2003).
153   Shiva (1989).
154   Westra (2004a).

CHAPTER 2

The Status of the Preborn
in Civil Law Instruments

INTRODUCTION

In order to be able to make policy recommendations (*lex ferenda*), it is important not to limit the research to present international instruments, but to extend it to single countries where one may be able to discover helpful trends for the protection of the child in law. The first question to be raised is whether there is any regulatory infrastructure that acknowledges any rights to the pre-birth child, as a juridical person. One of the most thorough discussions of this question I have found is 'Abortion and the Law' by Dolores Dooley-Clark of Ireland.[1] It is not necessary to enter into the details of her argument, but it is important to acknowledge that, political correctness aside, strong arguments can be made and I will return to those points below.

The research outlined in the previous chapter shows that advances in science should correspond to similar advances in public policy instruments and the law. From the standpoint of the environment, the United Nations Environment Programme (UNEP) initiative[2] is intent to ensure that Supreme Court Justices, faced with novel scientific and public policy issues regarding the environment, should be 'retrained' so that they could give better, more informed judgments. To my knowledge, no such initiative has been initiated simply for public health and the protection of the preborn, although the UNEP mandate may also fit well this area of research and advances. The most logical place to find some reference to child protection might be in the existing instruments for the protection of women, and several have come to be in the last decades. The main instrument referring to the protection of women is the *Convention on the Elimination of All Forms of Discrimination against Women*.[3] Nevertheless the rights (if any) of a pre-birth child, are obscured by the language used, referring to 'women's reproductive health' or to the lack of women's political or decision-making rights, rather than to abortion. The General Recommendation No 19 of CEDAW Committee, 11th Sess., 199,[4] under 'General Comment' 7.(a), lists 'The Right to Life' as the first of eight rights. But that right is not extended to the unborn, except in a report on China, for specific circumstances.

Under 'Concluding Observations of CEDAW Committee on Third and Fourth Periodic Reports of China',[5] under 49.(d), and under 51, concern is expressed for 'illegal practices of sex-selective abortion' in the former, and specifically for states where 'the government should enforce laws against sex-selective abortion', in the latter

(51). At best, therefore, some concern is expressed for the rights of female foetuses, *provided* that there is evidence of specific intent to abort them *qua* females. A general desire to abort any foetus, therefore, does not appear to be viewed as problematic, as long as it is not gender specific. There is no mention of the fact that at least 50 per cent of all viable, normal foetuses may well be female, nor any argument as to why the gender of the aborted should make any difference, morally or legally.

Hence neither the specific convention on the rights of the child, as was noted in the previous chapter, nor the legal instrument aimed at the protection of women demonstrates any concern with the preborn (except as indicated) nor does it offer any moral or legal argument why concern should exist at all. Yet there is a novel area of research where a strong concern is shown for the juridical status of the preborn: the area of technologically assisted reproduction. I will consider a study of the issues related to assisted reproduction in the next section.

THE JURIDICAL STATUS OF THE PREBORN: *INFANS CONCEPTUS* IN CIVIL LAW

Infans Conceptus pro iam nato habetur quoties de commodis eius agitur.[6]

It might be best to start with this issue in civil law, because (1) many of the OECD countries are civil law regimes; and (2) the concern with the status of the preborn can indeed be traced back to Roman law, as at that time the status of the conceived infant (*infans conceptus*) was well established in the classic rule cited above.[7] If any hope can be entertained of extending present law instruments to accommodate recent scientific advances and technological innovations, it is essential to recognize that *all* human beings should possess juridical personhood. Nathalie Massager says:

> *Il ne subsiste, à l'heure actuelle, qu'une seule limitation à la regle selon laquelle tous les etres humains sont dotés de la personnalite juridique: La personnalité suppose un minimum d'existence physique, c'est pourqoui il n'a pas été estimé pertinent d'ocroyer la personnalité juridique à ceu qui ne sont pas nés vivant et viable.*[8,9]

Despite this basic handicap, from ancient times, there has been a concern with how juridical personhood is to be granted, to whom and why, as it is, as Massager remarks, 'un don de la loi'.[10] A connection may be found with the last chapter's discussion on the preconditions of agency, as juridical personhood may be defined as 'a person's capacity to perform valid legal acts', although the traditional distinction between the ability to enjoy subjective rights, and the ability to act upon them or to exercise such rights to be secondary to the preconditions of agency, discussed above.

These rights (as preconditions of agency) are indeed biological and physical, whereas the former are purely the product of legislative fiat, 'le produit d'une décision legislative'.[11] But, aside from the biological, physical recognition of the human beings' person as juridical, the legal fiction aspect of personhood is extremely valuable as well:

it is sufficient to be able to *have* these rights (here understanding rights in the sense of possible ability to exercise them or act upon them), *not* just to be presently capable of their exercise. In other words, one may be a right-holder independently of whether one may have the ability (at present) to exercise the right, as a legal representative may be appointed to speak or act on behalf of whoever cannot – at this time – do either (e.g. a comatose person).

There is an obvious contrast between positive law, not only in civil regimes, but also in common law, with the Latin citation at the start if this section. This conflict is one that, as Massager affirms, merits to be resolved, *de lege ferenda*.[12] Massager's main concern is with the insufficient laws dealing with various aspects of artificial insemination (whether intra-conjugal or with a donor) and *in vitro* fertilization, as the present positive law is as incapable of dealing with these issues as it is unable and unwilling to confront the newest of the results of the WHO's research on the vulnerability of the preborn to environmental hazards from the moment of conception.[13] Both areas are novel and have become highly controversial because of recent scientific research findings; both need laws that are capable of meeting their challenges.

Unlike Massager, my interest is focused on the right of the child to health, but I intend to benefit from Massager's research as its premises and goal are fully compatible with mine.

The historical background of the rule of *infans conceptus*

One must return to antiquity and even to philosophy, in order to truly understand the status of human embryos and foetuses in its historical context. Aristotle's work offers the best starting point: 'becoming' is the passage from mere possibility to reality. But 'possibility' does not exist in itself, whereas the truly Aristotelian notion of 'potency' passing to actuality, best explains the status of the preborn.[14] Potency, in fact, exists as such, as the acorn is real, although it is not yet the oak tree it will become. Not a mere conceptual possibility, the embryo after conception is in potency the infant it will eventually be. That of course is precisely what modern science indicates as well. But this understanding of the preborn is bypassed by Latin Stoic thinkers, such as Plutarchus and Tertullian, even Ulpian and Plotinus himself is concerned with the infant's acquisition of the soul, something he believes happens only upon leaving the mother's body. Thus the doctrine that is viewed today as 'religious' dogma, has its basis in pagan, Stoic thinking.

Later, this belief is picked up by the Christian St Augustine, while St Thomas Aquinas held quite a novel (Aristotelian) position in this regard. Human life indeed started with conception, but after that, first the developing entity possessed only a vegetal existence, then animal, and only later in its development, these characteristics were joined by the incorruptible human soul, 28 days after conception for the female foetus, 40 days after conception for the male.[15] St Thomas, as usual, relies on Aristotelian doctrine, as this explanation repeats, in some sense, the *ergon* argument found in Aristotle.[16] It is unfortunate that a sound argument about the initial absence of a rational soul (something that is of little or no concern today to either legal scholars or philosophers), should somehow have been changed in modern times to the absence of humanity instead.

So, aside from religion none of the thinkers from either antiquity, or the Roman or medieval periods, would have thought to question the *humanity* of the foetus, even under the category of 'personhood', surely as vague and imprecise a notion as that of possessing a 'rational, immortal soul' after the requisite number of days after conception. Roman legislators, fully aware of the imprecisions and difficulties pertaining to the passage from the potency of conception to the actuality of live birth, to use Aristotelian terminology, designed the juridical personhood of *infans conceptus* with the laudable aim of ensuring that the child's rights to both economic inheritance and other benefits would be protected. Thus, although the expression *infans conceptus pro iam nato habetur quoties de commodis eius agitur*, never appears as a clear rule in any Roman text, the rule is often used and applied to the appropriate circumstances.[17]

Plutarch relates an example of the rule's application in *Lycurgus*.[18] He recounts that when Polydectus died everyone thought that Lycurgus would become king. But the queen, Polydectus's wife, was pregnant at the time, and the infant to be born was declared to be the rightful heir to the crown, relegating Lycurgus (his uncle), to the role of administrator on behalf of the infant to be. Another application of his rule can be found in the possibility of inheriting not only a title, but the social position of the father. Ulpian refers to the position of senator, but also to that of a freed slave, both of which are said to accrue to the preborn for his future life, even if the *pater familias* no longer exists: once again this use of the rule would be in the child's interest.[19]

That said, Massager argues that the time has come to extend the rule, because the progress of biology and of medical sciences demands it, beyond the presence of purely social and inheritance related advantages. The necessity to intervene *in utero*, whether or not the parents consent to such intervention, as it happens for instance in the case of Jehovah's Witness parents who refuse intervention for their unborn child who needs a transfusion to save his life, fully supports Massager's argument and that of other scholars.[20]

Although some authors only use the maxim *infans conceptus* in anticipation of a live birth, rather than in general recognition of a present juridical status, some acknowledge a status capable of generating immediate obligations.[21] Speaking of *lex ferenda*, Massager suggests that the present uses of the rule conditionally and in anticipatory fashion only, is not rational, and would prefer to see instead a 'uniform juridical regime', able to 'recognize a non-conditional form of personhood to the conceived infant' instead, albeit admitting the possibility of waivers in certain cases:

> De lege ferenda, *nous estimons qu'il serait plus rationnel de substituer au mécanisme de la fiction juridique infans conceptus, qui constitue désormais en realité, une anticipation assortie d'une condition résoltoire, un régime juridique uniforme, qui reconnait à l'enfant conçu une personnalité non conditionelle, sauf dérogations apportées par des textes particuliers.*[22]

After all, one must keep in mind that the consideration of the preborn as 'born' only applies when it is in her interest, so that – for instance – economic advantages may be attributed to the preborn, not debts.[23]

The right to inherit is indeed present in common law countries as well and, in the US, it is possible for a child or young adult to sue either parents or obstetrician for either 'wrongful life', if the child is born with severe, irreversible damage, or for damages as compensation for an injury that occurred pre-birth, but produced ill effects later.[24] Thus it is possible to acknowledge harms received by the preborn, even view them as criminal in some cases. Nevertheless it is not a commonly accepted approach, in common law countries. Even in civil law, although regulatory measures may deal with the conceived infant, legislators continue to require the precondition of live birth.[25]

Massager disagrees strongly with the conditions prevailing in civil law, and her conclusion on this point supports the argument of my work as a whole:

> *A vrai dire, la situation de l'enfant à naitre ne doit pas, selon nous, etre distinguée de celle du mineur, en ce qui concerne le contenu à réserver à la notion d'intérêt de l'enfant: ils sont tous deux incapable d'exprimer leur volonté, tout en étant susceptible de devenir le premier toutefois de façon conditionelle – titulaires de droits subjectifs.*[26]

Her approach is even more desirable as based on real biological conditions, when we consider the health concerns of the previous chapter rather than economic or status issues: the latter could – presumably – be dealt with in later life, when the child or adolescent might consider the need for legal action, or his parents/guardians might. But the health damage received pre-birth may well be irreversible and thus incompensable even in later years. Thus it is far more important to consider the preborn simply as minors in law.

Although earlier Latin uses of the rule *infans conceptus* were merely applicable to specific circumstances (some of which were alluded to earlier), there are now a large number of issues to which it is (or should be) applied, hence the need to re-establish it as a general rule instead, as the circumstances now envisaged may range from family issues, to social and economic ones, but also to the concern for health and normal function.

The major obstacle to this project, that is to the recognition of juridical personhood for the preborn, remains the increasing liberalization of abortion laws. For the most part this trend has been supported by a parallel trend emphasizing women's rights (including the right to decide on the death of the preborn), that is, at the expense of the conceived infant. By denying any human value or juridical personhood to the preborn, one eliminates the necessity to defend the woman's decisions, or to find valid reasons to justify such decisions in most cases.

In contrast, Massager argues that this step need not be taken as penal law indeed recognizes that there are possible derogations of the right to life (such as legitimate self-defence, or the state of necessity). Thus the conceived infant should have the right not to life, but to physical integrity, to 'moral integrity' or dignity, as well as the right to a name and a nationality, as argued in the previous chapter, as well as the right to inherit both financial and social advantages, such as a title or even a crown.

That said, *pace* Massager, it would seem that simple choice or preference should no longer be sufficient to set aside all those rights, except in cases where a woman's rights are of equal seriousness (again, such as self-defence or necessity), not simply issues of convenience or privacy, and there is copious literature in bioethics debating precisely those points.

But, unless we accept the seriousness of the 'minor's rights' that logically ought to accrue to the preborn, there will be almost no opportunity to redress the grave injuries children of all ages suffer, as shown by the work of the WHO and that of other scientists.[27]

To further emphasize this point, the next section will deal with the reality of positive (civil) law in a case where the preborn's death was caused by a physician's negligence and incompetence, without the consent of the pregnant woman, yet – according to the European Court of Human Rights – no crime was committed.

FROM *LEX FERENDA* TO *LEX LATA*: THE CASE OF *VO V. FRANCE* AND SOME OTHER 'LIFE' CASES

The previous sections set the stage, through an examination of Roman Law and its antecedents, for a strong argument for the rule of *infans conceptus*, thus for the possession of juridical personhood for the unborn, through the history of the doctrine, and the arguments for its preservation in Civil Law. The author is careful to repeat that the whole effort represents only *lege ferenda* at this time. She also explains that this examination of present law instruments is required because novel technological and scientific practices may benefit from being viewed under a new approach. Present regulatory instruments were not originally designed and hence presently able to deal with technologically assisted reproduction, intra-conjugal, donor assisted or *in vitro*. Yet, whatever the historical or juridical reasons for integrating the preborn into the general category of minors, even if conditionally in anticipation of live births, the reality in positive law is quite different.

A clear and extreme example of this difference may be found in the recent case of *Vo v. France*.[28]

> *Procedure*
> *3. The applicant alleged in particular, a violation of Article 2 of the Convention on the ground that the conduct of a doctor who was responsible for the death of her child* in utero *was not classified as unintentional homicide.*

The case revolves around a series of terrible mistakes that took place in the Lyon General Hospital, mostly at the hand of Dr G, involving the applicant in the case, Mrs Thin-Nho Vo, who attended the hospital for a regularly scheduled medical examination during the sixth month of pregnancy, and a Mrs Thi Thanh Van Vo who was at the same hospital to have a coil removed. Both women were of Vietnamese descent and their command of French was extremely limited. On 27 November Dr G. called for Mrs Vo as his next patient, and when Mrs Thin-Nho Vo came into his office, he attempted to remove a coil from her uterus, without previous examination, and in so doing he pierced the amniotic sac, causing a substantial loss of amniotic fluid. Her fluid was not replaced normally and, on 5 December 1991, her pregnancy was terminated on health grounds. On 11 December Mrs Vo and her partner lodged a criminal complaint that included not only unfitness for work up to three months, because of her ordeal, but also for the 'unintentional homicide of her child'. The details of the charge were as follows:

> *17. On January 25, 1992, following supplemental admissions by the prosecution on 26 April 1994, Dr G. was charged with causing unintentional injury at Lyons on 27 November 1991 by: (i) through his inadvertence, negligent act of inattention, perforating the amniotic sac in which the applicant's live and viable fetus was developing, thereby unintentionally causing the child's death,*[29]
> *(ii) through his inadvertence, negligent act, inattention negligent omission or breach of a statutory or regulatory duty of protection or care, causing the applicant's bodily injury that resulted in her total unfitness for a period not exceeding three months.*[30]
> *18. By an order of 31 August 1995, Dr G. was committed to stand trial in Lyons Criminal Court on counts of unintentional homicide and unintentionally causing injuries.*[31]

Despite the clear indictment of Dr G. on two crimes, the one concerning the applicant's injuries could not be pursued, because of an Amnesty pertaining to that offence in 1995. But that was not the most controversial issue, the charge of homicide was:

> *The issue before the court is whether the offence of unintentional homicide or the unintentional taking of the fetus's life is made out when the life concerned is that of a fetus, if a 20 to 21 weeks' old fetus is a human person.*[32,33]

A discussion follows about the definition of human being, but the only clear fact was acknowledged to be that 'the life process starts with impregnation', although it is not clear when an embryo becomes a foetus, or even when a zygote becomes an embryo.

Several points are particularly noteworthy in the setting out of this case. On the practical level, because of a special Amnesty, the harm to the mother went unpunished. The second difficulty was primarily theoretical: because of the difficulty of accepting the multiple legal definitions of a human being that state, for instance, 'the law guarantees respect of every human being, from the beginning of life ... this principle may only be derogated from the event of necessity and in accordance with the conditions set out in this statute'.[34,35]

Article 16 of the Civil Code states:

> *The law secures the primacy of the person, any assault on human dignity and guarantees the respect of every human being from the beginning of its life.*

Although these excerpts from the civil law of France appear clear on the question of the right to life, they appear to be superseded by the Law on the *Voluntary Termination of Pregnancy*. For instance, the discussion in the Vo case shows the extent of this primacy. When France signed the *convention on the Rights of the Child*, on 26 January 1990 in New York, it declared that the Convention would not be viewed as 'any obstacle to the implementation of the provisions of the French legislation on the voluntary termination of pregnancy'.[36]

Nevertheless, the paragraph that follows offers a glimmer of hope for the defence of the health of the preborn:

> *It follows that, subject to the provisions on the voluntary termination of pregnancy and therapeutic abortions, the right to respect for every human being from the beginning of life is guaranteed by law, without any requirement that the child be born as a viable human being, provided it was alive when the injury occurred.*[37]

Had this approach to pre-birth injuries prevailed, the case would have ended quite differently than it did, with the Court holding by 14 votes to 3 that 'there had been no violation of Article 2 of the Convention [right to life article]'.[38]

Beyond the cited paragraph, there were several arguments used throughout the case, which might have supported the right of the foetus to life and health. In the next section these arguments as well as the appropriate case law will be listed. We will also present the dissenting opinions and the counter arguments these Judges propose instead.

THE VO CASE CONTINUED: ARGUMENTS FOR AND AGAINST THE RIGHT TO LIFE OF THE PREBORN IN CIVIL LAW

In its survey of the relevant law, the Vo decision cites Article 223-10 of the (French) Criminal Code:

> *Article 223-10*
> *It shall be an offence punishable by five years imprisonment and a fine of 50,000 francs to terminate a pregnancy without a mother's consent.*

In addition, Section III, entitled 'Protection of the Embryo',[39] prohibits various activities on medical ethics ground, including 'the conception of human embryos *in vitro* for research or experimental purposes'.[40]

The Public Health Code,[41] 4 March 2002, also seems to protect all individuals against medical malpractice:

> *Article L.1142-1*
> *Save when they incur liability as a result of a defect in health product, the medical practitioners mentioned in the Fourth Part of this Code and all hospitals, clinics, departments and organizations in which preventive medicine, diagnosis or treatment is performed on individuals shall only be liable for damage caused by preventive medicine, diagnoses or treatment if they have been at fault.*[42]

> *Article L.2211-1*
> *As stated in Article 16 of the Civil Code as hereinafter reproduced: 'the law secures the primacy of the person, prohibits any assault on human dignity and guarantees the respect of every human being from the beginning of its life.*[43]

The French Court of Cassation followed its judgement in the Vo case in another two cases, one in 2001 concerned a drunk driver who hit the car Mrs X was driving, with the consequence that Mrs X, who was 6 months' pregnant, lost her unborn child. The Court of Appeal stated that 'unintentionally causing the death of an unborn child constitutes the offence of unintentional homicide of the unborn child if the unborn child was viable at the material time, irrespective of whether or not it breathed when it was separated from the mother'.[44]

The 25 June 2002 case dealt with both negligence and errors on the part of a midwife and a doctor, which resulted in a viable child being born but dying shortly thereafter. In both cases listed, the Court of Cassation decided against 'extending' in this way the relevant articles of the Criminal Code against unintentional homicide.[45] Returning now to Vo, at para. 31, the Court of Cassation criticizes some of the case law approaches,[46] noting that at this time, '28 out of 34 Articles' that discuss these decisions by the Court of Cassation do so in a critical vein. The critique include the following points:

> the laconic reasoning of the Court of Cassation judgments and the incoherence of the protection afforded, as a person causing unintentional injury is liable to criminal prosecution while a person who unintentionally causes the death of the fetus goes unpunished; the fact that a child who has lived for a few minutes is recognized as having standing as a victim, whereas a child who dies in utero is ignored by the law; and the fact that the freedom to procreate is less well protected than the freedom to have an abortion.[47]

This critique recalls some of the arguments, both theoretical and historical, made earlier in the chapter, and it clearly outlines the undeniable contradictions inherent in all these decisions. In order to help with these difficulties, the National Assembly of France in 2003 proposed the 'Garraud amendment', creating 'an offence of involuntary termination of pregnancy (ITP)'. However, after giving rise to fierce debate in the legislature and elsewhere, the amendment was declared 'unanimously deleted' by the Minister of Justice, Mr Preben on 5 December 2003.

It might be useful to pause here in order to assess what has been discovered so far: essentially the case law is not favourable to the possibility of giving due consideration to the life, let alone the health, of the preborn. The cases we have considered, as well as several others,[48] deal specifically with a single death, where the causal chain of events leading to the injury or death is not in question, it leads directly to one or more individuals, and it hinges on the commission of errors or the omission of appropriate treatment, leading to foetal death.

It seems clear that if even the cases where at least one unintentional or negligent homicide has been committed, or – according to the courts and the case law, it would have been committed if the infant had been already born – then it is difficult if not impossible to expect that negligent, widespread hazardous practices causing injury, loss of normal function or death, could be viewed as criminal, thus proscribed, under present legal regimes. What we have considered are primarily civil law instruments and cases, but I believe that the situation is no better and in fact might even be worse, in common law, and we will see the evidence in the next chapter.

As Massager indicated (see the first section of this chapter) the only hope for a wider appreciation of foetal harms, should be based on the biolaw connected with assisted procreation. An example of such a document in the law of Council of Europe, is the *Convention for the Protection of Human Rights and Dignity of the Human Being with Regard to the Application of Biology and Medicine: Convention on Human Rights and Biomedicine*,[49] where both Article 1 and Article 2 express the beliefs that are absolutely necessary to move forward to the protection of the preborn:

> *Article 1 – Purpose and Object*
> *Parties to this Convention shall protect the dignity and identity of all human beings and guarantee everyone, without discrimination, respect for their integrity and other rights and fundamental freedoms with regard to the application of biology and medicine.*

> *Article 2 – Primacy of the Human Being*
> *The interests and welfare of the human being shall prevail over the sole interests of society or science.*

Both the Vo case and *Calvelli and Ciglio*[50] would have benefited from the use of this convention, as both involved negligence, carelessness and poor judgement on the part of medical personnel. Nevertheless, although this convention was indeed cited by the Court of Cassation in the Vo case, as was its 'Explanatory report', the question of the human beings to which it applies still remains undecided. In the 'Report', Article I's commentary refers to the 'integrity', and to the 'dignity and identity' of a human being.[51] The Report continues:

> *18. The Convention does not define the terms 'everyone' (in French 'toute personne').*
> *These two terms are equivalent and found in the English and French versions of the European Convention on Human Rights, which however, does not define them. In the absence of unanimous agreement on the definition of these terms among member states of the Council of Europe, it was decided to allow domestic law to define them for the purpose of the application of the present Convention.*

Hence, although the convention repeats that 'the human dignity and identity of the human being had to be respected as soon as life began ...', states could and do debate these definitions when dealing with the embryo *in vitro*.[52]

The two major positions are present both in law and biomedicine: either the human embryos (and the foetus) is not considered a human being and therefore has a diminished right ('a relative worth of protection'), or it has the same status as other human beings, and is therefore equally worthy of protection. The legal treatment of both novel reproductive technologies and the health of the preborn will depend on the resolution of this quandary. From an environmental and health point of view, it is not sufficient to simply leave both debate and final decision to each individual state. Transboundary pollution, by definition knows no border, and hazardous practices and products are distributed globally, with the support of the WTO.

If we turn to a consideration of transboundary harms, one must also turn to the International Law Commission (ILC) international liability study. Article 19 of the state responsibility draft articles was dropped, environmental crimes *of state* along with it.

The international liability study continued and was in many respects generally regarded as a development of a specific legal regime for transboundary environmental harm even as its abstract language allowed it to cover other fields as well. It had – and has – much potential to provide the framework for liability without fault, and, I wish to argue, ultimately to assist in resurrecting the notion of certain institutional crimes – state crimes – that no more should require fault than so-called civil liability should.

Much that has preceded this section and the remainder of this work make the case, in various ways, for non-fault-based crime by institutions, with a more challenging task to render individuals criminally responsible without some element of fault, which need not, however, involve classic criminal *mens rea* standards.

However, even the ILC liability study seems, in my view, to shirk from dealing with the ultimate implication of non-fault-based harm, namely, that even some activities that in themselves are lawful, and are conducted without any failures of due diligence, should be stopped for the simple fact of causing serious harm. At the moment, the ILC is content with 'compensation' as the only consequence of harm caused by lawful activity faultlessly carried out. The same disregard for the gravity of environmental harms, whether caused by legal or illegal activities, is still apparent in the ILC Reports in the following years. It is Special Rapporteur Rao who writes the 'First Report on the legal regime for allocation of loss in the case of transboundary harm arising out of hazardous activities'.[53]

Six major points emerge and are worthy of note. First, there is no mention of criminal prosecution as only 'civil liability' and 'compensation' are mentioned throughout the report. Second, while 'serious harm' is viewed as 'significant adverse change'[54] in the environment, the extent of 'damage' is nonetheless left essentially underfined.[55] It is true that elsewhere in the report, Rao states that it is not speaking of *de minimis* damage, and the harm considered should be:

> more than 'detectable' and 'appreciable', and need not be at the level of 'serious' or 'substantial'. Further, the harm must lead to real detrimental effects on such aspects as human health, industry, property, the environment or agriculture in other States which could be measured by factual and objective standards.[56]

However, this advances matters very little: this confused and confusing statement is taken from the work of the 1996 ILC Working Group, and Rao adds that it could not be endorsed at that time (or since that time apparently) because, among other reasons, there was a lack of agreement on the emphasis on 'State liability' and the 'treatment of prevention as part of a regime of liability'.[57] Third, the question of whose 'factual and objective standards' would prevail in final decisions is never addressed. Fourth, the connection between environment and human health is never made as the two areas are treated as separate, despite the presence of abundant scientific evidence.[58] Fifth, there is no mention throughout the document of *erga omnes* obligations. In fact even the possibility, in case of severe damage, of demanding 'cessation or *restitutio in integrum*' is viewed as excessive. Rao adds, 'in those cases where harm cannot reasonably be avoided, since otherwise such activities would have to be closed down'.[59] Finally, the articles are described as dealing only with activities posing a risk of 'transboundary harm', with 'physical consequences'; but they do not deal with 'creeping pollution, pollution from multiple sources and harm to the global commons'.[60]

Hence it is clear that no move has been made to return to a more serious considera-tion of the criminality of grave environmental harms, nor to the imposition of limits and obligations based on the increasingly well-documented connection between all that is omitted *a priori* from consideration by the ILC, and human health, thus human rights, globally. So is it sufficient to claim that the activities giving rise to the described consequences were legal at the time they occurred, and might even be legal today? Article 3 of the International Law Commission,[61] is short and to the point on this issue: '*Prevention.* States shall take all appropriate measures to prevent, or to minimize the risk of, significant transboundary harm.' Special Rapporteur Srenivasa Rao (8 May 1998), says:

> *The objective of prevention of transboundary damages arising from hazardous activi-ties had been emphasized in principle 2 of the Rio Declaration ... and confirmed by ICJ in its advisory opinion on the* Legality of the Threat or Use of Nuclear Weapons, *as forming part of the corpus of international law.*[62]

That said, it might be best to devote all possible efforts to a reconsideration of the preborn in domestic, and international, law as the environment as such is far from being protected under the current regimes.

Although in preambles and other introductory language, it is clearly stated that life is entitled to full protection, in most European member states, there is presently no definition of the human embryo or foetus (Belgium, Denmark, Finland, France, Greece, Ireland, Italy, Luxembourg, The Netherlands, Portugal and Sweden) or the existing definitions vary a great deal (Austria, Germany, Spain and the UK). Nevertheless the opinion submitted by the *European Group on Ethics in Science and New Technologies*, is repeated in various instruments: progress of knowledge in life sciences cannot 'prevail over fundamental human rights'. *A fortiori* then, it would seem that when there is no question of scientific research or advancement as in the cases cited, the courts should be able to come down clearly on the side of the unborn. This is not the case, as we have seen, because of the problems of defining humans and human beings.

On the side of environmental/health hazards, the 'research and progress' aspect again should be clearly stated but viewed at best as secondary. For the most part haz-ardous processes, products and practices may be economically or otherwise useful, but even if they are, the notion of treating children and the preborn as subjects in indus-try's experiments, and for *their* (industries') economic advantage, should be viewed as repugnant by all humankind. Thus we are left with the stark contrast between a morally unacceptable *status quo* versus the possibility of acquiring a changed mindset that truly respects life at all its stages.

What should be changed in law, is the very issue under consideration in this research: the rights of the child to health, a question usually addressed only in the con-text of the rights to abortion instead:

> *For example, the Austrian and Netherlands Constitutional Courts had held that Article 2 should not be interpreted as protecting the unborn child, and the French Constitutional Council had found no conflict between legislation on the voluntary termination of pregnancy and the constitutional protection of the child's right to health.*[63] *That reading was consistent with the relevant legislation throughout Europe:*

thirty-nine member states of the Council of Europe – the exceptions being Andorra, Ireland, Liechtenstein, Malta, Poland and San Marino, which had maintained severe restrictions on abortion (with only very narrow therapeutic exceptions) – permitted a woman to terminate a pregnancy without restriction during the first trimester or on very broad therapeutic grounds.[64]

This is the crux of the problem. As long as governments' instruments are written with vague sentiments about the rights of the child, the protection of health of the unborn and the like, but the courts decide all cases with the understanding that women's rights to autonomy and privacy supersede the basic right to life and health of the preborn, then even cases that do not concern pregnancies will be treated in the same manner. Hence the health of the child, especially at the earliest times of her existence, will not be seriously considered. The Vo case had several dissenting opinions, and the next section will present their arguments against the Vo decision.

Dissenting opinions in the Vo case

In sum, I see no good legal reason or decisive policy consideration for not applying Article 2 in the present case. On a general level, I believe (in company with many serious judicial bodies in Europe) that there is life before birth, within the meaning of Article 2, that the law must, therefore protect such life, and if a national legislature considers that such protection cannot be absolute, then it should only derogate from it, particularly as regards the voluntary termination of pregnancy, within a regulated framework that limits the scope of derogation.[65]

Although the Vo case was one of medical negligence amounting to malpractice, and not the voluntary termination of a pregnancy, it is the latter concern that clearly restrains the Court and the majority from reaching a decision that is untainted by public policy and even political considerations. In his dissenting opinion, Judge G. Ress advances arguments that supports some of the theoretical points discussed in Chapter 1. France, he says, has a positive obligation to protect children against unintentional homicide, hence it needs effective procedures in place to prevent the recurrence of such acts. Further, tort actions, even when culminating in a favourable decision, cannot be sufficient when a life has been lost, not only as a matter of principle, but because, 'It is not retribution that makes protection by the criminal law desirable, but deterrence'.[66]

The criminal law itself has life as its main concern but, in the present case, there was 'no effective protection' either of the mother, or the foetus. The *Vienna Convention on the Law of Treaties*[67] 'requires treaties to be interpreted in accordance with the ordinary meaning to be given to the terms of the treaty …'[68] The question of the meaning of 'everyone' ('toute personne'), therefore, is easily understood as it has been, traditionally, by lawyers, as human life begins with conception, at which point, 'an *independent existence* develops until it ends with death, birth being but a stage in that development'.[69]

Although almost all contracting states in Europe permit abortion, the fact is that they all had 'constitutional problems [with that issue] because, in principle, the protection of life under constitutional law also extends to the prenatal stage'.[70]

So, even if the meaning of the terms in Article 2, hence the right to life is not totally clear, and there is no one unanimous interpretation of that meaning, Article 2 remains applicable in most cases, and the burden should be on the courts to explain why they must derogate from it, without reference to abortion policies and cases. In addition, this understanding of Article 2 is compatible with the Approach of the Charter of Fundamental Rights of the European Union. In the Vo case, the issue was the life of a 21-week-old foetus who is viable at that stage, although Judge Ress does not even agree with the present standards of viability. Thus Judge Ress concludes that France 'does not afford sufficient protection to the fetus against negligent acts by third parties'.[71]

This position is similar to that taken in the dissent of Judge Mularoni.[72] They argue that Mrs Vo chose a criminal action against a civil one, precisely to establish responsibility for her loss, as 'most victims of crime do'.[73] *Calvelli and Ciglio* is repeatedly referred to by the court in this case, but there, 'the father and mother of a newborn child who died two days after birth – had brought criminal proceedings which ended when the offence of involuntary manslaughter with which the obstetrician was charged, became statute-barred'.

In this case, Mrs Vo was not permitted at least to establish criminal responsibility in the same manner. In this dissenting opinion as well as the opinion of Judge Ress, Article 2 was taken to be applicable to the case at issue, especially because of the 'considerable advances made in science, biology and medicine, including the prenatal stage'.[74] *The Oviedo Convention on Human Rights and Biomedicine*[75] aims:

> to protect the dignity and identity of human beings and to guarantee everyone without discrimination respect for their integrity and other rights and fundamental freedoms with regard to the applications of biology and medicine.[76]

Judges Mularoni and Stra' Nicka' add that this convention protects the dignity of everyone, including the unborn, and that its main concern is explicitly the protection of the dignity and identity of human beings, and the primacy of the latter over *all* other scientific, social and political concerns.

The Oviedo Convention does not define either 'human being' or 'life', but given its concern with extending presently available legal instruments to cover novel technologies, it is fair, I believe, to concur with the interpretation of the dissenting judges. This understanding of a European Convention will be particularly relevant when we turn from civil to common law in the next chapter, not only because several of the cases cited in *Vo v. France* are common law cases, but also because, in general, the common law also 'borrows' from civil law the concept of the juridical presence of the preborn.[77]

TWO OTHER EUROPEAN CASES: *BRÜGGEMANN AND SCHEUTEN V. GERMANY* AND *IRELAND V. GROGAN*

In the previous chapter the definition of 'human life' taken from the case above was cited in full.[78] Now we return to the case where the Federal Republic of Germany defended its Basic Law[79] governing abortion. This law is viewed as too restrictive according to the two applicants, and as interfering 'in particular with their right to respect for their private life under Article 8(1) of the European Convention of Human Rights …'. In German law, according to the Fifth Criminal Law Reform Act, promulgated on 21 June 1974, there were several new provisions introduced in Article 218, as well as Articles 18a, 18b, 18c, and Article 219.

Article 218 – Termination of Pregnancy
1 *Whoever terminates a pregnancy later than on the thirteenth day after conception shall be punished by imprisonment for a term not exceeding three years or a fine.*
2 *The penalty shall be imprisonment for a term of between six months and five years where the perpetrator*
   1. Acts against the will of the pregnant woman, or
   2. Frivolously causes the risk of death or of a serious injury to the health of the pregnant woman.
   The court may order the supervision of conduct.[80]
3 *If the act is committed by the pregnant woman herself, the penalty shall be imprisonment for a term not exceeding one year or a fine.*
   The attempt shall be punishable. The woman shall not be punished for the attempt.

In the other articles mentioned, there are provisions to allow termination (1) 'on specific grounds (indications) after 12 weeks … provided that no more than 22 weeks have elapsed after conception';[81] (2) 'in the absence of information and advice being given to the pregnant woman …';[82] and (3) 'without a medical opinion'.[83] Highly relevant is also Article 219 d. 'Definition', which limits 'termination' to acts that occur after 'the termination of the implantation of the fertilized egg in the uterus'.[84]

Article 8(1) of the *European Convention on Human Rights* defends the right to respect for 'private life'. The Commission's response in this case is enlightening, especially in relation to the logic of the Vo case. Indeed all the arguments of that case hinge on the policy issue: to recognize juridical personhood to the foetus would be detrimental to women's rights to autonomy and privacy, and might prevent a woman's choices within that which is deemed to be her 'private sphere'. But para. 56 of the present case responds to that argument:

56. However, there are limits to the personal sphere. While a large proportion of the law in a given state has some immediate or remote effect on the individual's possibility of developing his personality by doing what he wants to do, not all of these can be considered to constitute an interference with private life in the sense of Article 8 of the Convention.

The truth of this statement is obvious. Of course not all state interference may limit a woman's liberty the way pregnancy does, but it is indisputable that, in general, anyone's liberty is limited by that of others to have and to exercise their own rights. Criminal convictions can be expected by anyone who puts another's life and health at risk by her own choices, hence by the exercise of her autonomy. This is true, for instance, of a drunk driver, even if she has not – so far – actually harmed anyone. It is hard to condemn as injust the prevention of offering more than just harm, but deciding on death for a child, unless immediate self-defence is at issue. This would remain true if the attacker were a stranger instead, and her ability to think, to reason, even to be fully functional in the normal sense, ought not to make a difference.

It is unclear why a different, closer relation to the possible 'attacker', even its presence in one's own body, should make a difference. Self-defence to the point of taking a life, when one's life is in danger, is justified, otherwise a very powerful reason needs to be advanced in its stead: a 'threat' to lifestyle, financial advantage, let alone the abstract protection of autonomy or of privacy, cannot justify killing in any other circumstances. The Commission's discussion refers to interference with private and public life in these cases:

> *58. In two further cases the Commission has taken account of the element of public life in connection with Article 8 of the Convention. It held that subsequent communication of statements made in the course of public proceedings*[85] *did not amount to interference with private life.*

> *59. The termination of an unwanted pregnancy is not comparable with the situation in any of the above cases. However pregnancy cannot be said to pertain uniquely to the sphere of private life. Whenever a woman is pregnant, her private life becomes closely connected with the developing fetus.*[86]

It is impossible to find a situation that is analogous to the relation of the pregnant woman to the foetus, as the latter is entirely *sui generis*. Nevertheless, broadly speaking, a comparison of sorts may be made with the relation between a woman and her incapacitated elderly parents, say her mother. A mother with dementia or Alzheimer's represents an even worse infringement of a woman's rights to privacy, autonomy and freedom of choice. If the care of such a person falls to her, a woman's rights may not prevail over her obligation to provide for care (not entirely or necessarily her own), as long as needed, which may well extend beyond nine months. A number of difficult, costly and emotionally wrenching options may be available to the woman, but death of the difficult parent is not one of those options. So, even moving beyond the mundane rights to privacy/autonomy described above in the case, the total elimination of the problem, even when the elderly disabled mother is no longer a rational person, and there is no reason to hope that, in time, she might be again, is not permitted.

The German Commission does not digress with other examples, but it does recognize that 'certain rights relating to pregnancy are legally protected'. In addition, 'certain rights are attributed to the conceived but unborn child, in particular the right to inherit'[87] and it is significant that the *International Convenant on Civil and Political Rights* does not permit the execution of a pregnant woman. The decision therefore states that to propose limits to abortion rights is not contrary to the provisions of Article 8(1) of the *European Convention on Human Rights*, as it does not interfere unduly with women's freedoms.

The main concern of this work is not to debate abortion, but to uncover the obstacles in the path of securing explicit rights of children to health and the environment. This goal cannot be achieved, I believe, without addressing the main issue: children *can* be and regularly are harmed pre-birth by environmental factors.[88] Unless it is possible to establish in law that at that most vulnerable stage, pre-birth, children have a right to be considered as human beings and to be protected by their own state as well as internationally, while *in utero*, from harms that manifest themselves after birth as genetic abnormalities, and mental and physical diseases, that goal cannot be achieved.

It is extremely difficult, to 'swim upstream' against the increasingly widespread liberalization of women's rights in most countries of the world. Perhaps it is even more difficult to do that, than it is to try and condemn the proliferation of corporate rights and the power of such organizations as the WTO over both health and environmental rights of citizens of all ages everywhere,[89] and I will return to this topic in a later chapter.

For now there is one more case in European law that addresses the issue of the reach of Article 8(1): *Society for the Protection of Unborn Children (Ireland) Limited v. Stephen Grogan and Others*. Grogan discusses abortion, not foetal harms, but it does so in two ways that render it particularly useful for our purpose. First, it treats abortion as a 'service' provided to pregnant women, hence an activity that should be covered by the European Trade regulatory infrastructure. Second, it brings in the issue of 'public interest'. The background of the case is the Irish legislation regarding abortion; the Union of Students of Ireland, the Dublin Students Union and the Trinity College Dublin Students Union all publish guidebooks for entering students, including information for pregnant students. These booklets discuss the possibility of having an abortion elsewhere, such as the UK, where the procedure is not forbidden by law. *The Irish Constitution*, however, says:

> *Section 58 of the Offences against the person Act 1861, makes it a criminal offence for the pregnant woman herself or another to unlawfully attempt to procure her miscarriage. Section 59 of that Act also makes it a criminal offence to provide unlawful assistance to that end. On the basis of, inter alia, those provisions the Irish courts have recognized the right to life of the unborn as from the moment of conception. Following a referendum in 1983 and express acknowledgment of the right to life of the unborn was inserted in the Irish Constitution. The new third subsection of Article 40, Section 3, of the Constitution reads as follows:*
>
> *'The State acknowledges the right to life of the unborn and, with due regard to the equal right to life of the mother, guarantees in its laws to defend and vindicate that right'.*[90]

The question, ostensibly, is whether 'the activities of abortion clinics constitute services within the meaning of Article 60 of the EEC Treaty[91] and, if so, can they do so in a country that criminalizes such services. The Community law dimension of the issue is that to eliminate the information available to the students, 'may have an adverse effect on Intra-Community trade'.[92]

Nevertheless, it is not sufficient to view this specific case simply as a case concerning the exchange of goods and services, as judgement continues, there are 'Imperative requirements of the Public Interest which may justify limitations on the freedom to supply services'.[93] The main point that emerges is when such 'fundamental rights' as the 'freedom of expression' and 'public policy and public morality' (in the view of one state, Ireland) come into conflict.[94] For the latter, in Ireland, the right to life is also applied to the unborn, but this is not equally true of the European Court of Human Rights, 'in the absence of a uniform European concept of morals'.[95] It is for each Member State to define those concepts in accordance with its own 'scale of values',[96] and the proposed 'answer' is that there is no reason why a Member State that recognizes the protection of unborn life as a 'fundamental principle',[97] should not impose limits on the provision of services its own Constitution condemns as criminal.

The *Grogan* decision is at best an acknowledgement that a country that supports the right to life of the preborn may do so, but there is no move towards incorporating their principles as equally fundamental in the jurisprudence of the European Court of Justice. Nor is there any evidence of an effort to debate the issue at the level of principles: essentially, that which the Constitution of Ireland views as a 'fundamental right' is simply reduced to a preference on the part of a Member State. Why Ireland views it as such is not even questioned and the debate moves the issue either to a simply procedural level, or to simply equate the right to life to that of freedom of expression, neither of which advances the cause of global consideration for the health of the preborn.

THE CASE OF THALIDOMIDE AS 'A SIGNIFIER OR A CHEMICAL COMPOUND THAT HAS TAKEN ON A MULTIFACETED CULTURAL IDENTITY'[98]

In the previous section the focus remained firmly on the status of the foetus in law, aside from the legal status of the environmental harms that may befall it. The approach appeared to be warranted as, in cases of clear negligence or even medical malpractice, neither tort nor criminal prosecution ensued, primarily because of the lack of status and rights on the part of the preborn. If these lacks represent the greatest obstacle to the quest for and the implementation of an appropriate regulative framework able to protect and save human health then, I believe, those are indeed the first problems that must be tackled.

However, there has been a health disaster giving rise to cases of mass torts, where the fact that foetal damages in the first trimester did not hold back the recognition that the harms produced were grave and their effects disastrous for the born alive infant. Hence, there has been an 'ideal' case for epidemiology and for law, as 'only a few toxins can meet' the high standards of causation manifested by the result of thalidomide exposure in the preborn:[99]

> *Unfortunately toxic substance injury cases cannot produce mechanistic, deductively derived causal evidence, and a corpuscolarian judge cannot process the available probabilistic evidence.*[100]

But thalidomide meets several 'qualifications' to enable litigants to succeed in the courts as: (1) 'Thalidomide, a sufficient causal antecedent by itself, easily fulfills the high standard; while other toxins would require a modified standard of cause-in-fact in order to support a finding of liability in tort';[101] (2) 'as a matter of tort history, it existed'; and (3) 'its harms formed a basis of worldwide litigation'.[102]

But the mass tort actions that followed the findings about thalidomide were not successful as the settlements that were produced were inadequate in most countries;

in the US, claimants obtained 'next to nothing'.[103] Thus Bernstein concludes that, 'Mass torts are a false cure for toxic exposure not because tort liability is pernicious, but because it is inadequate'.[104] I have argued that such exposures, when caused by environmental causes including chemicals and toxic substances, should be treated as crimes, rather than torts.[105] Both the proven effects of thalidomide and the procedural results of tortious claims, I believe, reinforce my argument: tort claims are necessary but not sufficient in such cases.

For the most part, both scientists and various government institutions are inclined to be sceptical about toxic risks, a highly irresponsible position, as Mark Hertsgaard says: 'Innocent until proven guilty may sound fine in theory, but it lets the bodies pile up before the truth gets written.'[106] When one considers that the 'innocent until proven guilty' approach now applies also to wealthy corporate criminals, and 'environmental culprits', rather than the vulnerable impoverished individuals for which it was originally intended, perhaps my argument for 'ecocrimes' may appear credible.[107]

In general, studies consider one substance at a time, and do not look at cumulative and synergistic effects. Low dose exposures are seldom considered, and the time of the exposure is hardly ever an issue.[108] Yet the possible sources of harm are, at present, immense:

> in 1989 the United States made and imported 5.9 trillion pounds of industrial chemicals, excluding pesticides, pharmaceuticals and food additives, to say nothing of natural poisons and alleged toxins, such as Gulf War exposure, that implicate sources beyond the list – and the conclusion of 'proven guilty' becomes even more impossible.[109]

It is also worthy of note to realize that many diseases are not even considered, as cancer is viewed as primary, for instance, according to the *Delaney Clause*, which bans food additives that cause cancer in animal species.[110]

Thus the horrors of a teratogenic substance like thalidomide can be accompanied by some benefits. For instance, it can be viewed as a 'new signifier',[111] as it showed clearly the potential ability of chemical substances to cross the placenta, hence the need to recognize the right of protection to the preborn. The right of the child to have normal function and health at birth is therefore based, inescapably, on foetal protection. Thalidomide has also spurred the development of institutional watchdogs especially in Europe; and in law, it has demonstrated the failure of regular tort procedures, despite the fact that, unlike the trials for tobacco exposure or other adult exposures where corporate representatives attempted to blame the lifestyle and personal habits of the victims, all thalidomide victims were clearly innocent.

The European Medicine Evaluation System and the US Legal Instruments

I believe that both the thalidomide example of mass torts and its most important result as causative of new institutions and standards both play out primarily in Europe, hence the addition of this example to the chapter devoted to civil law. But the comparison of US and European approaches to allowing the use of pharmaceuticals may provide a bridge to the next chapter and the discussion of common law. The US Food and

Drug Administration (FDA) was, in 1960, the employer of Dr Frances Kelsey who, as an FDA examiner, did not approve the use of thalidomide, because of the lack of significant information about its safety.[112] The FDA has been targeted by critics intent on deregulation, and disturbed by the power of that agency over a large range of products, particularly because of the Republican Congress's efforts 'to challenge traditional patterns of administrative activity'.[113]

But it is vital to note that the fact that neither patients nor managed health care insurers, nor even doctors, are well able to replace the research the FDA provides prior to granting an approval.[114,115]

However, critics argue that the FDA is very slow to approve, and that, although the results following upon the approval of a potentially harmful drug are highly visible, the consequences for ill people of lengthy delays with the possible deprivation of helpful medications, are hidden from the public eye, for the most part.

I have noted elsewhere the disasters that follow upon deregulation in general, such as the E. coli epidemic in Walkerton, Ontario, after the conservative government of Mike Harris enacted its 'Common Sense Revolution', which included the deregulation and privatization of local water controls and extensive cuts to both administrative bodies and environmental protection, with disastrous results.[116] The public interest should be protected by those entrusted with that task and publicly supported to perform their job for the common good, not for the optimization of corporate and political interests. The courts themselves may be used after the fact, and as we noted in the case of thalidomide, the ensuing tort litigation did very little for the severely affected victims.

However, the European Community has established a centralized agency in order to combine both safety and efficiency in the approval process.[117,118] The European Community has created a new body at a time when the awareness of recent public health threats is emerging as a danger that cannot be ignored, whereas the US may be tied to older paradigms of legal protection. Professor Wendy Parnet, for instance, speaks of the 'deconstitutionalization of public health'. She adds:

> *The Supreme Court has had difficulty making the transition from early years of American history, when the pre-eminent threats were epidemics of infectious diseases, to the present, when the threats are broader in scope and include chronic diseases caused by industrial activities.*[119]

The 'disassociation of public health and constitutional theory' is highly problematic for the future of public health protection, as the loss of a 'constitutional foundation' means that no such rights are entrenched in US laws, and the same appears to be true of the Canadian Charter of Rights and Freedoms, where s.7 on the security of persons has never been extended to the protection of public health or the prevention of environmental harms.

The European Medicines Agency (EMEA) is a supranational agency: its rulings are intended to be binding on the entire European community. These rulings are to be given within 300 days after applicants submit new drug considerations for the agency's approval.[120] A cooperative international approach, subject to supranational controls, however, appears to conflict with the present US administration's goals and practices, whereas, ideally, it is only through a supranational approach that public health and safety can be truly protected. The present trend to protectionism for corporate 'freedoms' at the expense of public health affect us all in various degrees, starting with the 'canaries', the children whose normal function and development is under attack in as many ways as there are pervasive, untested chemicals in our habitat.

In the next chapter we will turn to an examination of common law cases and instruments. Although they clearly take different approaches than the cases mentioned so far, a common thread can be discerned in both groups: the expressed belief either by the majority or by the dissenting judges, that the issue of the life of the preborn is a grave one, and that it should be dealt with in detail by the legislature, *not* by lawyers or even by the courts.[121]

In sum, so far we have noted the vast gulf separating the well-argued and well-researched theory[122] from the total abandonment of theoretical or historical justification for the political/public policy led decisions reached by the court in Vo, only barely supported by existing law instruments. It must be acknowledged that the same dichotomy will be found to prevail in the decisions and the arguments of common law cases.

NOTES

1 Dooley-Clark (1982), pp31–46.
2 The Judges' Portal; see Westra (2004a).
3 CEDAW, effective 1981, 165 State Parties in March 2000.
4 *UN Doc A/47/38*,1 Int. Hum. Rts. Rep. 25, 1994.
5 CEDAW/C/1999/1/L.1/Add.7,1999.
6 L'enfant simplement concu est repute ne chaque fois qu'il s'agit de ses interets; Massager (1996).
7 Massager (1996).
8 Massager (1996).
9 Meulders-Klein (1975), p20.
10 Massager (1996), p4.
11 Christian Atias (1985), no4.
12 Massager (1996), p9.
13 Tamburlini et al (2002); Wigle (2003).
14 Aristotle *De Generatione Animalium II*, 1731b 24–1732a 3; see also Aristotle *De Anima II*, 4.415a25–b7.
15 Massager (1996), p16.
16 Aristotle, *Nicomachean Ethics X*, chapters 7–8.
17 Massager (1996), pp17–19.
18 Plutarch, *Lycurgus*, t.1, p8, Garnier ed.
19 Massager (1996), p21.
20 Meyer (1987), p578.
21 Mémenteau (1983), p332.
22 Massager (1996), p33.
23 Labbée (1984), pp401–404.
24 Murray (1996), pp464–472.
25 *Doc. Parl. Ch.S.O. 1989–1990*, No.1033/1p.11; see also full citation and discussion in Massager (1996), p395.
26 Massager (1996), p44.
27 Tamburlini et al (2002); Wigle (2003).

28 European Convention on Human Rights (ECHR), Strasbourg, 8 July 2004.
29 A criminal offence under Article 319 of the former Criminal Code – which was applicable at the material time – now Article 221-6 of the Criminal Code.
30 A criminal offence under Article R.40, subparagraph 4, of the former Criminal Code – which was applicable at the material time – now Article R. 625-2 and R.625-4 of the Criminal Code.
31 The Criminal Code, p5.
32 'Another' within the meaning of Article 221-6 of the Criminal Code.
33 The Criminal Code.
34 *Voluntary Termination of Pregnancy Act* of 17 January 1975 (Law no. 75-17).
35 Law no. 94-653 of 29 July 1994 on the *Respect for the Human Body* (Article 16 of the Civil Code).
36 *Vo*, p7.
37 *Vo*, p7.
38 *Vo*, p41.
39 Ch.1, Public Offences – Book V.
40 Article 511-18 (*Vo*, p10).
41 Under the *Patient's Rights and Quality of Health Services Act* (Law No. 2002-203).
42 *Vo*, p10.
43 *Vo*, p11.
44 *Vo*, p12.
45 Article 221-6.
46 'Unintentional violence on pregnant women and the offence of unintentional homicide', Receuil Daloz (2004), p449.
47 *Vo*, p13, para. 31.
48 *Calvelli and another v. Italy* [2001] ECHR 3296/96.
49 Oviedo, 4 April 1997, in force December 1, 1999.
50 *Calvelli and another v. Italy* [2001]ECHR 3296/96.
51 Vo case, Commentary, para. 17.
52 See for instance the debates in the work of the *European Group on Ethics in Science and New Technologies at the European Commission*, 5th Framework Program, 23 November, 1998.
53 *International Law Commission (ILC) Fifty-fifth Session*, Geneva 5 May–6 June and 7 July–8 August, 2003.
54 *ILC Fifty-fifth Session* (see note 53 above), p27.
55 *ILC Fifty-fifth Session* (see note 53 above), p27.
56 *ILC Fifty-fifth Session* (see note 53 above), p15, para. 31.
57 *ILC Fifty-fifth Session* (see note 53 above), p16.
58 See Chapter 1 of this work
59 *ILC Fifty-fifth Session* (see note 53 above), p15, ft. 59.
60 *ILC Fifty-fifth Session* (see note 53 above), p16, para. 35
61 ILC Rep. (1988), Ch. 4, at www.un.org/law/ilc/reports/1998/chp4.html
62 ILC 1 X.B. I.L.C. 61 (1998)
63 *Decision no. 74054* of January 15, 1975.
64 *Vo*, pp2–29, para. 62.
65 Separate Opinion of Judge Costa joined by Judge Traja, p49, para.17.
66 Dissenting Opinion of Judge Ress, p50, para. 1.
67 Article 31, no.1.
68 Article 31, p51, para. 3.
69 Article 31, para. 4.
70 Article 31, p52, para. 5
71 Article 31, p53, para. 9.

72 Judge V. Stra' Nicka' concurring.

73 Article 31, p55.

74 Article 31, p57; see also Massager (1996) and chapter 1.

75 4 April 1997, came into force 1 December, 1999.

76 Article 31, p57.

77 *Dobson (Litigation Guardian of) v. Dobson*, [1999] 2 S.C.R. 753.

78 *Brüggemann and Scheuten v. Federal Republic of Germany*, ECHR Appl. No. 6959;3 E.H.R.R. 244/245

79 *Grundgesetz*

80 Article 68 (1) (2).

81 Article 218b (2).

82 Article 218c.

83 Article 219.

84 Article 219, p215.

85 App. no. 3868/68, *X v. U.K.* (1970) 34 C.D. 10,18) or the taking of photographs of a person participating in a public incident (App. no. 5877/7 *X v. UK.* (1974) 45 C.D. 90.93.

86 3E. H. R. R. 244,2530.

87 At para. 60.

88 Tamburlini et al (2002); Wigle (2003).

89 Westra (2004a); Barlow and Clarke (2002).

90 1991 *ECJ Celex Lexis* 6962, p2.

91 1991 *ECJ Celex Lexis* 6962, p4, para. 8.

92 1991 *ECJ Celex Lexis* 6962.

93 1991 *ECJ Celex Lexis* 6962, p8.

94 1991 *ECJ Celex Lexis* 6962, pp15–16, para. 37.

95 1991 *ECJ Celex Lexis* 6962.

96 1991 *ECJ Celex Lexis* 6962.

97 1991 *ECJ Celex Lexis* 6962, p17, para. 41.2.

98 Bernstein (1997).

99 Bernstein (1997).

100 Brennan (1988), pp469, 491.

101 Bernstein (1997).

102 Bernstein (1997).

103 Bernstein (1997).

104 Bernstein (1997), p7.

105 Westra (2004a), see Chapters 2 and 7.

106 Hertsgaard (1996), p10.

107 Westra (2004a).

108 Colborn et al (1996); Tamburlini et al (2002).

109 Bernstein (1997), p7; Zeeman (1996), p542.

110 *Delanewy Clause* U.S.C. 348 (C) (3)(A), 1994.

111 Bernstein (1997), p3.

112 *Harvard Law Review* (1995).

113 *Harvard Law Review* (1995).

114 Hutt (1993), pp216–217.

115 Burley et al (1993).

116 Westra (2004a), chapter 4.

117 Kingham et al (1994).

118 Katz (1993).

119 Parnet (1996).

120 Kingham et al (1994), pp304–312.

121   *Stenberg v. Carhart* 530 U.S. 914; Apr. 25, 2000 Argued June 28, 2000 Decided; 2000 U.S. Lexis 4484.

122   Massager (1996).

CHAPTER 3

The Status of the Child and the Preborn in Common Law Instruments and Cases

INTRODUCTION: HUMAN RIGHTS IN THE CONTEXT OF NEO-LIBERAL GLOBALIZATION

> *Matters involving their rights, you will have noticed – or so-called rights – are more readily voiced by consumers than those involving duties or agonizing choices ... It is indeed my opinion that this self-assertingness, this harping on limitless rights, the disregard for the rights of other people that characterize these consumers' liberation movements constitute one aspect of the moving-spirit, the* Weltanschauung, *of our times.*[1]

When the rights of the child are considered in theory, even those of the preborn, it is easier to find and use arguments that are favourable to the protection of these children from environmental harm. But there is a vast gulf between theory and the practical results that ensue when theories, including definitions of the child or the preborn are tested in the courts of law. The rights of the child are, like many other rights, victims of a spreading, ever more powerful, neo-liberal globalization, and that is harmful in itself:

> *neo-liberal globalization is incompatible with globalization of human rights.*[2]

In 1948 the *Universal Declaration of Human Rights* required justice in all human dealings, including the distribution of material and non-material advantages. Article 25 reads, in part, as follows:

> *Everyone has the right to a standard of living adequate for the health and well-being of himself and his family, including food, clothing, housing and medical care and the necessary social services, and the right to security in the case of unemployment, sickness, disability, widowhood, old age or other lack of livelihood.*

Children are not named specifically but surely their health and well-being ought to be protected at least as well as those of other vulnerable groups named. John O'Neill argues that the child is 'missing ... in liberal theory'. He also argues against 'putting a market price upon the staples of a good society', and against 'irresponsible greed' and the 'privatization of the commons'. Speaking of the situation in Canada, he says:

> *It is time for Canadians to re-think the grounds of child, youth and family security,*
> *and to refurbish the institutions of civic sustainability that are richer than the forced*
> *choices of a market or welfare-state provisions. The sustainability of civic institutions*
> *is enriched through an embodied tradition of obligations to one another that cannot be*
> *limited to contracts any more than it can be captured in the device of a safety net.*[3]

The presence of globalization then, as George argues, does not involve everyone in an 'integrated and unified world ... from which all earth's inhabitants will somehow benefit'.[4] Instead it can be demonstrated that globalization is a phenomenon that ensures the triumph of the world's market economy, at the expense of the weak, the impoverished and the vulnerable everywhere. George adds:

> *If neo-liberal globalization is allowed to endure politics will concern primarily the*
> *deadly issue of survival. This is the bottom line issue of human rights: who has the*
> *right to live and who does not?*[5]

No doubt here George addresses the issue of poverty and non-participation. But we can easily see the connection if we consider that children too neither produce nor consume, much like poverty-stricken peoples, so that advocates for their rights are few and far between.

When this reality is understood together with the fact that – in general – preferences and choices in society are routinely used by the powerful to neglect or even eliminate the rights of those who are not able to fight for themselves, we see that while corporate rights and power expand, others' ability to defend themselves does not. This expansion of power also accrues to those whose preferences and choices can mobilize support, but children, let alone the preborn, do not appear to have gained in the decades since the 1924 Geneva *Declaration of the Rights of the Child*; if anything, they have receded in the public consciousness, as they are bypassed even by public morality. It is not the rights of the future, but advantage here and now that drives public policy, and this reality will manifest itself once again as one considers common law countries as well as those where civil law prevails. In general, human rights to health are viewed as secondary to trade advantage, as it is evident for instance in the battle between the WTO and the European Community in the Hormones case.[6,7]

If no trade or economic advantage would accrue, then the motivation of groups and individuals to pursue a moral course of protection on behalf of the most vulnerable is sadly lacking. Even the recent WHO/EU Ministerial Conference,[8] tended more to precaution and negotiation, where those who impose harm (e.g. chemical companies) were 'at the table', heard as equals with the scientists and the WHO representatives, whose extensive research clearly indicts their practices.

The precautionary principle was indeed invoked, but even that move appeared dictated more by a desire to continue a dialogue with the powerful harm imposers than by logic. When a large number of scientists have been able to demonstrate the significant, often irreversible harms inflicted on children by practices and products, it is no longer a question of 'scientific uncertainty', which might perhaps have been justified many years ago, but which makes little sense today, other than as tool of appeasement, when the volume of research is too extensive to be doubted.[9]

These issues will be addressed in more detail in later sections, as it is not necessary now to establish whether common law countries follow the same patterns of 'political correctness' over logic and human rights that was evident in the civil law cases. Hence the next section will follow the pattern of the previous chapter: it will address first the theoretical arguments found in common law, for and against the possibility of acknowledging legal personhood, hence rights to the preborn.

SOME ARGUMENTS REGARDING THE RIGHT TO LIFE OF THE PREBORN IN COMMON LAW

The case is not the measure of the principle . . . thus, . . . one by one, important principles become recognized through adjudications which illustrated them, and which constitute authoritative evidence of what law is when other cases shall arise.[10,11]

Although common law draws strictly from civil law in its consideration of the preborn, the arguments provided for the status of the *infans conceptus,* are viewed from a somewhat different perspective. Rather than harking back in time to Ancient Rome, Greece and the traditional values and arguments present in the scholarly work of those times and then tracing their historical development, common law relies primarily on decided cases.

Thus its main disadvantage is the lack of requirements to consider seriously legal tradition and, especially, scholarly argument. Its main advantage, however, is the fact that, as Mr Justice Holmes suggested, 'the life of the law has not been logic: it has been experience'.[12] As Mr Justice McGuire put it: 'The common law is not an arid and sterile thing, and it is anything but static and inert.'[13] Mr Justice McGuire continues by recognizing the existence of 'the process of judicial lawmaking', as common law is intended to be more than a sterile exercise of the consideration of precedents, but that process permits 'extracting a rule of law' from that judicial process.

In contrast with civil law, common law judges are expected to appraise and compare 'social values'. This, I believe, is a significant part of both its weakness and its strength. It is its weakness because then it must rely on the 'social values' of a specific state or nation, and it does so no matter what the logical or factual basis of these values, at times. In this respect then, it skirts very close to unrestrained cultural relativism. Yet if judges are allowed, even encouraged, to reason out the arguments supporting precedent, they might also do so by rejecting positions that do not fit recently discovered scientific facts, for instance, or by embracing positions that better respect extended human rights.

This comparative analysis must be preformed, according to Mr Justice McGuire, by '. . .weigh(ing) competing demands of social advantage, not unmindful that continuity and symmetry of the law are themselves such advantages. . .'[14] Through this exercise the 'vitality of the common law system' and its capacity for growth is advanced.

The case of *Dietrich v. Inhabitants of North Hampton*[15] has been relied upon and its main position, that is, the 'fact' that the unborn child is part of the mother, accepted without question, despite the presence of conflicting decisions and dissents, such as *Allaire v. St. Luke Hospital et al*, decided after Dietrich, at the turn of the century,[16] where the strong dissent of Boggs, J. introduced another more logical point of view:

> *Medical science and skill and experience have demonstrated that a period of gestation in advance of the period of parturition, the fetus is capable of independent and separate life, and that, though within the body of the mother, it is not merely a part of her body, for her body may die in all its parts and the child remain alive, and capable of maintaining life, when separated from the dead body of its mother.*[17]

This position and approach is basic to moving forward to a more serious consideration of the rights of the child to health and the environment, our main quest in this work. It is this medical reality that permits Ron Beal to argue that, 'It would be difficult to set fourth an argument that a child does not have the right to the fullest extent possible to be born with a sound mind and body'.[18]

Beal's argument goes to the heart of the matter as it deals with the most intractable of topics: not only the possibility of tortious action for harm to the foetus because of negligent acts or omissions by third parties, but also the possibility of such action being brought against the mother herself.

If accepted, this position would effectively reverse the 'correct' policy that gives, in most countries, effective life/death power to the mother, in regard to her conceived infant. But scientific research has increasingly been able to demonstrate the connection between early embryonic stage and foetal exposure, and harm to the child: 'In fact, the medical profession recognizes the fetus as an individual patient, in addition to its mother, as it relates to prenatal care.'[19] But the US Supreme Court decided that the mother's right to privacy supersedes the child's right to life before birth. Yet, 'It appears then that society may still recognize the right of a child to begin life with a sound mind and body, the right to be well-born'.[20] The intractable conflict between the US Supreme Court Decision and even the mere possibility of acknowledging the preborn's rights to health, to be 'well-born', is not often recognized in any of the treatments of this topic I have come across.

Its lack of logic is not addressed, although it is especially obvious when it is possible for a child to sue her mother for 'wrongful life' or pre-birth negligence. How can a mother who has not exercised her absolute power of life/death over the foetus (a right held by the Roman *pater familias* in ancient times), be sued subsequently, if after granting the foetus a 'stay of execution', later she does not fully direct her energies and efforts to its well-being? Clearly this conceptual conflict is not a major component of this work's research, but the US Supreme Court decision in *Roe v. Wade*[21] (which allowed only some consideration to the foetus at viability), certainly is, as no case or instrument escapes at least one reference to that landmark decision. Thus we can benefit, for instance, from Beal's arguments without getting fully involved in the specific focus of possible actions for negligence by the born child, against its mother.

Acts and omissions by third parties are clearly much easier to handle, if we accept the child's right to be 'well-born', that is to have health and normal function. One significant aspect of Dietrich must be emphasized. Although the judgement was intended to make clear the fact that the preborn does not have legal personhood, hence that prenatal injuries caused by negligence were not actionable, in that case the infant actually survived for ten or fifteen minutes 'in the sense that the child exhibited motion in its limbs for that period of time'.[22] Hence there was a point when the infant was (a) not 'part of his mother's body' (as Justice Oliver Wendell Holmes maintained); and (b) alive; hence the decision was biologically as well as logically unsound, and its 'rejection of the civil law "birth for benefit" approach'[23], was equally unsound, in this case.

Tort law aims to allow a remedy when a wrong has occurred as Bonbrest clearly indicates.[24] Criminal law, as was noted in the previous chapter in *Vo. v. France*, aims at bringing to justice those who commit crimes. Both realms of law are not well-served by the Holmes decision, which has been set aside and superseded by later cases as we shall see.

It is unfortunate, however, that the *Roe v. Wade* decision has not been viewed as equally obsolete in recent times, as I believe it might be that decision, single-handedly, that has blocked the possibility of advances in the recognition of human rights, that was one of the touted advantages available to common law decisions.

Arguments about the possible introduction of 'human life amendments' into law

Following the *Roe v. Wade* Decision (1973), the US Congress received several proposals for 'human life statutes' and for 'constitutional amendments', to reserve the decision that held that:

> *the constitutionally protected right to privacy includes the right of women to terminate pregnancies free of state interference until the fetus is viable...*[25]

This decision prompted no less than 'three proposed constitutional amendments and the Helms-Hyde Bill'.[26,27,28,29,30]

The first thing to note is that David Westfall writes on the topic from a pro-abortion perspective, a routinely found position in most writings on this subject. Thus his analysis of the problems that might follow the acceptance of a human life amendment considers first all the difficulties without offering a balanced list of possible advantages that might also result. He does recognize that there are 'fundamental ethical and religious views on the value of human life', as well as considerations about 'society's high regard for individual privacy and autonomy'.[31] Yet to characterize the value of human life as 'ethical and religious', mistakes the issue. It prompts the question, 'whose ethics', and 'whose religion', thus providing a mistaken analysis of the issue from the start. The human right to life is entrenched in international law instruments, and not open to contrary 'evidence' based on religious or culturally bound beliefs.

In the previous chapter, the difference between the question of 'ensoulment' of the *infans conceptus*, and her humanity, was discussed. The former is clearly a religious question, the latter is based on biology and the medical sciences. To attempt to reduce it to a religious question is simply to embrace the neo-liberal approach that gives primacy to preferences, however based, over principled and thus defensible choices; and that is the true mark of relativism. But the value of all human life is a basic principle of both law and morality. For instance the (human) rights of women are so viewed, and appeals to religious dogma do not excuse depriving women of their human rights, either in domestic or international law.

Similarly, support based on a religious stance that does not recognize and respect humanity in the preborn, should not be used as a final argument in support of her non-humanity. Many recognize the conflict as one of rights. For instance Section 2 of *The Garn-Rhodes proposal* (see n. 27), says:

> *Section 2. No unborn person shall be deprived of life by any person. Provided however that nothing in this article shall prohibit a law permitting only those medical procedures required to prevent the death of the mother.*

It is worthy of note that this and other proposed amendments use the highly controversial expression 'person', a position on which much has been written in biomedical ethics, specifically on the abortion issue. Instead, *The Helles-Dorman Proposal* (see n.28) reads as follows:

> *The paramount right to life is vested in each human being from the moment of fertilization without regard to age, health or condition of dependency.*

This proposal starts with a biological fact, thus avoiding the controversial issue of what a person is, and when, precisely, an infant becomes one, a subject treated for instance by Mary-Ann Warren, and Michael Tooley, the latter in relation to infanticide.[32]

The *conceptus*, however, is undeniably human, thus not feline, porcine, or representing the embyonic or foetal state of any other animal. That said, the next argument advanced by Westfall is a sound one: it would be extremely difficult, once one of the proposed amendments became law, to ensure that its only effect would limit abortion to conflicts with the right to life of the mother, as other laws would be affected as well, in various realms, from voting to taxation, all of which depend on live birth being the start of life.[33] If an 'abortion only' application of a 'life proposal' would not be possible, there are two other possible interpretations: it might be used to ensure (2) 'Protection from Bodily Injury', or even ensure (3) 'Equal Protection with other Persons'.[34]

I believe that any attempt to characterize foetuses and embryos as persons is doomed from the start, because it lacks both logical and scientific support. In fact, a 'full panoply' of rights, comparable to those adults enjoy, even if available to born infants is not defensible; instead for the *infans conceptus*, civil law's proposal of accepting 'rights as minors' then, is a lot closer to a defensible position as we saw above (Chapter 1). But the second possibility, if combined with the first, has a much stronger, more defensible sound than the paradoxical inclusion of 'full rights' or 'personhood', positions that can easily be attacked and defeated. In contrast:

> *It would be possible to weigh the potential detriment to the* conceptus *from given forms of conduct by the woman, against the potential interference with her privacy and autonomy interests.*[35]

Aside from the obvious disanalogy between the potential limitation of 'privacy and autonomy' for a specified time, and, on the side of the *conceptus*, the elimination of all potential life experiences through the irreversible termination of all life processes,[36] another possibility is not even envisaged: that of third parties inducing bodily injury, a common occurrence, as we noted in the work of the WHO and others (see Chapter 1).

In fact a parallel situation exists with another group that is strongly demanding and powerfully defending its almost unlimited present 'rights': the group of corporate legal persons. As Dr John Bradshaw says as he laments the lack of reflective interventions in biomedical public policy by the laity:

> *Matters involving their rights, you will have noticed – or so-called rights – are more readily voiced by consumers than those involving duties or agonizing choices... It is indeed my opinion, that this self-assertiveness, the harping on limitless rights, the disregard for the rights of other people that characterizes these consumers' liberation movements constitute one aspect of the moving spirit, the* Weltanschauung *of our time.*[37]

Bradshaw contrasts the consumerist approach with the reflective soul-searching needed instead, to understand these issues. He also argues that what has happened in America and Britain in abortion laws, did so 'in clear contravention variously of the expressed intention of the legislators, the judges and the doctors'.[38]

The evidence of events contrary to the public interest in those countries is also surprising: 'Washington, DC now has more abortions than live births'.[39] With widely available contraceptives, in the late 1970s, the number of sexually active girls aged 15 and under doubled; in England and Wales, abortions among 15 year olds has tripled; and freely available contraception (the 'pill', as Bradshaw has it) 'now kill more women than did all forms of abortion in the 1960s'.[40]

Thus, simply citing 'privacy and autonomy' as unequivocally superior 'goods', capable of superseding all other choices, is incorrect even if the only referents are the women involved. Figures regarding the result of sexual activities with multiple partners, regarding sexually transmitted disease and cancer of the womb, bear out this analysis, thus any 'balancing' should include other effects of abortion on demand (based on the foetus's status, that is, on no legal personality), as it now exists in most common law countries.

In addition, *infans conceptus* can also be seen as a member of a politically helpless and highly vulnerable minority, a minority that has endured a history of discrimination matched by few other groups.[41] But the recognition of the preborn as a minority, suffering from unparalleled discrimination, as they are, legally, 'as a class, unlike any other human beings... made subject to death at the convenience of others'[42], is not yet acknowledged.

From the standpoint of the present work, however, it is important to note that to continue to grant 'consumerist', preference-based rights to women, carries with it the overwhelming presence of similarly oppressing, harm-imposing rights, to other legal persons, that is, to the corporate bodies whose interests, as we shall see in Chapter 4, supersede even those of adult citizens to be free from interference in their physical integrity and normal function because of harms caused by products and processes that are presently legal.[43]

Nevertheless Westfall cautions about possible problems that may arise if a 'life amendment' were adopted. Some of the issues he names include the interests of a whole new class in federal elections, the 'allocation of voting rights' which may be of critical interest to the preborn, thus demanding guardians to speak on their behalf;[44] another issue is 'the distribution of fiscal benefits' if the term 'dependent child' were to include the preborn;[45] as well as possible effects on capital punishment. But by far the most controversial effects would be those that affect the civil liberties of women, and that will be the topic of the next section, together with a consideration of some of the legal instruments that may also be affected by the adoption of a human life amendment.

Women's rights to privacy and autonomy: Instruments and cases

If the preborn are to be protected, then many fully fledged legal persons will need to curtail some of their rights, and the implications of this possibility for born children will be discussed in Chapters 4 and 5. What is clear, however, is that to expect voluntary compliance without legal implications, from either group (that is either feminists or corporate groups), is – to say the least – naive. In general, for instance, although after *Roe v. Wade* US states could impose criminal liability for terminations after the point of viability, most did not, and do not to this day, despite the advances in scientific knowledge that show the need to consider the preborn during the first trimester.

Because of the limitations imposed by that precedent, and because of the general climate of society, law did not keep pace with science. There is, however, a trend toward accepting tortious actions to recover for 'direct injury to a viable conceptus subsequently born alive. Today a conceptus born alive, generally is allowed to sue for prenatal injuries'.[46]

This of course is the main point of this research, as the rights of the child to health and the environment can only be protected by third parties (self-limiting corporate activities or government instruments) although they can be breached by pregnant women as well as by third parties. At this time, there seems to be no agreement in common law cases on whether the preborn should have been viable at the time of the injury. *Allaire v. St. Luke Hospital et al,*[47] provides the precedent for reliance upon viability, through the forceful dissent of Justice Boggs:

> *A fetus in the womb of the mother may well be regarded as but a part of the mother during a portion of the period of gestation; but if, while in the womb, it reaches that prenatal age of viability when the destruction of the life of the mother does not necessarily end its existence also, and when, if separated prematurely and by artificial means from the mother, it would be so far a matured human being as that it would live and grow . . .*

But Boggs, J. also recognizes that:

> *A child en ventre sa mère was regarded in common law as in esse from the time of conception for the purpose of taking any estate, whether by descent or devise or under the statute of distribution, if the infant was born alive after such a period of fetal existence that its continuance in life was or might reasonably be expected.*[48,49]

By 1946, in *Bonbrest et al v. Kotz et al,*[50] the truth is affirmed that, although the foetus cannot exist separate from the mother prior to viability, it is 'a separate entity biologically distinct from its mother, throughout pregnancy'.[51,52] In addition, in *Smith v. Brennan,*[53] Justice Proctor argues that, 'viable or not at the time of injury, the child sustains the same injury after birth...'

It is the subsequently born child then, who is injured and must at least be able to recover for such injury. In *Bonbrest v. Kotz* the born alive child could recover from injuries inflicted by the attending physician, contrary to what happened in the Vo case (see Chapter 2). It is unclear why a physician who inflicts injuries serious enough to warrant the death of a viable child, should escape prosecution altogether, because the injuries were so serious that the child in perfect health prior to the doctor's 'intervention', could not be born alive but died in the womb.

Several cases point to a gradual acceptance of pre-birth injuries as actionable. For instance in *Montreal Tramways v. Leveille,*[54] the Supreme Court of Canada affirmed an award for prenatal injuries on the prenatal rights of the injured preborn, not on having reached viability prior to the injury. This approach is reaffirmed in *Kelly v. Gregory,*[55] as Bergen, J.'s opinion states in regard to foetal injuries sustained as the mother (in her third month of pregnancy) was knocked down by a car, while walking over a crosswalk:

> *We ought to be safe in this respect in saying that legal separability should begin when there is biological separability. We know something more of the actual process of conception and fetal development now than when some common-law cases were decided; and what we know makes it possible to demonstrate clearly that separability begins at conception (at para. 543–544).*

To demonstrate the progression toward increasing the consideration of pre-birth harms, one need only consider such cases as *Jorgensen v. Meade Johnson Laboratories.*[56] Twin daughters were born to Andrew and Kimberly Jorgensen, both with Down's Syndrome, and one of these died because of the difficulties associated with that condition at age three and a half. The claim was that the oral contraceptive Oracon, produced by Meade Laboratories, caused the condition and the death, and that 'the company (was) liable under the principle of strict liability in tort negligence and breach of express and implied warrantees (Opinion by Holloway, Circuit Judge).

This is a case where a product was used before conception and still judged to have been harmful to the future infants. Although at first the plea appeared to apply to circumstances prior to conception, effectively 'the pleading should not be construed as being limited to effects on development before conception' (at para. 239). This is the crux of the issue addressed here, and the disposition of the case lists a number of cases that are equally based on negligently inflicted prenatal injuries.[57,58,59,60,61,62] If the causal connection between the product and the results that eventually followed its use could be proven in fact, they convinced Holloway, J. to allow the complaint to go forward.[63]

In contrast, in *Grodin v. Grodin,*[64] the case concerned a woman who continued to take a harmful antibiotic (tetracycline) as she was repeatedly assured by her physician that she was unable to get pregnant. Only when a different doctor told her she was indeed pregnant, in her seventh month, did she discontinue the practice, with subsequent harm to the child. This case raises another controversial issue: if women were to be treated as responsible in law for prenatal harms, the fact that pregnancies are often not discovered immediately, would pose a grave problem, perhaps limiting the reach of their responsibility. This case is only peripheral to our main concern, but it is still an important issue, because it concerns a woman's civil liberties, the very basis for the lack of standing for the foetus today in most common law and civil law countries.

Specifically, the possible curtailment of the civil liberties of women who are, or could become pregnant is relevant for two reasons: first, it is foundational to the demands of women's movements in regard to their freedom, privacy and autonomy, and the popular support almost worldwide of this position and these goals without either nuance or the possibility of some limitations is the one major obstacle to the thoughtful, serious consideration of the status of the preborn through the lenses of biology, medicine and even logic. This position has also been instrumental in viewing the question of women's absolute rights in regard to the foetus as a settled question, beyond re-examination or dispute.

The second point, already alluded to, is that there is another group globally present and even more powerful, that of corporate legal persons who, in contrast, today have achieved 'rights' that are almost unlimited vis-á-vis individual human beings who are routinely victimized through the environment by their products and processes. The profits that accrue to these 'persons' through those harmful practices, simply serve to increase their already excessive power, at the expense of all human beings, but particularly of women, children and infants and the preborn as well.

Both groups, I suggest, already have too much power over the most vulnerable individuals and peoples: the former on the life of the preborn, and on its health and normal function; the latter on the life health and function of all living beings particularly the most vulnerable. As Bradshaw indicated, the 'consumerist' affirmation of rights, without reflection or consideration of those whose own rights are disregarded in the process, that is, without consideration of corresponding obligations, is typical of the approach to life and its difficult issues in both cases. As long as a member of group A benefits, the question of who pays for the benefit from another group recedes to almost non-existence.

In the case of women, the issue becomes increasingly complicated as science discovers all possible choices and activities that may have negative impacts on the *infans conceptus*, even before such conception may take place. Corporations take advantage of their rights and freedoms and, I am persuaded, will continue to do so unless some status is granted to the preborn and more emphasis is placed on the well child as limits to their freedom. As an example, the tobacco companies could not have been attacked, and forced to some compliance with the rights of others, unless the 'others' that were proven to be and have been harmed *had* such rights. In another example, in the early days when the US South permitted slave ownership, no 'master' could have been taken to court for ill-treatment or other gross abuses of slaves at a time when these were considered no better than disposable tools.

WOMEN'S CIVIL RIGHTS AND PRESENT LAWS (US)

The social determination of how the legal system should view the fetus, should be informed by a careful consideration of the implications.[65]

This brief analysis of presently existing laws can be viewed as an example, as Canada, for instance, has similar laws, and we will review some other cases from Canada, New Zealand and Australia below. The main problem is that gender-based protection can be viewed and often is viewed as 'employment discrimination'. In 1964 women acquired the right to secure equal employment opportunities in the US.[66] But some companies exclude women from jobs where they might come into contact with chemicals that destroy the cells of the *conceptus* beyond possible regeneration.[67]

Women's responses have varied from choosing to be sterilized, in order to retain a high-paying job, to suing employers for discrimination. Westfall states that so far there is no case law specifically on this issue, although, 'The Equal Employment Opportunity Commission (EEOC) estimates that as many as 20 million jobs may involve exposure to alleged reproductive hazards'.[68]

Thus preborn harms enter the arena of rights by the back door – so to speak – because of women's rights, although, as science has clearly shown, women are exposed to hazardous substances both in and out of the workplace (air fresheners and deodorants are an example of in-home hazards). The problem is complicated by the additional existence of racial and ethnic discrimination. If any kind of 'discrimination' is tolerated on 'protective' grounds, it can also be used to encompass other grounds.[69,70]

The main point is that if one allows grounds that are not directly related to job qualifications to exclude some from employment, this practice, even if well-intended in regard to foetal protection, may give rise to a host of other discriminatory practices that are not so well-founded. The US 1978 *Pregnancy Amendment to Title VII*,[71] in response to a Supreme Court decision regarding a health insurance plan that 'covered almost everything except pregnancy', was held to be non-discriminatory.[72] The Amendment refers to all matters concerning childbearing.[73]

It is not only chemical exposure, but also exposure of the *conceptus* to high altitudes in travel, as in cases involving pregnant flight attendants, that has come to the attention of the courts.[74,75] Most of all, there have been cases about toxic exposure, affecting men, women and the *conceptus* in varying degrees, especially exposure to 'mutagens, teratogens and transplacental carcinogens'.[76] The medical literature shows that teratogens pass through the placenta to cause cancer.[77]

The *Occupational Safety and Health Act*,[78] is intended to protect the health of both men and women in the workplace. OSHA seeks also to protect the *conceptus* by ensuring that women do not suffer from 'diminished … functional capacity' regarding reproduction, but does not go so far as to protect the preborn from the same harm or from harms even greater. Thus the introduction and acceptance of a human life amendment would certainly strengthen what is already germinally present in workplace protective regulatory instruments.

Nevertheless, even if these products continue to proliferate, even through the labour of males aware of the possible dangers to their fertility, their very presence in homes might suffice to harm both women and the preborn, although they might have been 'protected' by being taken out of the hazardous workplace.

These problems are all real enough, but they are magnified exponentially by those who continue to view all regulations exclusively from the standpoint of the woman, as we saw in the brief but telling paragraph by Dawn Johnsen at the start of this section. Why is it entirely, or primarily, a 'social determination of how the legal system should view the fetus' that must be determinant? Johnsen comments further that 'the decision is a social one, not dictated by biology'.[79]

Yet many grave issues in law are decided by biological/medical facts, not social fiat. This is true of all life and death issues. The very 'born alive' evidentiary rule is entirely a medical, not a social one:[80] it is a rule of medical jurisprudence,[81] following upon the limited medical knowledge about pregnancies, including questions about the role of 'quickening' and 'live birth'.[82,83]

'Quickening', or the effect of increasingly forceful foetal movement (10th–11th week) is felt differently by different women; for instance, a woman's weight may influence the time when such movement is clearly detected and, appropriately enough, 'quickening' has little legal significance today, although 'prior to the 20th century, quickening remained the first reliable proof that the mother was pregnant'.[84] In contrast, the 'born alive' rule is still in existence today, despite having outlived its usefulness to allow the courts a certainty that today is available at much earlier times through various tests and procedures including ultrasound. Like the existence of human *infans conceptus*, 'live birth' is a medically, not socially, determined event:

> *Live birth ... is the objective, clinical observation that a fetus, upon coming out of the womb, is alive. Whenever the infant at or after birth breathes spontaneously or shows any other sign of life such as heartbeat, or definite spontaneous movement of voluntary muscles, a live birth is recorded.[85] ... Live birth is not synonymous with pregnancy brought to full term. Nor does live birth imply a viable fetus.[86]*

A final medical term needs some attention because of its continuing importance in modern jurisprudence: 'viability'. Although the concept was not particularly significant in earlier times, today it has a determinant role, a highly problematic one, given the fact that it is a highly evaluative term in itself, although today in North America it is viewed as present between 24 and 28 weeks of gestation.[87] Practically, viability depends on race, geographical location, economic status of the pregnant woman and the availability of medical facilities and even medical expertise at the place of the birth's occurrence. A foetus that is 'viable' in Toronto, Canada, at a local hospital, may not survive in a Zimbabwe village hut, even at the same gestational age. Nevertheless, the concept itself means 'the capacity to live' independently although even the historical dimensions of the concept, as Taylor has it, for instance in the late 19th century,[88] are worthy of note.

The reasons for the emphasis on various medical events in order to ensure the presence of a pregnancy and the existence of a foetus, was to be able to trace the causality required for the commission of a crime. In cases of alleged child murder, the courts needed to be sure that a 'child' had existed before the crime could have been committed. Hence, when an alleged crime had been committed in early times, before technologies and medical science were able to prove a pregnancy, long before birth,

> *live birth was required to prove that the unborn child was alive and that the material acts were the proximate cause of death, because it could not otherwise be established if the child was alive in the womb at the time of the material acts[89]*

The technologies that exist to assist the 'scientific revolution' in both obstetrics and foetology, did not exist before 1965. Today these advances can ensure that the unborn child is viewed as 'the second patient'.[90]

Thus the 'born alive' rule was simply adopted as evidentiary.[91] It was never intended to deny 'humanity' to a fetus who, as conceived by human beings, could only be human as well. In fact, its separate life from conception was recognized by several cases, including *Bonbrest v. Kotz*,[92,93] and although many US courts have been reluctant to reconsider the 'born alive' rule and to declare it obsolete, this is a desirable move today.[94] Nevertheless, a modern common law case, *Keeler v. Superior Court of Amador County*,[95] after tracing a detailed history of the 'born alive' rule, did not question its validity nor its original purpose: in the dissent, Justice Burke stated that in common law the unborn child is indeed a 'human being', and that the 'born alive rule' served only to differentiate between life and non-life, before later scientific advances made it easy to do so.

As the Supreme Court of Massachusetts in 1984 decided that killing an unborn child constituted a homicide (a vehicular crime), the rule was effectively set aside later. In *Commonwealth v. Cass*, Chief Justice Hennessey said:

> *an offspring of human parents cannot reasonably be considered to be other than a human being, and therefore a person, first within, and then in the normal course of events, outside the womb.*[96]

Thus, despite many arguments to the contrary by several groups, because of modern science's ability to discern, even picture the unborn, the trend appears to be toward acknowledging the humanity of the foetus: both Minnesota and Illinois legislations apply to the unborn child from conception and the California legislation added the phrase 'or a fetus' to the expression 'human being'.[97,98,99]

The question that arises then is how so much of feminist literature ignores altogether all arguments other than those about the 'privacy, autonomy' and the 'equality' of women, and view all developments of foetal rights as 'threatening women's fundamental rights', ignoring legal, moral and even medical arguments, as well as the fact that at least 50 per cent of pregnancies result in the birth of a female.[100] Dawn Johnsen is indicative of the kind of assumptions that underlie feminist arguments.[101]

It will be instructive to examine some of these assumptions, as they will also be basic to the arguments of the corporate harm imposers that permit the continuation of the status quo in ecoviolence[102] and corporate crimes that are foundational to the harms perpetrated against the child's health through environmental means.

The first assumption has already been noted: the claim is that there is no need to consult medicine, biology or treatises on gynecology, foetology or pediatrics, in order to understand what a foetus is. Even when citing a case like *Commonwealth v. Cass*, where it is acknowledged that killing a viable foetus constitutes vehicular homicide, Johnsen says that the case is decided 'to protect the interests of a woman who has chosen to carry her pregnancy to term'.[103] Johnsen does not explain why such a case then should have been decided about a viable foetus, as the woman's decision might render any foetus eligible to have the right to life, if that decision were the major determinant factor in the court's decision.

Another assumption is the conceptual move toward 'granting' rights to a foetus. Note the terminology: not speaking of 'recognizing' or 'acknowledging' such rights, but 'granting', that is assuming without argument that such rights can be 'granted' or not, at will a kind of language that would be deemed unacceptable if the newly acknowledged 'right-holder' was someone belonging to a minority in society, or to a woman herself. The rights of women to liberty, privacy and autonomy are deemed to be placed especially at risk by any regulation or court decision intended to protect the foetus:

> *Perhaps most alarmingly states have taken direct injunctive action against pregnant women. Courts have seized custody of fetuses (i.e. of pregnant women) in order to enjoin women from taking drugs that are potentially harmful to fetuses. They have ordered women to submit to blood transfusions to benefit the fetus, and have even compelled women against their wishes to undergo cesarean sections.*[104]

What is left out of the equation is a candid comparison not only of the person (the woman) and the foetus (variously defined as 'human being', 'human creature' or even 'conceptus'), but the relative losses of each. Consider some of the examples Johnsen proposes: drug abuse, for instance. In *Winnipeg Child and Family Services*,[105] where a woman addicted to glue sniffing since age 18 produced two severely handicapped children, presently in the custody of Child and Family Services, before becoming pregnant once again, while still addicted. Note the implications of her 'freedom' beyond the irreversible damage to three children: the financial responsibility for her choices fell each time on the provincial government's institutions, not the woman herself; or consider alcohol abuse;[106] blood transfusions as in the cases of refusal of treatment by a Jehovah's Witness, without which the infant would be born with severe irreversible impairment.[107]

When neither morality nor decency or an ethic of care suggest a path that would protect the unborn, the state must step in to protect. Let us take the case of the Canadian 'glue sniffer'. Her mind was seriously affected by the glue sniffing, as was her general health and she was hospitalized twice (her choice) for that condition in the early stages of her pregnancy. What must be considered is what would give her the right to gravely and irreversibly affect the life and health of three children, and why would a court's decision to halt her destructive path be judged excessive or unfair. Yet that is precisely what the court's decision amounted to, in the protection of the woman's rights. It was only in dissent that Sopinka J. advanced the arguments:

> *Having chosen to bring a life into the world, that woman must accept some responsibility for its well-being. In my view that responsibility entails, at the least, the requirement that the pregnant woman refrain from the abuse of substances that have, on proof to the civil standard, a reasonable probability of causing serious and irreparable damage to the fetus (at para.116).*

See also at para. 120:

> *The 'born alive' rule should be abandoned, for the purposes of this case, as it is medically out-of-date. . . . The fetus should be considered within the class of persons whose interests can be protected through the exercise of the* parens patriae *jurisdiction.*

Johnsen and others consider this sort of interference unacceptable given the primacy of women's freedom rights. But let us consider a man who also has an addiction problem, say alcohol. If he drives under the influence of drink he can be stopped by police. If his alcohol level is high enough (let alone high enough to require hospitalization), he can be 'inconvenienced', his 'privacy' and 'autonomy' can be taken from him for a period of time, ranging from a temporary loss of his driving licence, for a day or so, to much longer periods. This may happen even if he has not harmed anyone at the time, or if someone is actually harmed, the restraints, including jail time, can be much more serious.[108,109,110,111,112]

In comparison, a woman may be restrained for short periods of time, at most a few months (that is, to delivery), never for years; for a transfusion, certainly a day or less. In contrast, the harms imposed on the foetus would be fatal or at least severe enough to represent permanent impairment. Thus it is not sufficient to compare those whose freedom is affected. It is also necessary to compare the degree of inconvenience, loss of liberty or loss of autonomy, and the duration of such restraints.

Aside from alcohol addiction and restraints to prevent vehicular homicides and severe harms, there is another class of persons that is legally (and morally) restrained in their freedom and autonomy for the common good: those who suffer from contagious diseases, from measles and rubella, to more serious ailments. Children are prevented from attending school or day-care centres, no matter what the inconvenience to their parents. In addition, people suffering from serious adult infectious diseases, such as TB, may be restrained under the direction of the *Health Protection and Promotion Act*.[113,114] For instance persons may be required 'to isolate' themselves (22.(4) (c), in fact, in case a communicable disease is present:

> *22.(1) A medical officer of health, in the circumstances mentioned in subsection (2), by a written order may require a person to take or refrain from taking any action that is specified in the order in respect of a communicable disease.*[115]

Thus the imposition of temporary restraints for the common good can be taken for granted for both men and women, and it is compatible with the presence of democratic institutions as well as that of rights of persons, be they male or female, clearly identifiable at the time the restraint is imposed, or not. That is, one does not need to be able to pinpoint exactly who will be harmed and where; in fact there is no need to be certain that harm will occur, before restraints may be imposed.

If we hold fast to both (1) the primacy of everyone's rights, especially the right to life and to freedom from harm and (2) the risk thesis itself, then we need to seek another avenue to ensure that rights are protected, given the failure of present democratic institutions to guarantee appropriate restraints to risk imposers. The resurgence of many infectious diseases assumed to have been conquered and eliminated, such as tuberculosis, may indicate a possible avenue for public policy. Tuberculosis is making a comeback in North America and other parts of the world; resistant now to most antibiotics, and harder than ever to control because of population density and other modern conditions, it brings with it threat of the 'White Death'. Tuberculosis is highly contagious and requires very little contact to spread, unlike, for instance, sexually transmitted diseases such as AIDS. It is sufficient to sit next to an infected person or to breathe the same air in order to be infected. Tuberculosis is curable, but it requires a lengthy course of treatment. Many people who want to get well decide to abandon the treatment when the worst symptoms subside, even though they are still highly contagious. If these persons are not prepared to persevere with their treatment and yet want to continue to lead normal lives, interacting with others, they are endangering not only their close associates but also the general public.[116,117,118,119,120] The question is what to do when the course, treatment and hazards of the disease are fully explained to contagious persons, and they understand and yet refuse to comply with either treatment or restraints. It appears that some action must be taken in defence of public safety.

As in the case of contagious childhood diseases, what is necessary is the use of quarantines and other forms of involuntary restraints and treatment.[121] The starting point is the realization that tuberculosis is a threat to public health par excellence. As far as I know, however, only New York City has clear-cut legislation in this regard. The following course of action is supported by this new legislation:

> *The City Department of Public Health may order a person removed to a hospital or detained for treatment there only if two conditions are met. First, the Department must have found the tuberculosis to be active and without treatment likely to be transmitted to others... Second, the Department must have found the subject of the order unable or unwilling to undergo less restrictive treatment.*[122]

These requirements are based on 'epidemiological or clinical evidence, X-rays or laboratory tests', and the final decision to commit rests with the courts, as it does with the commitment procedures for the mentally ill. Note that in order to restrain the liberty of risk imposers in this context, it is not necessary to 'prove' in a court of law that they have harmed someone: it is sufficient to demonstrate that they and their activities are hazardous and potentially harmful to the public. Depending on the response of the infectious person to requests that he be treated, the interests of public health may be served by civil confinement for treatment, which in turn may be justified as preventing harm to the public through 'reckless endangerment'. In fact, jail could justifiably be used for anyone who might resist the suggested civil confinement for treatment.

How can this situation help us to conceptualize the problem of imposing restraints on those endangering the public through environmentally hazardous practices? First, we need to note that there are public threats that cannot be controlled through democratic institutions, that is, through voluntary public choices. One may counter that even the imposition of forced restraints is embedded in a general system of individual rights and democratic institutions. That is, of course, correct. But it is important to understand that rights to life and health are primary and should be put ahead of other choices. This perspective allows us to view environmental endangerment as something that needs to be controlled directly, and even by coercive means, rather than as something that is simply to be limited only by cost/benefit analyses or by a counting of heads and a weighing of preferences. In order to explain detention in medical cases, M. Davis says 'The alternative to detention is the moral equivalent of letting someone, without adequate justification, walk crowded streets with a large bomb that could go off at any moment.'[123]

In the White Death threat, we are not sure of the gravity of the harm imposed; we cannot anticipate with any certainty just who is at risk from the infected person; we cannot be sure of precise numbers of potentially affected persons. We have information about risks and harms, but we cannot present a specific infected person or persons as 'proof' to justify placing the risk imposer under criminal restraints. The only reason we can offer for imposing criminal or civil restraints is reckless endangerment, without being able to point to any one person who might have been harmed.

In fact, it is in order *not* to have victims that we are justified in invoking civil and criminal restraints. Contrast this preventive approach with that of corporate bodies who expose persons in the immediate vicinity of their hazardous operations to risks of harm, yet demand not proof of endangerment but clear proof of actual harm before they are even prepared to compensate for, let alone to consider discontinuing, their hazardous activities.

Hence the question, often asked in feminist literature, why a woman should be restrained, even coerced on behalf of anyone else or even the common good or the interests of the state, can be answered by considering legal and moral aspects of the issue. In general, proximity and the exclusive capacity to remedy the hazardous situation, are strongly determinant. One need only consider the parallel arguments of corporate legal persons, their focus is invariably that their self-interest is paramount, in fact that it is their mission to preserve their 'freedom' to act for that interest;[124] that rethinking their activities infringes their rights to freedom and autonomy; that any desire to limit their freedom to advertise curtails their right to free speech (recall tobacco companies' arguments in this regard); and that all requests to disclose the details of the harms they impose through their products and activities infringe their right to privacy. One then recognizes a very familiar litany of objections, by adducing positions that clearly place corporate risk/harm imposers against the public interest of all, men and women alike.

Business ethics literature, in contrast, has responded with vigorous arguments, starting with the well-known 'Kew Gardens Principles', that clearly indicate that those who can best help to redress these wrongs, must do so.[125] In the next section we will survey some other cases of third-party foetal harms, from various common law countries, before turning to a discussion of workplace hazards for women workers, and the latter's reaction to the regulation of these hazards.

THIRD-PARTY FOETAL HARMS IN COMMON LAW: CASES AND INSTRUMENTS

it is of the utmost importance to define the precise nature of the duty involved in the tort of negligence in such a case. In our opinion, the duty is not simply one to take reasonable care in the abstract, but to take reasonable care not to injure a person whom it should reasonably have been foreseen may be injured by the act or neglect if such care is not taken.[126]

This Australian case, *Watt v. Rama,* which also cites many of the cases already referred to in the previous sections, concludes that a man who, through his negligent conduct, drives his car and hits the car driven by a pregnant woman, is indeed at fault. The women was rendered a paraplegic through his negligence, and eventually delivered the plaintiff (the infant Sylvia Watt), suffering from brain damage and epilepsy. The defendant argued that although he had been negligent in the collision, he owed no duty of care to the unborn (at the time) plaintiff, and that the father of the paraplegic woman, seeking to recover damages, was also 'too remote in law'. The judgement was expected to answer three main points of law:

> *(a) whether in the circumstances set out in the statement of claim the defendant owed a duty of care not to cause injury to the plaintiff who was then unborn; (b) whether in the circumstances set out in the statement of claim the defendant owed a duty of care to the infant plaintiff not to injure her mother; (c) whether in the circumstances set out in the statement of claim the damages sought to be recovered by the plaintiffs are in law too remote.*[127]

The court eventually answered as follows: (a) yes; (b) unnecessary to answer; (c) no. Clearly the evidence of the defendant's negligence and the harm suffered were compelling enough, although the basic question of the rights (if any) of the preborn was avoided rather than answered. The pregnancy and the results that followed the collision indicated that the defendant, whether or not he owed a specific duty to the preborn at the time of injury,

> *would be bound to take the woman as he found her, if sued by her, and the pregnancy would be as much a physical condition in his victim as would the case of a person having an eggshell skull.*[128]

Citing the 'thin skull' rule, entrenched in criminal law, however, Winneke, CJ remained within the limits of the harms caused to the woman, although in the following paragraph (at para.26), he argues that there was, if not a potential child, at least, 'a potential relationship capable of imposing a duty on the defendant in relation to the child if and when born', as birth would then serve to 'crystallize the relative duty at that time'.

   Gillard, J. cites Lamont, J. in the Supreme Court of Canada in *Montreal Tramways v. Leveille*,[129]

> *where for the first time it was accepted in a Superior Court that an infant plaintiff should be able at birth to recover damages for prenatal injuries.*
>
> . . .
>
> *If a right to action be denied to the child, it will be compelled without any fault on its part, to go through life carrying the seal of another's fault and bearing a heavy burden of infirmity without any compensation therefore. To my mind, it is but natural justice that a child, if born alive and viable, should be allowed to maintain an action in the courts for injuries wrongfully committed upon his person while in the womb of its mother.*

Gillard, J. does remark that appealing, as Lamont, J. does, to natural justice, implies appealing to principles *de lege ferenda*, which will not actually yield principles and precedents to assist in the present case.

   However, in another country, New Zealand, in the *New Zealand Bill of Rights Act* 1990, s.8, 'the right to life' of the foetus may apply in part to the preborn, although there is no present case law, to my knowledge. Although most of the 'guaranteed rights and freedoms are inapplicable to the pre-born', the right not to be deprived of life without the observance of fundamental justice (s.8), the right not to be subject to medical or scientific experimentation may potentially apply (s.9, s.10). If we also consider the Preamble to the *United Nations Convention on the Rights of the Child*, 1989,[130] we should accept that, 'the child ... needs special safeguards and care, including appropriate legal protection before as well as after birth', although no reference is made to this act in any of the cases in common law I have examined.

The reference to 'cruel treatment' in the New Zealand Act, as well as the reference to protection before birth, are once again more about what the law should be, than about what the law is, at the present time, as Gillard, J. indicated. However, the New Zealand commentary on the act remarks that the 14th Amendment of the US Constitution,[131,132] deny the preborn to be a 'person', or 'everyone', so that, even under the *New Zealand Bill of Rights Act* 1990, it could be the case that 'fundamental justice' would permit abortion in certain circumstances, in the interest of the bodily integrity of the mother or for other reasons. All these instruments then appear to leave the door open to the defence of the preborn from third-party attacks, as no 'reason' can be given or accepted for such attacks.

In fact, the *New Zealand Children, Young Persons and Their Families Act*,[133] and the *New Zealand Guardianship Act*[134] include unborn children; and the *Crimes Act* 1961[135] say that, 'unborn children may be the victims of manslaughter'. Even the *New Zealand Contraception, Sterilization and Abortion Act* 1977, has as its purpose, 'inter alia (to) provide for the circumstances and procedures under which abortions may be authorized after having full regard to the rights of the unborn child'. Nevertheless it appears that even in this regard New Zealand laws have not been tested in the courts.

However, no mention is made of the preborn's health. Our concern is not abortion per se of course, but its influence on policies that might address the right of the preborn to have its health and normal development protected, so the language of these instruments at least would permit an interpretation that might allow courts to be sympathetic to future claims asking for that protection. In addition, the *New Zealand Resource Management Act* 1991, s.5 (2) states that:

> *The Act recognizes that people and communities need to provide for their social, economic and cultural well-being, and **for their health and safety**.* [emphasis added]

Without mentioning children specifically, this act seems to connect environment and resource issues to public health, a distinct advantage. The *Biosecurity Act* 1993, and the *Hazardous Substances and New Organisms Act* 1996, further addresses public health questions, especially in paras. 110–114 of the latter. Finally, on the meaning of the right not to be 'deprived' of life, the New Zealand Bill of Rights act 1990, in a commentary on s.8 states:

> *If 'deprived' does cover accidental killing, it is likely that accidental death caused by acts falling within s.3 of the New Zealand Bill of Rights Act will always amount to a violation of s.8 because few accidental deaths are permitted by law (and therefore they could not meet the requirement of being in accordance with law). Equally very few laws 'authorize' state officials to ignore specific known threats of harm to individuals when the state is aware of the potential for harm. Accordingly, if the failure of the state to*

*intervene amounts to a deprivation of life, then a finding of breach of s.8 of the 1990
Act will follow.*

This approach would be very useful for our purpose, as harms to the preborn are often
deemed to be part of business, caused by 'externalities' at most, although some times
negligence might be invoked, but for the most part, it is legal activities that impose
the harms. As already argued, the other problem is that common law is based on case
and precedent, in order to decide on the proper legal treatment of harmful events.
We can look briefly at the cause of some other prenatal harms, caused by medical
negligence, but, to my knowledge, environmental/health cases have not been tried in
Canada or elsewhere, although the Walkerton case (deaths and illness caused by E. coli
contamination of the water supply) comes as close as any to this issue, despite the fact
that it has not been so far the basis for any lawsuit. The grave harms that were imposed,
affected primarily infants, children and the elderly.[136]

Some medical negligence cases

These cases may have some causes for our research only in two senses: (1) the all-
important definitions of the foetus/preborn they use, and the references to the 'born
alive' rule; and (2) the way negligence is included without the need for the presence of
intent and the way they appeal to standards of causation.

In *Cherry (Guardian ad litem of) v. Borsman*[137] the tort involves both medical negligence, abortion and a wrongful life suit. An attempted 'therapeutic abortion' by Dr
Borsman, failed and the infant was eventually born. The 'dilation and currettage' was
improperly performed, so that placental tissue was found in the evacuated material.
The woman experienced three weeks of heavy vaginal discharge, and later was found to
remain pregnant. On 20 January 1982, Elizabeth Roseanne Cherry was born, 'afflicted
by a number of congenital defects', including brain damage, cerebral palsy, spasticity in
the lower legs and other problems.

The starting point for the legal analysis of the case was the principle in *Donaghue
v. Stevenson,*[138] that one must not do injury to one's neighbour. But, it was argued, it
must also be taken that the foetus has rights before birth, at least in the law of torts and
property, involving either inheritance of prenatal injury, but not unless it was born alive.
Thus Skipp, J.: 'I find the defendant doctor was negligent both in his performance and
in his post-operative care.'

The question of causation in malpractice cases is also discussed. Courts are forced
to evaluate difficult scientific evidence, and Skipp, J. cites Sopinka, J. in *Snell v. Farrell*:

> Snell v. Farrell *mandates a return to traditional negligence principles in the field of
> medical malpractice. This requires that the plaintiff establish on balance of probabili-
> ties that the defendant's negligent act caused or materially contributed to the injury.
> As stated previously inferences may be drawn; the standard is proof on balance of
> probabilities, not proof beyond the shadow of a doubt.*

An earlier reference to the effects of the drug thalidomide is also relevant.[139] In that case, negligent, or incomplete research, rather than medical negligence is the issue, but the results are also severe enough that I would even term them crimes, rather than merely torts, as the harm to those born without limbs is not entirely a compensable harm.

Another interesting case is one of harm at birth,[140] as it deals with an improper delivery resulting in pre-birth harms. Another case, this one in British Columbia,[141] deals with the case of informed consent of the part of the mother to a procedure that proved harmful, once the foetus was born. Garson, J. says:

> *33. The crux of the issue here is whether a live born infant may bring suit against a doctor in negligence by relying on a lack of informed consent on the part of the mother. Given the principles outlined above, there is at least an arguable case that it is.*

Essentially therefore, the courts appear to reach the fundamental principle that follows from civil law, that is, that a born alive foetus can be found to have had rights that may have been infringed by medical malpractice or by other corporate negligence or in general negligence by third parties, and that her harms may be compensated separately, aside from the possible compensation due to the mother. This is indeed helpful from our point of view, although it is also clearly a paradoxical finding. Should the pre-birth harm be severe enough to cause the foetus' demise, no cause for action remains. The fact that for reasons we have noted, as well as for other policy reasons (see next section), the killing remains 'lawful' as non-actionable in many circumstances beyond abortion, gives rise to a number of serious disadvantages. John O'Neill for instance, lists no less than eight serious disadvantages accruing to the status quo in his country (New Zealand), despite the well-worded and well thought out instruments we have described in the previous section.[142]

REPRODUCTIVE HAZARDS OR DISCRIMINATION IN THE WORKPLACE?

While corporations continue to produce, use and market hazardous materials, harmful 'from cradle to grave', that is, from the time they are produced to when they are ultimately eliminated as waste,[143] feminists are busy defending themselves from 'paternalistic' state protection, scarce and incomplete though that protection is.

For instance, Sally Kenney says:

> *The Employment Act gives the secretary of state for employment (in consultation with the Equal Employment Opportunity Commission (EEOC)), broad powers to determine whether treating men and women differently is protective or discriminatory.*[144]

On this issue, the feminist argument that highly toxic products are most likely to be equally toxic to males, is well-taken. In *Page v. Freight Hire*,[145] a 23-year-old woman was told that she could not continue to haul dimethylformamide (DMF), because the substance was known to be embryotoxic. The hazards of the substance have been reviewed and found to be the source of testicular lesions as well as embryolethal and highly teratogenic in rodents, according to several sources.[146,147,148]

Thus the obvious question that should be pursued is not why women are being discriminated against by being told not to haul such a substance, but why it is manufactured at all, and where and how is it eventually used and sold, and to whose detriment. According to the textbook analysis of the substance, it is fair to assume that it is indeed harmful to the preborn,[149,150,151] although there are to date no cases that prove the extent of those harms conclusively. Kenney, however, is far more concerned with reporting the way various local British newspapers referred to the story, describing the driver as 'attractive', or as a 'pretty divorcee', and concluding that:

> *Page illustrates the comparative approach in practice and shoes the problems with so-called protective policies. A close inspection of Freight-Hire's policy reveals that it is based on unexamined assumptions about physical differences between the sexes and may be based on judgments about the appropriate role for women in society.*[152]

But Kenney comes close to the heart of the matter as she notes that:

> *Page's union, the Transport and General Workers, has not made health and safety a high priority in general, nor has it been actively concerned with reproductive hazards in the workplace.*[153,154]

Kenney also notes that men, too, may be at risk, but she finds far more significant the fact that women's childbearing may be viewed as their primary role, rather than viewing women as equal to men in their role as breadwinners.[155]

This discussion, and others like it, are clearly based on the assumption that the foetus, let alone the state's obligation to protect it, should not be considered, in line with the arguments of the previous section. Another author, Joan E. Bertin, even questions the reality of 'Fetal Hypersusceptibility', as she notes that this circumstance is often cited without specific support.[156] Nevertheless most of her argument is for equal protection of men and women in the workplace, as 'health effects of toxic chemicals are rarely confined to the fetus in utero'.[157,158]

A case in point is that of Occidental Chemical Company in California. In 1977 it was found to have exposed its male workers to pesticide DBCP, a known carcinogen, capable of shrinking testes in laboratory animals and causing genetic damage, as well as causing either sterility or very low sperm count in males.[159] In the US, unlike the UK, the Pregnancy Discrimination Act[160] allows judges to examine both science and policy issues to decide on difficult discrimination cases.[161] But in the US, as in most other countries, public opinion and the political focus of feminist groups is to militate against 'discrimination' on the job, a focus which may help them to bring actions for losing well-paying jobs, on the basis of traditional, even 'Victorian' beliefs about 'women's place' in society.[162]

Kenney, however, recognizes another anomaly in the law:

> *The development of the law on exclusionary policies, then, reflects the fact that workers find it easier to challenge a health and safety policy as discriminatory than*

not protective of their health and safety. It is easier for women to demand access to hazardous work, than to demand that employers not require them to perform tasks that expose them to hazardous substances.[163]

That said, it might be important to reconsider positions that have solidified in a hostile stance over the years. Perhaps both feminists and neo-liberal supporters, if they were not so intent on arguing against discrimination, might join forces with modern sciences and with the defenders of foetal rights, and focus instead on demanding the cessation of manufacture/use/disposal of hazardous substances, and major changes in the operation of 'risky business'.

The first chapter of this book argued that children are today's 'canaries', and that the especially vulnerable preborn is the very first 'canary' to succumb to harmful and inappropriate exposures. This implies, as did the canary in relation to mineworkers, that after the canary has been affected, adult persons both male and female, will be the next to be harmed, although in different ways, in different degrees, and most important, often by different substances.[164] This biological reality indicates that for women, as well as for men, the 'enemy' is not the traditionalist, the male 'Victorian' mentality, but the powerful corporate persons who, unlike the foetus, enjoy all rights and freedoms and consider no one's rights to health and normal function in their path to 'success'. The tobacco companies are a good example to keep in mind in that regard.

But, unless the preborn is understood not as a full person with rights to free speech, education, a passport and so on, but simply as a human being, with minimal rights to be 'well-born', it will be much more difficult to insist, legally and morally, on full protection from harm imposers. What of the 'right' to abortion though? Self-defence is morally and legally permissible, if it is understood in its full sense of the defence of one's life, or from the infliction of grave harms: the same conditions that would permit the killing of any assailant, whether or not intent was part of the attack. For instance, one may envision a mentally challenged 'person' attacking, without the ability to understand the gravity of her action or to formulate a reason for the attack itself. Self-defence appears to be permissible and fair even in this case.

Understanding the preborn as a particularly vulnerable human being would simply force the woman to formulate for herself and for society's representatives the reasons why killing is the only answer in this case, something that one needs to do even before a dog that has attacked someone already, is put to death. The inconvenience of having to either (a) possess a clear and convincing reason for such an act; or (b) to bear the intrusion, and possibly a somewhat modified or restricted lifestyle for a few months, before giving away a healthy born infant, would be fully offset by the advantages that both women and men would gain. If society is allowed to recognize that the hazards to which most of us are exposed need not be tolerated, but that a unified society without polarized gender-based adversaries, who would instead demand that the research of the WHO, not corporate/institutional interests, should set the standards for both industrial operations, terms of employment, and in general civil life. Recent work published by the Archives of Pediatric and Adolescent Medicine,[165]show that not only is the workplace hazardous to pregnant women, and to the children that result from these pregnancies, but that all solvents and like chemicals are as hazardous when used as parts of products in the home, as they are when used in manufacture, in the workplace:

> *Organic solvents are a huge group of disparate chemicals. Toluene, for example, is an ingredient in polyurethane, as well as in paints, glues and gasoline. Hexane is used in pesticides, wood stains and printing ... Solvents are also ingredients in many household products, including cleaners, polishers and deodorizers.*[166]

Therefore demanding 'equal opportunity' to be harmed, even aside from the possibility of pregnancy, is no more productive than withdrawing from the workplace altogether: what is important is to demand that health mandated changes be made not only to manufacture/production and shipping procedures, but that the onus to demonstrate their safety before use should be placed squarely on the corporate risk imposers that are guilty of exposing all to 'equal opportunity' harms.

NOTES

1   Bradshaw (1982).
2   George (2003), p15.
3   O'Neill (1994), p4.
4   George (2003), p16.
5   George (2003), p23.
6   *Appellate Body Hormones Decision*, EC Measures Concerning Meat and Meat Products (Hormones) AB-1997-4WT/DS 26 AB/R, WT/DS48 AB/R.
7   Westra (2004a), chapter 6.
8   Budapest, Hungary, 23–25 June 2004.
9   Tamburlini et al (2002).
10   *Allaire v. St. Luke Hospital et al*, 184 I11.359, 56 N.E. 638.
11   Boggs, J. dissenting.
12   Holmes (1881).
13   *Bonbrest et al v. Kotz et al*, 1946, 65 F.Supp.138; 1946 U.S. Dist. *Lexis* 2712, p.2.
14   *Bonbrest et al v. Kotz et al*, 1946, p3.
15   *Dietrich v. Inhabitants of North Hampton*, 1884, 138 Mass.14, 52 Am. Rep. 242.
16   *Allaire v. St. Luke Hospital et al*, 184 I11.356,56 N.E. 638, Feb. 19, 1990.
17   *Allaire v. St. Luke Hospital et al*, 184 I11.356,56 N.E. 638, Feb. 19, 1990, p6.
18   Beal (1984).
19   Pritchard and MacDonald (1980).
20   Ament (1974), p24.
21   *Roe v. Wade*, 410 U.S. 113 (1973).
22   *Roe v. Wade*, 410 U.S. 113 (1973), p327.
23   *Roe v. Wade*, 410 U.S. 113 (1973), p328.
24   65 F. Supp. 138 (D.D.C. 1946).
25   Westfall (1982), p98.
26   *The Ashbrook proposal*, H.R.J. Res. 13, 97th Cong., 1st Sess. (1981).
27   *The Garn-Rhodes proposal*, S.J. Res. 17, 97th Cong., 1st Sess. (1981).
28   *The Helles-Dorman proposal*, S.J. Res. 19, 97th Cong., 1st Sess (1981).
29   *The Helms-Hyde human life bill*, S. 158, 97th Cong., 1st Sess. (1981).
30   *The Ashbrook Proposal*, H.R. 900, 97th Cong. 1st Sess (1981).
31   *The Ashbrook Proposal*, H.R. 900, 97th Cong. 1st Sess (1981), p97.
32   Warren (1991), pp438–444; Tooley (1983).
33   Westfall (1982).

34   Westfall (1982), p104.
35   Westfall (1982).
36   Marquis (1989).
37   Bradshaw (1982), pp85–86.
38   Bradshaw (1982), p86.
39   Bradshaw (1982), p89.
40   Bradshaw (1982).
41   *United States v. Carolene Prod. Co.*, 304 U.S. 144, 152-53, n.4 (1938) (dictum).
42   Westfall(1982), p106.
43   Westra (2004a), Chapters 4 and 6.
44   Westfall (1982), p108.
45   Westfall (1982), p110.
46   Westfall (1982), p115.
47   56 N.E. 138, Feb. 19, 1990.
48   10 Am. and Eng. Enc. Law,624.
49   *Allaire v. St. Luke Hosp. et al.*
50   65 F. Supp.138, March 6, 1946.
51   Steinbock (1992), p92.
52   *Kelly v. Gregory*, 282 A.D. 542,125 N.Y.S. 2d 696 (1953).
53   31 N.J. 353,157 A.2d 497(1960).
54   4 D.L.R. 337 [1933].
55   282 A.D. 542,125 N.Y.S. 2d 696, Nov.12, 1953.
56   483 F.2d 237, July 25,1973.
57   *Jackson v. Cushing Coca-Cola Bottling Co.*, 445 P.2d 797,799 (Okla.).
58   *Barnhart v. Freeman Equipment Co.*, 441 P.2d 993,999 (Okla.).
59   *Marathon Battery Co. v. Kilpatrick*, 418 P.2d 900, 914–915 (Okla.).
60   *White Motor Corporation v. Stewart*, 465 F.2d 1085, 1088-1089 (10th Cir.).
61   *Marshall v. Ford Motor Co.*, 446 F.2d 712,714 (10th Cir.).
62   Gordon (1965).
63   *Conlay v. Gibson*, 355 U.S. 41, 45-46, 2 L.Ed.2d 80, 78 S. Ct. 99.
64   102 Mich. App.396; 301 N.W. 2d 869, Dec. 15, 1980.
65   Johnsen (1986), p599.
66   *Title VII of the Civil Rights*, 42 U.S.C. §§ 20000e to 2000e17 (1976 and Supp.1980).
67   Westfall (1982), p120.
68   EEOC Interpretive Guidelines on Employment Discrimination and Reproductive Hazards, 45 Fed. Reg. 7514 (Feb.1, 1980) (corrected in 45 Fed. Reg.16, 501 (1980)).
69   *Griggs v. Duke Power Co*, 401 U.S. 424.
70   *Nashville Gas Co. v. Satty*, 434 U.S. 136 (1977).
71   42 U.S.C.§ 2000e - (k) (Supp.1980).
72   429 U.S. 125 (1976).
73   H.R.Rep. No.948, 95th Cong., 2d Sess. 5, reprinted in U.S. Code Cong.Ad.News 4749, 4753.
74   *Burwell v. Eastern Airlines, Inc.*,458 F. Supp.
75   *Hamiss v. Pan Am World Airways, Inc.*, 437 F. Supp.
76   Manson (1978), pp322, 326.
77   Westfall (1982).
78   29 U.S.C. §651–678 (1976).
79   Leff (1997).
80   Forsythe (1987), pp563, 567.
81   Forsythe (1987), p567.
82   *Dorland's Illustrated Medical Dictionary* (1985), p1105.

83   Beck (1860), p253.
84   Forsythe (1987), p568.
85   Pritchard et al (1985).
86   Forsythe (1987), p568.
87   Forsythe (1987), p569.
88   Taylor (1861).
89   Forsythe (1987), p575.
90   *Williams Obstetrics* (1985), p267.
91   *Commonwealth v. Cass*, 392 Mass. 799, 467 N.E. 2d 1324 (1984).
92   *Bonbrest v. Kotz*, 65 F. Supp.138 (D.D.C. 1946).
93   *Sinkler v. Kneale*, 401 Pa.267,164 A.2d 93 (1960).
94   Forsythe (1987), p603.
95   2 Cal.3d 619,470 P.2d 617 87 Cal.Rptr.481 (1970).
96   392 Mass.at 801, 467 N.E. 2d at1235.
97   *Cal.Penal Code* §187 (a), West Supp. 1986.
98   *Minn.Stat. Ann.* § 609.266 (1987 Supp.).
99   *Ill. Rev. Stat.*, Ch. 38, 9-1.2, 12-3.1 (1986 Supp.).
100 O'Neill (1976).
101 Johnsen (1986); Gallagher (1989), pp185–236.
102 Westra (2004a).
103 Johnsen (1986), p603.
104 Johnsen (1986), p605.
105 *Northwest Area v. D.F.G.* [1997] 3 S.C.R. 926.
106 Moffatt (no date).
107 *Raleigh Fitken Paul Morgan Memorial Hospital v. Anderson*, 42 N.J. 421, 201 A.2d 537,cert.
     denied, 377 U.S. 985 (1964).
108 *R.v. Phelan* (1982), 41 A.R. 28, 1982 Carswell, Alta 457, C.A.
109 *R. v. Pineau* (1980), 50 A.R. 278.
110 *R. v. Harton* (1983), 23 M.V.R. 223, (1983), 23.
111 *M.V.R. 2231R. v. Muise* (1990).
112 25 M.V.R. (2d) 298, 99 N.S.R. (2d) 186, 270 A.P.R.
113 R.S.O. 1990, chapter H.7.
114 Part III (Community Health Protection), and Part IV (Communicable Diseases).
115 R.S.O. 1990, ch.7, s.22 (1).
116 American Philosophical Association Central Meeting, April 1995; Davis (1995). 'Reckless
     endangerment' and 'endangerment' are terms used in laws. M. Davis, my authority on
     these issues, cites the New York City Health Code (3-31-93), ch. 11.47 (RCNY:103039-
     10312); the Illinois Criminal Code, ch. 38, secs. 4–6 and 12–5 (in 'Reckless Conduct');
     and the N.Y. Penal Law 120.25. In Canada, the strongest legislation on consent is
     under the heading of 'Suicide' (Martin's Criminal Code, 1996; 241s.14): 'no person is
     entitled to have death inflicted upon him, and such consent does not affect the criminal
     responsibility of any person on whom death may be inflicted'. 'Criminal negligence' is
     defined in the same code, Part VIII, 5.219(1), as 'wanton or reckless disregard for the
     lives or safety of other persons'. This is also discussed under 'Causing Harm by Criminal
     Negligence' (Y21). 'Everyone who by criminal negligence causes bodily harm to another
     person is guilty of an indictable offense.' This may cause 'culpable homicide', defined
     in 5.222(1) as 'when a person causes the death, indirectly, directly, of another person'.
     Finally, 'Murder, Manslaughter and Infanticide' (5.229), under 'Liability of Party', refers
     inter alia to 'the perpetrator ... cause[s] bodily harm of a kind likely to result in death
     and be reckless whether death ensues or not'. The *Health Promotion and Protection Act*
     (Ontario Law) permits 'confinement' through loosely defined steps, and this includes,

for infectious diseases, 'known and suspected cases'. These might lead to court orders for detention and treatment.

117 New York City Health Code (3-31-93), Ch. 11.47 (RCNY:103039-10312).
118 *Illinois Criminal Code*, ch. 38, secs. 4–6 and 12–5 (in 'Reckless Conduct').
119 *Martin's Criminal Code*, 1996.
120 *N.Y. Penal Law* 120.25.
121 *Health Protection and Promotion Act*; R.S.O. 1990, Chapter H.7, Part III, 'Community Health Protection'; and Part IV Communicable Diseases.
122 Davis (1995).
123 Davis (1995).
124 Friedman (1993), pp249–254.
125 Simon et al (1972).
126 *Watt v. Rama*, Supreme Full Court of Victoria; 1971 Vic Lexis 143; Y1972U VR 3531 Dec. 14, 1971.
127 *Watt v. Rama,*, p2.
128 Winneke, CJ, at para. 25.
129 [1933] 4 DLR 337.
130 CRC, 20 November 1989, GA44/25.
131 *Roe v. Wade*, 410 U.S. 35 [1973].
132 *Constitution of the United States of America* (1787), Amendment XIV, ratified 1868.
133 1989 s.2 (1).
134 1968, s.7.
135 ss.182 and 187.
136 Westra (2004a), chapter 4.
137 [1990] B.C.J. No.2576, Vancouver Registry No.C845601; Judgment Dec.3, 1990.
138 [1932] A.C. 562.
139 Bennett (1965), p256.
140 *Keys v. Mistashia Regional Health Authority*, [2001] A.J. No.461, Action No.9703 14590, Judgment April 10, 2001.
141 *Forliti (Guardian ad litem of) v. Woolley*, [2003] B.C.J. No.1627, 2003 BCSC 1082; Judgment: July 10, 2003.
142 O'Neill (1976), p55.
143 Draper (1991).
144 Kenney (1992).
145 *Tank Haulage Ltd.*, Case no. 1381/80, March 26,1980; [1981] 1 RLR 13 (EAT).
146 Kenney (1992), p186.
147 Fletcher (1985).
148 Barlow and Sullivan (1982).
149 Tamburlini et al (2002).
150 'Ban on woman transporting DMF NOT unlawful discrimination', *Health and Safety Information Bulletin*, vol 62 February 1981, pp18–19.
151 'British EEO Agency warns employers that discharge for pregnancy is illegal', *Daily Labor Report*, (BA) vol 175, Sept. 11, 1987, pA5.
152 Kenney (1992), p185.
153 Kenney (1992), p198.
154 'TGW Action', *Hazards*, 11, (1986), p10.
155 'TGW Action', *Hazards*, 11, (1986), p301.
156 Bertin (1989), p279.
157 Bertin (1989), p280.
158 Bertin (1989), explanatory note 9, p301.
159 Bertin (1989), p280.

160   *A Report by the Majority Staff on EEOC, Title VII and Workplace Fetal Protection Policies in the 1980s,* House Education and Labor Committee 101st Cong., 2d sess., April 1990, p16.
161   Kenney (1992), p207.
162   Gallagher (1989), pp188–191.
163   Kenney (1992), p211.
164   Colborn et al (1996).
165   Kohn (2004), pF2.
166   Kohn (2004).

CHAPTER 4

Supranational Governance: The European Court of Human Rights, and the WTO–WHO Conflict

INTRODUCTION

Article 8
1 *Everyone has the right to respect for his private and family life, his home and his correspondence.*
2 *There shall be no interference by a public authority with the exercise of this right except such as is in accordance with the law and is necessary in a democratic society in the interests of national security, public order, or the economic well-being of the country, for the prevention of disorder or crime, for the protection of health or morals, or for the protection of the rights and freedoms of others. (European Convention on Human Rights)*

One of the most striking features of child's rights law is its global presence, however limited in its effects. Some of its principles are internationally accepted, for instance, the principle of 'the best interests of the child', although it does not appear explicitly in any legal document.[1] Another case of lack of specificity and of explicit direction, similar to that of this principle, is the question of definition: who is the child under international law?[2,3]

It is useful to start with the European law, because that represents a better example of a supranational regulatory regime, better in the sense that it incorporates traditional moral principles that are, for the most part, not open to negotiation and agreement, as happens with international treaties.[4]

Nevertheless, the question of whether unborn children have convention rights has not been authoritatively decided:

> While the UN Convention on the Rights of the Child provides some guidance as to who is a child under international law, the European Convention does not address specifically the age at which a person may enjoy its rights. Moreover, the line between ability and entitlement is blurred in children's rights given that the age at which a child is entitled to enjoy Convention Rights may be different from the age at which s/he is capable of enjoying them.[5]

The silence on these issues makes it unclear whether there is protection before birth, hence whether abortion, for instance, is even compatible with Article 2 and Article 8(2).[6] We noted in earlier chapters, the groundbreaking judgement in *Brüggemann and Scheuten v. Germany*,[7] which stated unequivocally that the absence of legal abortion rights was not a violation of Article 8(2), given the wide variety of beliefs in the European Community on that topic. The court, however, did not feel that it was necessary for it to decide,

> *... whether the unborn child was to be considered 'life' in the sense of Article 2 ... or whether it could be regarded as an entity which under Article 8(2) could justify interference for the protection of others.*[8]

In Chapter 1, we noted that only the *American Convention on Human Rights* (1969) is explicit in its protection of the right to life of the preborn, in contrast with the lack of position in most other instruments. In Paton, for instance, the absolute right to life is denied to the preborn, but whether any protection is available to the foetus remains unclear in that decision.[9] Thus, given the possibility that the right to life as in Article 2 is left deliberately vague, it becomes even more important to examine closely the implication of Article 8(2), in order to discover whether the 'best interests of the child' – a principle that surely should include the right to be 'well-born', that is born with health and normal function – has been applied in the European Court of Human Rights.

The first obstacle encountered is the lack of jurisprudence on the topic of this work. Cases involving the rights of the child to health and the environment are extremely rare. That said, it is important, especially under those circumstances, to look carefully at the three cases that use Article 8(2) in European case law.

THREE CASES IN THE EUROPEAN COURT OF HUMAN RIGHTS

In fact, only two of these cases, *Guerra v. Italy*, and *Lopez-Ostra v. Spain* involve children specifically, although their presence and their interests may be inferred in the third one, and the preborn is not an issue in any of these cases.[10,11]

These are cases that reaffirm the primacy of life and health of individuals explicitly, and the direct effect of Community law over national law, in cases where these are at issue.[12] Both cases were brought to the European Court of Justice (ECJ) after the plaintiffs failed to receive satisfaction from their respective countries. For the Guerra case, although at first the Italian government expressed a preliminary objection based on 'non-exhaustion of domestic remedies', the Court did not accept their argument: had they pursued such remedies, at best they might have caused a temporary closure of the plant, perhaps even a criminal conviction of the factory's managers. However, such a course of action would not have provided them with the information they sought, or any redress.

The court judged, in the merits of the complaint, that the state had failed to act:

> *Direct effect of basic emissions on applicant's right to respect for private and family life meant that Article 8 was applicable. Applicants complained not of an act of State, but of its failure to act – object of Article 8 was essentially that of protecting individuals against arbitrary interferences by public authority – it did not merely compel State to abstain from such interference: in addition to that primarily negative undertaking, there might be positive obligations inherent in effective respect for private or family life.*

This case concerns a group of citizens of Manfredonia, located one kilometre away from Erichem Agricoltura, a chemical factory, and involving the release of large quantities of flammable gas. Often the operation caused chemical explosions that spewed highly toxic substances into the air. In 1988 the factory was classified as 'high risk' according to European Union Directive (EEC) 82/501m, that is, the major accident hazard of industrial activities, 'dangerous to the environment and the well being of local populations'.[13]

Forty citizens complained to the European Commission of Human Rights that the action and especially the omissions of the Italian authorities had violated Article 10, as well as Articles 8 ('Respect for Family and Home') and 2 ('Right to Life') of the ECHR (*European Convention on Human Rights*). Article 10, Freedom of Expression, emphasizes something on which this book has focused: the exercise of freedom is and must be limited by responsibilities and duties:

> *Article 10(2) – Freedom of Expression*
> *The exercise of these freedoms, since it carries with it duties and responsibilities, may be subject to such formalities, conditions, restrictions and penalties as are prescribed by law and are necessary in a democratic society, in the interests of national security, territorial integrity or public safety, for the prevention of disorder or crime, for the protection of health or morals, for the protection of the reputation or rights of others, for preventing the disclosure of information received in confidence, or of maintaining the authority and impartiality of the judiciary.*

This article is outstanding among other international human rights instruments because of the thorough and painstaking way it outlines the 'duties and responsibilities' that balance and limit all 'freedoms' not only freedom of expression, but also 'freedom of thought, conscience and religion' (Article 9), 'public safety', 'the protection of health and morals' and, in Article 9(a), in addition, 'the protection of the public order'. Hence, the freedom of the corporate enterprise is by no means absolute, and it does not appear to extend as far as it does in North American instruments, as it is clearly limited even in the realm of legally sanctioned activities.

In turn, the freedom of citizens to be safe in their homes, and to retain their health, is openly considered to have been under attack. The right to protection extends, according to Article 8, to the right of respect for the 'well-being' of persons, and the 'respect for their private and family life'. The failure of the Italian authorities to protect the 'right to life' extends to the protection of 'physical integrity', as 'guaranteed by Article 2 of the *European Convention* (1950). Although this extension is not explicitly spelled out in the language of the convention, it appears to represent a juridical extension by analogy. The logic of this extension has also been argued as the necessity for microintegrity given its clear connection to ecological (macro)integrity, in my earlier work.[14]

Returning to Guerra (1998) 26 EHRR, 357, eventually several steps were taken to impose government restraints on the corporation, because of the status of the latter under Council Directive (EEC) 82/501 (under the *Seveso Directive*). In 1993, the Ministry of the Environment issued an order, jointly with the Ministry of Health, prescribing measures to be taken (at para. 17), and in 1994 the factory permanently stopped the production of fertilizer (at para. 18).

But already in 1985, 420 residents of Manfredonia had complained of the health effect of the air pollution, and criminal proceedings had been brought to bear against seven directors of the company (at para. 19). The court declared that 'a complaint is characterized by the facts alleged in it and not merely by the legal grounds or arguments relied on' (at para. 44), hence, despite objections on various legal points, it concluded: '46. Having regard to the foregoing and to the Commission's decision on admissibility, the Court holds that it has jurisdiction to consider the case under Articles 8 and 2 as well as under art.10.'

Aside from the disposition of the case ordered by the court in favour of Guerra and the other citizens, it is instructive to read a paragraph in the 'Concurring Opinion of Judge Jambrek' as he, as well as Judge Walsh, hold that this case clearly represents a violation under Article 2:

> *Article 2 states that 'Everyone's right to life shall be protected by law. No one shall be deprived of his life intentionally save …' The protection of health and physical integrity is, in my view as closely associated with the right to life as with 'respect for private and family life.' An analogy may be made with the court's case law on art 3 concerning the existence of 'foreseeable consequences' where* mutatis mutandis *substantial grounds can be shown for believing that the person(s) concerned face a real risk of being subjected to circumstances which endanger their health and physical integrity, and thereby put at serious risk their right to life, protected by law. If information is withheld by a government about circumstances which foreseeable, and on substantial grounds, present a real risk of danger to health and physical integrity, then such a situation may also be protected by art 2 of the convention: 'No one shall be deprived of his life intentionally.'*

This case, I believe, demonstrates, without a doubt, the strength of the *European Convention* and the position of the European Court of Human Rights, in contrast with other venues discussed above, both domestic and international, but also in the United States, based on the example of the *Constitution of Pennsylvania*. What is striking is the lack of any effort to 'balance interests', and the lack of any argument citing the 'economic and social interests' of the legal persons involved in maintaining a noxious operation, despite its effects on the health of citizens.

This is a major consideration in our quest for a blueprint for an improved regime, based on a supranational regulatory framework. Another case offers further evidence of the judicial superiority of the European Court of Human Rights: the case of *Lopez-Ostra v. Spain* (1995) 20 EHRR 277, (1994) ECHR 16798/90. Mrs Lopez-Ostra lived in Lorca (Murcia), a town with a high concentration of leather industries, all of which belonged to SACURSA, a company that also had a plant for the treatment of liquid and solid waste, built with a state subsidy on municipal land, 12 miles away from Lopez-Ostra's home, in July 1998 (at para. 8).

The gas fumes and other contamination, arising from the tanneries and the waste treatment operation, caused health problems to many in Lorca, and in September 1988 health authorities, and the Environmental and Nature Agency (Agencia para el Medio Ambiente y la Naturaleza), forced the company to cease some of its activities, and relocated a number of residents. However, some of the practices of the operation were allowed to continue, such as the treatment of waste water contaminated with chromium (at para. 9). Mrs Lopez-Ostra sought protection of her fundamental rights, and the language of her complaint is worthy of note (at para. 10):

> *She complained, inter alia, of an unlawful interference with her home and her peaceful enjoyment of it, a violation of her right to choose freely her place of residence; attacks on her physical and psychological integrity, and infringements of her liberty and her safety. (Articles 15,17(1), 18(2) and 19 of the (Spanish) Constitution)*

Despite the strong evidence available, both the Municipal and the Supreme Court of her country dismissed both her case and her appeal, respectively. Evidence was eventually accumulated by the National Toxicology Institute, the Ministry of Justice Institute of Forensic Medicine (Cartagena) and even by three police offices called to the home. The health effects were listed as 'a clinical picture of nausea, vomiting, allergic reactions, and anorexia', in addition to acute symptoms of 'bronchopulmonary infections' (at para. 19), all in clear conflict with Article 15 of the Spanish Constitution: 'Article 15: Everyone shall have the right to life and to physical and psychological integrity.'

Hence, once again, we see the protection of fundamental human rights and environmental protection provisions, coupled explicitly in a way that justifies the imposition of severe penalties, including imprisonment and hefty fines, and allows the temporary or permanent closure of the establishment in question. Under the European Court of Human Rights, the Court found that there had been a breach of Article 8 and awarded 4 million pesetas for damages, and 1.5 million for costs and expenses to Mrs Lopez-Ostra.

In sum, not only are the relevant articles of the *European Convention on Human Rights* progressively and analogically applied and understood, but there is little or no effort to view as comparable economic (corporate) rights on one hand, and health/life rights (individual or group based), on the other. Therefore, the Council of Europe appears to be far ahead of other similar courts. There has been a similar case argued in a similar way by Greek authorities, around 400BC, in a tannery edict, that is the target of the first environmental decree known (Rossetti, 2002).

Both cases show, first of all, that the right to life can be extended analogically to the right to health and to biological integrity, hence that the connection between the latter and the environment, possibly even environmental rights themselves, gain support, at least in principle. Second, those omissions to protect and to give information to citizens, on the part of a state, are perceived as culpable. Like direct interference, negligent omissions that support or enable operations that impose risks constitute a punishable harm, even if specific intent to harm is not present. Article 10(2) of the Convention may be viewed as prohibiting a government from preventing citizens from receiving information.[15]

The Council Directive of 7 June 1990 on the Freedom of Access to Information on the Environment states: 'Article 1 – The object of this directive is to ensure the freedom of access to and dissemination of information on the environment held by public authorities and to set out the basic terms and conditions on which such information should be made available.'

In addition, Article 4 enables whoever considers that the request for information has been unreasonably refused or ignored, or has been inadequately answered by a public authority, has the right to seek 'judicial or administrative review'. This position of the Court represents, in part, one of the bases for the successful conclusion of both cases cited.

Third, in the Lopez-Ostra case, the Court stated (at para. 52):

> *Admittedly, the Spanish authorities, and in particular the Lorca municipality were theoretically not directly responsible for the emissions in question. However, as the Commission pointed out, the town allowed the plant to be built on its land, and the State subsidized the plant's construction.*

Although there are no specific environmental rights in the *European Convention of Human Rights*, these cases come close to deriving such rights not only from Article 8, but also from Article 3. Kiss and Shelton (1997, p84), cite Article 45, para. 11 of the 1978 Spanish Constitution, which 'speaks of the right to enjoy an environment suitable for the development of the person'.

Principle 1 of the *Stockholm Declaration* says:

> *Man has the fundamental right to freedom, equality and adequate conditions of life, in an environment of a quality that permits a life of dignity and well-being, and he bears a solemn responsibility to protect and improve the environment for present and future generations.*

The link between the right to life and that to a 'suitable' environment is in the fact that both life and health depend upon environmental conditions.[16]

Fourth, Article 3, Prohibition of Torture, states: 'No one shall be subjected to torture or to inhuman or degrading treatment or punishment.' In Lopez-Ostra, the Court did not view the severe health effects suffered by the applicant and her family as sufficiently grave to be termed 'inhuman or degrading treatment' (at paras. 59 and 60), although Mrs Lopez-Ostra had so characterized her ordeal (at para. 30) (see also Birnie and Boyle, 2002, pp252–254, 287, n.10).. The Court's response appears to be less a rejection in principle of the possibility of viewing environmental harm in that light, than a matter of the gravity of a specific instance of harm. The Court's decision would allow the harm to be viewed as a difference of degree of 'inhumanity' or 'degradation,' rather than a difference in kind between environmental harms and torture.

Finally, moving from substantive to procedural matters, both cases support the choice of a supranational regulatory entity, as better able than either internal or international tribunals to restrain, and, if necessary, redress environmental harms.

The Supremacy of the *European Convention on Human Rights* over (European) state law is shown to be absolute, as is its ability to redress environmental human rights violations, rather than being hampered by economic agreements that might prescribe, and, in fact, demand a different course.

The final case of this environment/health trio also appeals to Article 8(2), but, like the other two cases, does not refer to the possibility of pre-birth injuries.[17] The conflict is a familiar one, the economic interests of an area, a region, or a group, aided by such NGOs as, for instance, Friends of the Earth.[18]

The judgement of the Grand Chamber acknowledged that there are, at this time, no 'environmental rights' guarantees in the convention, but added that:

> *Article 8 may apply in environmental cases whether the pollution is directly caused by the State or whether the State responsibility arises from the failure properly to regulate private industry.*[19]

It also cited Lopez-Ostra, but the judgement added that:

> *regard must be had to the balance that has to be struck between the competing interests of the individual and of the community as a whole; and in both contexts the State enjoys a certain margin of appreciation in determining the steps to be taken to ensure compliance with the Convention.*[20]

The question at issue was whether the number and frequency of night flights around Heathrow Airport should be limited, given the evidence presented of severe sleep disturbance affecting nearby resident families.

The situation in this case was somewhat different from the Guerra and Lopez-Ostra cases, because these involved regulatory breaches leading to illnesses and harms to the families and children in the vicinity, whereas the night-flight schedules were perfectly legal (since 1993). In addition, these flights, '... played a major role in the transportation infrastructure of the UK and contribute significantly to the UK economy and living standards of the UK citizens'.[21] It is significant that the court acknowledged that in matters concerning such 'complex issues of environmental and economic policy',[22] it is necessary to investigate all matters thoroughly, if only to reach 'a fair balance'. This is the position taken by the Portal initiative initiated by UNEP in September 2002.[23] This recent 'Portal' project is an effort to provide ecological and scientific information regarding the environment to Justices of the Supreme Courts of all countries, and the reform legal regimes from that standpoint. As Justice Arthur Chaskalson of South Africa says:

> *Our declaration and proposed program of work are, I believe, a crucial development in the quest to deliver development that respects people and that respects the planet for current and future generations and all living things.*[24]

Here the connection between 'environmental human rights' and future generations' rights is inescapable, especially when first generation's rights are at stake. Former International Court of Justice (ICJ) President Christopher Weeramantry makes the further connection between environmental rights and health:

> *The protection of the environment is likewise a vital part of contemporary human rights doctrine, for it is a* sine qua non *for numerous human rights, such as the right to health, and the right to life itself. It is scarcely necessary to elaborate on this, as damage to the environment can impair and undermine all human rights spoken of in the Universal Declaration of Human Rights and other human rights instruments.*[25]

Of course the *European Convention on Human Rights* does not explicitly enshrine 'environmental rights' as such, although the Judgment of the Grand Chamber in the Hatton case referred to 'environmental human rights' for the first time in the Court's jurisprudence.[26] That passage is worth citing in full for the connection it makes explicitly to health:

> *In the field of environmental human rights which was practically unknown in 1950, the Commission and the Court have increasingly taken the view that Article 8 embraces the right to a healthy environment, and therefore, to protection against pollution and nuisances caused by harmful chemicals, offensive smells, agents which precipitate respiratory ailments, noise and so on.*[27]

In the end, in Hatton, the Grand Chamber's decision was based on the doctrine of the 'margin of appreciation', despite its judicial critiques;[28] but the mere fact that environmental human rights could be discussed by a high court and even joined to the concept of health rights, demonstrates that perhaps Article 8(2) should be considered to be as basic as Article 2 for research on the rights of the child to health.

This list of other rights to which environmental rights are linked reinforces the argument of Prudence Taylor for 'ecological rights'.[29]

Perhaps when we acknowledge the right to a healthy environment and to protection against the effects of 'harmful chemicals', the right to life itself may need no special additional argument. In that case, perhaps we might be able to bypass the contentious issue of the 'right to life' (Article 2), and follow the supranational jurisprudence of the European Court of Human Rights, for a somewhat easier road to environmental harm protection.

THE PRINCIPLE OF THE 'BEST INTEREST OF THE CHILD' AND THE PROBLEM OF FREEDOM

This question was addressed briefly in Chapter 1. The main difficulties in adopting this principle as primary are two: the first concern is the view that the principle is primarily Western, that it embodies and represents a specific cultural tradition, one that it is argued, may appear to conflict with the 'practice of tradition' of other parts of the world.[30] The second difficulty is the question of who should decide on what might constitute the best interest of the child, and on what grounds.[31] Mnookin raises hard questions about making decisions according to a variety of perspectives. For instance, how does a judge compare the expected utility of one solution to a child's problem, with another possible solution? Does one consider the child's happiness or utility immediately or within a longer time frame?[32]

Most of the cases where the principle is invoked deal with interventions when either the biological parents or some other adults are to be weighed against one another, to select the best in the child's interest, using the principle as the primary consideration for adjudication.[33] But this is an exceedingly complex and uncertain judgement, at best:

> [N]o one ... can foresee just what experience, what events, what changes a child ... will encounter. Nor can anyone predict in detail how the unfolding development of a child and his family will be reflected in the long run in the child's personality and character formation. Thus the law will not act in the child's best interests but merely add to the uncertainties if it tries to do the impossible – guess the future and impose on the custodian special conditions for the child's care.[34]

Claire Breen argues in favour of a 'non-interventionist stance',[35] because of these uncertainties, taking the position that the protection of human rights starts with the defence of liberty.[36] Aside from the difficulties of this position, when John Stuart Mill himself argued that his doctrine applied only to those in full possession of their faculties and – in fact – even whole countries he judged to be not of age, were to be excluded from full rights to freedom, our argument is based on a quite different doctrine.

The position of this work as a whole is based on another understanding of the relation between human rights and freedom, and on the work of Alan Gewirth and Henry Shue instead (see Chapter 1, pp12–13). For Shue, freedom is important, but the 'basic rights' of individuals to security and subsistence are primary, to ensure that the most vulnerable people could be in a condition to exercise their right to freedom. Gewirth's emphasis on the 'pre-conditions of agency', which alone support human claims to rights, are also viewed as primary. Part of the reason for this contrasting point of view is that the main concern of this work is far less controversial than the choice of the preferable guardianship and residence for a child.

Our main focus is on the right of the child to be 'well-born', with both health and normal function, so that full agency, capabilities and free choices may be hers in the future. In this sense then, the preconditions of agency are equally preconditions of liberty, as the 'freedom to' achieve will be severely limited by any interference with the child's normal development. For instance, we considered the best known and most obvious of such prebirth intereferences, the case of thalidomide.

The main point is not how to best arrange care or guardianship so that the child my have the most free choices to seek fulfilment in her handicapped state, although this is important as well. The primary concern is to ensure that such environmentally caused harms be prevented by whatever means necessary, no matter how unacceptable such means may appear prima facie, to liberal, globalized lawmakers and courts. It is one of the aims of this work to show the two, related aspects of such means.

The first aspect is the restoring of value, hence the recognition of some rights to the preborn, a topic to which the first part of this book is devoted, including this chapter. The second is the quest to identify instruments and precedents to impose significant limitations to the freedom of corporate persons and their harmful enterprise, a topic that will be addressed in Chapters 5 to 8, below. As long as 'freedom' of all, including corporate persons is primary both in the public consciousness and in the law, and as long as each proposed restriction is viewed first as radically 'right wing' or conflicting with the most important values, it will not be possible to move forward toward a positive, empowering understanding of freedom.[37]

'Freedom' and 'free' are mostly used as simple concepts in both political and legal discourse, thus their inherent complexity is obscured. Joel Feinberg explains this hidden complexity well:

> *Since 'maximal freedom' (having as much freedom on balance as possible), is a notion that can be made sense of only by the application of independent standards for determining the relative worth or importance of different sorts of interests and areas of activity, it is by itself merely a formal ideal, one that cannot stand on its own feet without the help of other values. One person's freedom can conflict with another's; freedom in one dimension can conflict with another; and the conflicting dimensions cannot meaningfully be combined on one scale.*[38]

Thus appeals to 'freedom' per se to justify certain activities, practices or laws, remains vague and inchoate unless the other dimensions and values that underscore the support for these activities and practices is brought to light. In addition, Feinberg claims that, 'the study of kakapoeics', or the general theory and classification of harms, should be a central enterprise of legal philosophy.[39]

A fortiori then, the freedom from harm might be a pre-eminent topic in both law and philosophy. In the case of a young child or the preborn, the issue is rendered even more complex by the fact that children may not be aware that they are harmed, and the standard definition of being harmed as 'having someone invading or blocking ones interests'[40] is therefore inaccurate. Neither the thalidomide-damaged infant with flippers, not the young child exposed to harmful environmental conditions (say as in Guerra or Lopez-Ostra's cases) may be aware of having had their interests 'invaded', that is, of being harmed.

But the freedom to harm must be viewed as the most important factor to be eliminated, when any decisions are reached in the interests of the child. Claire Breen discusses the changing, 'emerging' tradition of the best interests of the child, in the context of guardianship issues and custody matters, with the possible conflicts between 'biological' and 'psychological' parents.[41,42,43]

The only health concern present in any of these cases is the emotional or psychological fragility of the child, hence the arrangements, no matter what the rights of the biological or foster parents involved.

One can therefore see the need to consider freedom/autonomy seriously in such cases. Our focus, however, demands a different perspective altogether: before a child can be asked to assert her autonomy or to exercise her freedom, she must have the required ability to normal intellectual function. For this to happen, her worth must be respected and whatever might eventually affect her ability to function, must be eliminated so that its harmful effects can be prevented. This will ensure that the physical preconditions of the normal exercise of her faculties will be protected. Joel Feinberg says:

> *In attributing human worth to everyone, we may be ascribing no property or set of properties, but rather expressing an attitude – the attitude of respect toward the humanity in each man's person. That attitude follows naturally from regarding everyone from the*

human point of view, but, it is not grounded in anything more ultimate than itself, and it is not ultimately justifiable.[44]

But is it sufficient to rely on 'having a human rights attitude'? Some argue that perhaps the dignity of human beings is basic to human rights, and that it is an inherent, basic, not contingent property of all humankind, one which does not depend on other conditions or abilities for its existence. According to the Preamble to the American *Convention on Human Rights* (1969), 'the essential rights of man ... are based upon attributes of the human personality', but the inescapable connection between humanity and their rights cannot simply depend on either 'acceptance' or the presence of a certain 'attitude'.

A Kantian position puts humanity first, with its abilities and capacities, even when these are not immediately present or exercised. Thus, pace Beylesveld and Brownsword, their argument that human beings have dignity 'on condition that they are agents',[45] could be modified to state that they have dignity because they in principle are able to be agents. This interpretation appears much closer to Kantian theory, where even the intoxicated, homeless man is worthy of the same respect due to all humanity not in virtue of his present ability for agency, but in virtue of possessing that capacity in principle and potentially, regardless of his present condition of incapacity.

THE PROTECTION OF FREEDOM AND ITS PRECONDITIONS IN A GLOBALIZED WORLD GOVERNED BY WESTERN ECONOMIC INTERESTS

Respect for humanity, for human dignity, and for the preconditions of free agency, are technically first in the rhetoric of every nation, group and individual. Yet the promotion of liberty understood mostly as 'freedom from'[46] or prevention of any interference with one's rights, neglects the basic interrelation and correlativity between rights and duties. Historically, it is easy to understand the primacy of rights to freedom from interference. The times when kings, noblemen and rulers had absolute powers, and in the absence of any procedural guarantees or protection mechanisms, the gravest danger to common people came precisely from the unrestrained and capricious power of these rulers.

But the proliferation of human rights instruments and regulations both domestic and international, as well as the development of constitutional, procedural guarantees, have worked together to diminish the need for that specific emphasis in the law. Today, it is increasingly the corporate rich and powerful institutions that are in the position of ruling the world,[47] hence they ought to be identified primarily with the absolute kings and rulers of old, rather than with the citizens and the ruled, as they currently are.

Like the kings and noblemen of the ancient and medieval world: (a) their power is absolute and hereditary, in the sense they have not been elected, cannot be recalled, work exclusively in their own interest, and their lifespan continues almost in perpetuity, as one CEO follows another (none are democratically chosen); (b) they are not accountable to the citizenry but, at most, to their shareholders and to an abstraction, in the 'market'; (c) they are, for the most part, beyond the reach of the law that restrains the freedom of biological persons to pursue their interests in most countries: for instance, whether criminal law may apply to the corporate criminal is a highly debated issue among legal scholars;[48] (d) although they do not govern directly any nation, through lobbies, political donations to various parties, and other forms of influence (more or less legal, depending on circumstances and the geographical location of these activities), they exert enough power to affect significantly elections and policies in most countries;[49] and (e) their powers (unlike those of a single citizen) extend across most borders, often globally, in the case of large multinational corporations.[50]

This final aspect is a very important basic one that demonstrates the difference between the corporate person and the biological person: the latter, at best, possesses some measure of political control within their own borders, as even democratic votes do not extend beyond one country's borders.[51] In contrast the influence of corporate persons is felt in different countries and all continents, not only through their economic activities, but also because of their presence (although not as full participants) at meetings from which various international instruments emerge, as well as 'free market' agreements such as GATT, NAFTA and the WTO. They cannot be signatories as are representatives of countries, but their manoeuvres insure they have a significant impact on all decisions.

It is clear that it is in the interest of corporate individuals to stand on their 'rights' to freedom, without considering the complexity of freedom,[52] and their impact on the rights and freedoms of others. This attitude is analogical to the attitude of many women's groups. Women were originally highly vulnerable and even oppressed, but gaining an ever increasing plethora of rights, at times, and clearly in relation to the preborn, can be identified with oppressors instead.

Corporate power as such is a grave direct threat to the health of the child at all stages of development, as we will see below. For now, if we consider briefly the points above, for (a) we can contrast the powerlessness of children at all stages of development. Children and their representatives do not normally band together for class actions, except perhaps in the thalidomide case, where the clear causal links eliminated a priori the standard corporate defence, that is, the claim that somehow the responsibility for the harms incurred by citizens rested on the affected parties themselves and their lifestyles or activities of choice.

The next point (b) is obvious: even when corporations are at times requested to eliminate a specific product or to modify a certain activity or practice, their research and development divisions are immediately hard at work to produce an equivalent substitute that is, most likely, just as harmful, although it may not yet have been named as such by specific laws at that time.[53] On the question of hazardous activities such as harmful waste disposal practices, the usual industry response is to move the whole hazardous operation to another location, most likely in a developing country, where the environmental regulatory regime is less 'restrictive', thus effectively transferring the harms from 'presently threatened populations' (PTP) in zone 1 to even more vulnerable populations in zone 2. The latter will be exposed to an even greater threat, and, more than likely, be given less information about the practice or product.[54]

For (c) the problem was the lack of appropriate legal structures and regimes to deal with corporate criminals, both in domestic and international law. For instance, G. P. Fletcher says:

Negligent motoring and negligent manufacturing significantly threaten the public interest, yet Western judges seem more comfortable punishing counterfeiters and prostitutes, than imposing sanctions against those who inadvertently take unreasonable risks.[55]

Most of us are also keenly aware of the recent proliferation of accounting-related corporate crime, which, attacking as it does the sanctity of the market and the pockets of the investors, is dealt with in a more severe manner. But 'Ecocrime'[56] has not been correspondingly pilloried, censured and even punished. Why this is so can be answered succinctly: it is the basic way of doing business, that is legal for the most part, and that provides these corporate persons' lifeblood, while at the same time it feeds its insatiable hunger for environments and resources, while trampling on humanity's 'ecological rights'.[57]

Most of the attacks on the children's health and function are part of this cycle of negligently harmful activities to which the first affected new 'canaries' bear witness. The next point, (d), is also an important one for our research goal: the questions it raises are basic indeed: business's main aim is protect its own well-being, not the well-being of affected children in its area of operation. It is the duty of the governments, both national and international to protect all natural humans, who, unlike corporate persons, can be harmed. By the time that citizens band together in desperation, to bring a case to the attention of a supranational court like the European Court of Human Rights, in most instances, the harm has been done and it is very often irreversible like it was in the case of thalidomide: the harm has long since been imposed, and the crime has been committed.

For the next point, (e), one could argue, as I have done,[58] that the transnational reach of corporate harms requires that such activities be publicly proclaimed to be 'attacks against the human person', by organs such as the UN and the WHO.[59]

Given the all-pervasive presence of harmful corporate activities globally, culminating in the powerful policies of the WTO, it is necessary that the UN should strike back through the only body able to do so in an authoritative manner, the WHO.

THE WTO AND THE WHO IN CONFLICT

In 1998, Gro Brundtland, a former Prime Minister of Norway, was appointed Director General, with wide support within the Organization. Under her leadership WHO began a period of major strategic and structural reform. Rapid change during the past 5 years and a ficys ib a few priorities under central leadership reinvigorated WHO and restored its international credibility. Many new programs and partnerships were established and the Organization has elevated health successfully on the international development agenda, for example, the Tobacco Free Initiative's work on the Framework Convention on Tobacco Control, which was approved by the World Health Assembly (WHA) in May 2003.[60]

The conflict between the economic motive and the protection of health and the environment that was noted in the last two sections , as well as in the first chapter of this book and in the case law of the European Court of Human Rights, is even more clearly in evidence when global trade and world health clash.

The WHO should work more actively not only to respond and advise in crises requiring its technical expertise, but in the general field of public health. Its mandate of 'Health for all in the 21st Century' indicates that the WHO 'should begin to develop international law more actively'; in fact, 'WHO has to pay more attention to the many and diverse areas of international law that relate to its global health mission'.[61] In contrast, some recognize the difficulties of an organization whose mandate is affected by so many variables outside their control and area of expertise, such as wars, poverty and global climate change. In addition, its State Members often do not have the financial resources or the political will to support major international plans, including drafting better common regulatory regimes.[62,63]

Many of the issues the WHO should regulate among those listed by Fidler as the major areas that should be covered under 'Health for All in the 21st Century', deal specifically with issues of concern for this world. Two are particularly worthy of mention, 'standards on the safety and purity, and potency of biological, pharmaceutical and similar products flowing in international commerce ...' and, most of all, 'diverse issues arising from the link between international trade and health' (e.g. tobacco, alcohol, food safety and the relationship of intellectual property protection to pharmaceuticals).[64]

These two areas, however, do not emphasize the gravest threat to children and everyone's health: the trade of chemicals other than pharmaceuticals, that are among the worst 'offenders' against children's health. What are at issue are international human rights law, international trade law and international environmental law, thus the lack of involvement in all these areas coupled with the grave problems present in those areas of law, 'demonstrates that the WHO's policy of ignoring other areas of international law has been a serious mistake'.[65]

We must acknowledge, however, that the WHO is in an invidious position being, like the UN itself, both a player and a stage at the same time. As a 'stage', it must negotiate and listen, but as a player, it must stand up for public health, as it is the only international organ competent and authoritative enough to do so. No other powerful organization steps up to help or support a position in defence of public health, although the 25 November 2004 decision of the International Union for the Conservation of Nature (IUCN) in Bangkok to adopt the *Earth Charter*, which will be integrated in the 2000 Draft International Covenant on Environment and Development, is a good step forward. In addition, we noted the ECHR case law in the previous section, and its clear defence of human rights to health and the environment, particularly when children are affected.

The vital importance of a possible WHO intervention becomes obvious when one considers the most powerful global organization in international relations, the WTO. It will be best to start by looking at the important Article XX where questions of health and environment area addressed:

Article XX

General Exceptions

Subject to the requirements that such measures are not applied in a manner which would constitute a means of arbitrary or unjustifiable discrimination between countries where the same conditions prevail, or a disguised restriction on international trade, nothing in this Agreement shall be construed to prevent the adoption or enforcement of any contracting parties of measures . . .

(1)   necessary to protect human, animal, or plant life or health; . . .

(2)   relating to the conservation of exhaustible natural resources if such measures are made effective in conjunction with restrictions on domestic production or consumption.[66]

This document, like the *Agreement on the Application of Sanitary and Phytosanitary Measures* (SPS Agreement; 1994), is entirely oriented to trade, not to the protection of health and the environment.[67] In the *Hormones* case, as in the other cases (the Australian *Measures Affecting the Importation of Salmon* and the Japanese *Measures Affecting Agricultural Products*), the government that was appealing the use of substances or products judged to be harmful to human health lost its case.

These decisions may represent violations of human rights, but they are defended purely on economic grounds, although clearly there are other values at stake, including democratic values, such as the right to due process. For instance, Robert Howse raises the obvious question: because of their role as transnational organizations with power over individual states, what of democracy in this context? Howse claims that democracy is not implemented by responding 'to widespread fears of citizens about risks'; instead, the WTO decisions 'can and should be understood not as usurping legitimate democratic choices for stricter regulations, but as enhancing the quality of rational democratic deliberations about risk and its control'.[68] Howse adds that 'popular choices should be respected,' but only 'if the choices have been made in awareness of the facts'.[69] But that is precisely the point raised here: the facts provided by the corporate interests who wish to avoid regulation and their hired experts may be far removed from the true facts of the case. Right decisions are only taken after all scientific sides of a debate are heard, with those affected by the decision casting the deciding vote and the precautionary principle is brought into the decision.[70]

Perhaps the basic error lies in expecting these documents, specifically and openly oriented to deal with trade, to also provide health and environmental protection that we all require, and that humanity should have a 'basic' right to have. However, given the lack of other instruments of equal or superior enforcement and implementation power designed for our protection, it is hard to see why we should reduce our expectations of fairness and justice, principles that govern all laws, including civil laws pertaining to trade. We need to be aware of this cardinal problem: 'free trade' has been described as a 'Corporate Charter of Rights and Freedoms' for Canada,[71] and the notion of an 'economic Constitution for North America' was proposed by then President Ronald Reagan.[72] For a country less rich and powerful than the United States, such as Canada, the effect of WTO judgements may include 'trading away one's national sovereignty',[73] and may include a number of consequences far beyond 'trade' issues.[74] In some sense, what is at stake is the existence of sovereignty itself.

Part of what is at issue is the increasing dissonance between the proliferation of explicit 'green' 'soft law' instruments that give primacy to our habitat and to humanity, and the even greater proliferation of 'trade-as-sovereign' documents. These, for the most part, express a few green sentiments in their nonbinding Preambles perhaps, but continue to view cases and issues as 'business first'. In the first group, we can include such documents as the UN *Agreement Governing the Activities of States on the Moon* (1979); the *Convention on the Law of the Sea* (UNCLOS, 1982); the *Rio Declaration* (1992); the Vienna *Convention for the Protection of the Ozone Layer* (1985); the Montreal *Protocol on Substances that Deplete the Ozone Layer* (1987), as adjusted and amended in 1990, 1992 and 1995, and others pertaining to forests and to the 'Common Heritage of Mankind' principle.

These treaties are not primarily designed for the defence of human rights to health and the environment, let alone for a specific consideration of children's rights to supersede the primacy of trade interests. The European Community, however, stands alone in having rejected the WTO's mandates in the Hormones case; in fact, the protection of health is emphasized in their treaties:

> *Treaty Establishing the European Community (19. .) Article 30 (ex Article 36)*
> *The provisions of Articles 28 and 29 shall not preclude prohibitions or restrictions on imports, exports or goods in transit justified on grounds of public morality, public policy or public security; the protection of health and life of humans, animals or plants; the protection of national treasures possessing artistic, historic or archaeological value; or the protection of industrial or commercial property. Such prohibitions or restrictions shall not, however, constitute a means of arbitrary discrimination or a disguised restriction on trade between Member States.*

There are a fair number of EC cases that involve public health issues, and these involve Article 30,[75] where grounds are sought to validate measures that might otherwise be considered discriminatory.[76] For example in the Sandoz case,[77] the Dutch authorities 'refused to allow the sale of muesli bars that contained added vitamins', on the grounds that the vitamins were dangerous to health. Article 30 was also fundamental in Preussen–Elektra,[78] and doubts were even cast on whether the list of 'grounds' in Article 30 was truly exhaustive in Preussen–Elektra

> *Advocate General Jacobs re-examined the issue. He argued that the approach in the Walloon Waste case was flawed, in the sense that, whether a measure was discriminatory was logically distinct from whether it could be justified. He suggested however, that there could be good reasons for allowing environmental protection to be pleaded as a justification, even in cases where there was direct discrimination.[79]*

In the Cassis de Dijon case,[80] the ECJ, in contrast, deemed that the protection of public health was not (in this case) a 'decisive consideration'[81] to establish that the rejected import's alcohol content, although it was lower than that prevalent in Germany, was necessarily conducive to addiction or other harmful health effects. But the Simmenthal case[82] demonstrates that extraordinary health measures (e.g. a second veterinary opinion) may be necessary to protect the public in the case of transboundary movement of beef and beef products. Yet the case is viewed in the literature as an example of the affirmation of the supremacy of community law over national law, with some overtones of market protectionism for Italy's own beef producers.

At any rate, the combination of a forward-looking 'teleological' law, as exemplified for instance by Article 308 (ex Article 235), often used to introduce and justify measures for environmental protection or other normatively desirable outcomes, on one hand, and the presence of 'judicial activism' on the other,[83,84] together appear to distance EU Law from all other trade agreements, as we note in Chapter 6. Lord Howe cites Sir Thomas Bingham in *Customs and Excise v. Samex*:

> *The interpretation of Community Instruments invokes very often ... the creative process of supplying flesh to a spare and loosely constructed skeleton, and the taking of a broader view of what the orderly development of the Community requires.*[85]

This forward-looking approach to law, coupled with a supranational form of governance that is inherently (though not exclusively) normative, manifests a deep contrast with the approach of trade organizations such as the GATT or the WTO. The conflict between the two approaches comes to a head in the Hormones case.[86] In this case, the US tried without success to remove the EC import ban 'on meat raised with growth hormones',[87] which according to Fidler's report are at least five hormones. The case hinged upon several issues: (1) the use of the precautionary principle; (2) public health protection; and (3) the nature and import of risk assessment on the part of the European Community. All these issues were brought into question in the case the US brought to the WTO.

The Panel Report, issued 18 August 1997, (WTO Doc. WT/DS26/R/USA), is a lengthy and complex document, hence we will limit our discussion to the three areas listed above. The first difference between the EC and the WTO centres on the nature and the role of the precautionary principle. The EC viewed it as a 'general, customary rule of international law', or least, as 'a general principle of law'. Further, the EC believed that it was 'not necessary for all scientists around the world to agree on the possibility and the magnitude' of the risk, nor for all of the WTO members to perceive and evaluate the risk in the same way.[88] In the following paragraph the US position is outlined: 'The United States does not consider that the "precautionary principle" represents customary international law and suggests it is more "an approach" than a "principle".'

The implication here, of course, is that if it is not a principle of law, then its use does not have the legitimacy it might otherwise have; and, if the US position is accepted, the use of the principle might be termed 'arbitrary'.

The second problem concerns the nature of public health, based on international standards and the debate between the possible interpretations of Article 3.1 of the SPS Agreement, which states:

> *To harmonize sanitary and phytosanitary measures on as wide a basis as possible, Members shall base their sanitary or phytosanitary measures on international standards, guidelines or recommendations, where they exist, except as otherwise provided for in this Agreement, and in particular in paragraph 3.*

The question is whether it is possible to equate measures 'based on international standards', with 'measures which conform to such standard', therefore, whether one or the other interpretation is the basis of the EC's understanding of 'public health'.[89] It is clear that 'based on' certain standards is not the same as being in conformity or compliance with these standards. Hence, the scientific justification required by the EC may well be understood to exceed international standards, rather than simply to conform to them.

Finally, on the question of risk assessment, Paragraph 4 of Annex A of the SPS Agreement defines risk assessment as: 'the evaluation of the potential for adverse effects on human or animal health arising from the presence of additives, contaminants, toxins, or disease – causing organisms in food, beverages or feedstuffs.[90] The problem is that, although the Panel refers to 'potential' as an alternative to 'probability,' 'potential' is a concept much closer to 'possible' than to 'probable' and the European Community's understanding of risk assessment sees risk as present when the mere possibility of harm to human health is present. Five levels of protection of human health are required by the EC:

1 the level of protection in respect of natural hormones when used for growth promotion;
2 the level of protection in respect of natural hormones occurring endogenously in meat or other food;
3 the level of protection in respect of natural hormones when used for therapeutic or zoo technical purposes;
4 the level of protection in respect of synthetic hormones (zeranol and trenbolone) when used for growth promotion; and
5 the level of protection in respect to carbadox and olaquindox.

Aside from details pertaining to point(s), which are both technical and complex,[91] all other listed levels of protection indicate a perfectly understandable and scientifically supportable stance, which eliminated the possibility of an arbitrary position on the part of the EC. Even if the EC has economic interests in addition to the health concerns, that is, if it had an interest in protecting its own beef sources, the fact remains that there is a solid position in defence of public health, in the face of the cancer epidemic that exists.[92] Nor is this case unique. In the later case of *Portugal v. Council*,[93] the ECJ judgement stated:[94] 'It follows for all those considerations, that having regard to their nature and structure, the WTO agreements are not in principle among the rules in the light of which the Court is to review the legality of measures adopted by the Community institutions.'

Like the European Community, the WHO can and does stand up to trade and other harmful interests at times. A fine example of their ability to do so is the *WHO Framework Convention on Tobacco Control*.[95] The 'Preamble' is strongly worded as can be expected in defence of children's rights to health, and against trade interests. Inter alia, the 'Preamble' says:

> *The Parties of this Convention*
> *Determined to give priority to their right to protect public health*
> ...

Acknowledging that there is a clear scientific evidence prenatal exposure to tobacco smoke causes adverse health and developmental conditions for children,

...

Deeply concerned about the escalation in smoking and other forms of tobacco consumption by children and adolescents worldwide, particularly smoking at increasingly early ages...

Clearly in this instrument, the WHO goes beyond general commitments, both in the 'Preamble' and in the body of the instrument. Article 4(2) recommends 'strong political commitments' to develop measures that take into consideration, 'the need to take measures to address gender-specific risks when developing tobacco control strategies' (Article 4(2) (d)). Of course 'taking into consideration' is not a mandate to implement, as it goes perhaps too far in respecting the State Parties' sovereignty (in contrast with the language of ICISS, which views 'intervention' as the responsibility to protect instead, see Chapter 1).

The State Parties' sovereignty and the same respect for the Parties is in evidence in Article 5. Under 'General Obligations', the Article states that each Party 'shall develop, implement...' tobacco control strategies, and, equally strongly, Article 5 says:

Article 5.3.
In setting and implementing their public health policies with respect to tobacco control, Parties shall act to protect those policies from commercial and other vested interests of the tobacco industry in accordance with national law.

Given the WHO's own research finding, perhaps the compilation of a 'Framework Convention on the Control of Hazardous Chemicals', might be a desirable and even possible future development. After all, the 2000 *Basel Protocol on Liability and Compensation for Damage Resulting from Transboundary Movements of Hazardous Wastes and their Disposal* states that the Parties to the Protocol have agreed to:

Article 1
Objective
The Objective of the Protocol is to provide for a comprehensive regime for liability and for adequate and prompt compensation for damage resulting from the transboundary movement of hazardous waste and other wastes and their disposal including illegal traffic in those wastes.

And in the introductory language, they acknowledge they are 'Aware of the risks of damage to human health, property and the environment caused by hazardous wastes and other wastes and the transboundary movement and disposal thereof.' It is highly unlikely that the production of the materials and the processes that give rise to 'hazardous wastes' will be risk-free from the standpoint of health.

The *Stockholm Convention on Persistent Organic Pollutants*, under Article 1, 'Objectives' states:

> *Mindful of the precautionary approach as set forth in Principle 15 of the Rio Declaration on Environment and Development, the objective of this Convention is to protect human health and the environment from persistent organic pollutants.*

It is important to note that only the Tobacco Convention refers explicitly to children, and obliquely (through a reference to 'gender specific policies') to pre-birth exposures, whereas the other documents, which are not produced by the WHO, are far less comprehensive and thorough in their approach.

Perhaps one can hope that the WHO will use its own findings for a third major convention or even for the request, once again, for an Opinion from the ICJ (or the UN itself). I am referring not only to the Tobacco Convention, but to the first occasion when the WHO submitted a question requesting an advisory opinion on 'the legality of the use by a state of Nuclear Weapons in an armed conflict', to the ICJ, as follows: 'In view of the health and environmental effects would the use of nuclear weapons by a state in war or other armed conflict be a breach of its obligations under international law including the WHO constitution?'[96]

Several states argued that the question went beyond 'the WHO's proper activities'. The Court added (at para. 10) that:

> *three conditions must be satisfied in order to found the jurisdiction of the Court when a request for an advisory opinion is submitted to it by a specialized agency: the agency requesting the opinion must be duly authorized, under the Charter, to request opinions from the Court; the opinion requested must be one arising within the scope of the activities of the requesting agency.*[97]

Despite the interest and the competence of the WHO to assess and evaluate the health effects of the use of nuclear weapons, at first the Court judged that the final condition had not been met, as the WHO was not a state able to wage a war, or enter into a conflict, and it did not use these weapons.

Hence, the UN General Assembly had to bring the question to the Court once again. The Court held that neither 'customary' nor 'conventional' international law authorizes specifically the use of nuclear weapons (by 11 votes to 3); and that the threat or use of nuclear weapons is also not specifically permitted, and that:

> *it follows from the above-mentioned requirements that the threat or use of nuclear weapons would generally be contrary to the rules of international law applicable in armed conflict, and in particular the principles and rules of humanitarian law; however, in view of the current state of international law, and of the elements of facts at its disposal, the Court cannot conclude definitively whether the threat or use of nuclear weapons would be lawful or unlawful in an extreme circumstance of self-defence, in which the very survival of a State would be at stake (the President casting his vote to break the 7 to 7 tie).*

This opinion, despite its ambiguous tone, was viewed as an important decision, and it shows the transition from state treaties as sole arbiters of the status of nuclear armaments, to an opinion whose history and background served to bring a normative issue to the forefront of public opinion.[98]

Falk traces the history of the movement that culminated in that request, from several groups in civil society, as 'the push to achieve elimination [of nuclear weapons] often merges with the view that weapons of mass destruction cannot be reconciled with international humanitarian law'.[99]

Falk shows how world opinion as well as the work of many committed non-governmental organizations prepared the ground work for the very possibility of asking for an opinion, from the time of the London Nuclear Warfare Tribunal (1985), where those weapons were defined as 'unconditionally illegal', hence, that even a threat of their use would amount to a 'crime against humanity'.[100]

The main point that emerges is that neither politics nor economic factors, nor even the advantage of groups of nuclear states, could be allowed to decide on the use of these weapons. Hence, at first the UN General Assembly and the WHO referred a difficult question to the World Court, and although the question could be evaded on the grounds that 'health', narrowly construed, would not include the use of weapons, later, an opinion was given. Implicit in both the original request by the WHO and the eventual opinion is the fact that, 'Nuclear Weaponry, with its global implications, raises question of legality that affect not just the citizenry of the nuclear weapons states, but the entire world'.[101] This position supports, once again, the *erga omnes* status of the question at least in principle, given the careful phrasing of the Court's statements. Falk does not use this language in regard to either the question or the Opinion itself, but he adds:

> *Although not so formulated, the radical element in this request was to transfer the question of nuclear weapons policy from the domain of geopolitics, where it had remained since the first attacks on Hiroshima and Nagasaki, to the domain of international law.*[102]

And if it has not transferred the question to treaty law – clearly both incomplete and insufficient to deal with this global threat – then Ragazzi's argument for placing its normative aspect among the few *jus cogens* norms generating an *erga omnes* obligation appears to be correct.[103]

In sum, the WHO may not have armies at its command to save health and to protect human rights, especially those of children. But it does have the clout and the status to ensure that when it speaks people do listen; it also can (as it has already done) influence legal scholarship and public policy. It is the only UN organ that has the ability to do so in response to the increasing attacks by globalized trade on public health, to the detriment of children everywhere today, and of future generations.

NOTES

1 Breen (2002).
2 Kilkenny (1999), pp18–21.
3 Van Beuren (1995), pp33–38.
4 Koskenniemi (1992), pp123–128.
5 Kilkenny (1992), p18.

6   Kilkenny (1992), p19.
7   *Brüggemann and Scheuten v. Federal Republic of Germany*, ECHR Appl. No 6959/75, Comm. Rep. 12.7.77, DR 10.
8   E.H.R.R. 244/245, at para. §60.
9   *Paton v. UK*, No841b/78 Dec.13.5.80, DR 19,p.244, 3 EHRR 408.
10 *Guerra v. Italy* (1998) Rep. 1998-I, no.64, p.21026 EHRR 357.
11 *Lopez-Ostra v. Spain* (1994) Series A, no 303, 20 EHRR 330.
12 *Guerra v. Italy* (1998) 26 EHRR, 357 and *Lopez-Ostra v. Spain* (1995) 20 EHRR 277, (1994) ECHR 16798/90).
13 *Guerra v. Italy*, 'Head note'.
14 Westra (1998).
15 *Lender v. Sweden*, A/116 (1987) 9 E.HR.R. 433.
16 Kiss and Shelton (1997), p85; compare Soskolne and Bertollini (1999).
17 *Hatton and Others v. United Kingdom*, 37 EHRR 28(2003) Grand Chamber Judgment; see also 34 EHRR 1 (2002).
18 Mowbray (2004), pp151–152.
19 *Hatton and Others v. United Kingdom*, at para § 98.
20 *Hatton and Others v. United Kingdom*.
21 Mowbray (2004), p154.
22 *Hatton and Others v. United Kingdom*, at para. 128.
23 Westra (2003), p136; see also U.C. *Davis Law Review*, Vol. 37, No.1.
24 Justice A. Chaskalson, Address at the Summit for the Johannesburg Principles on the Role of Law and Sustainable Development, 27 August 2002.
25 *Gabcikovo-Nagymaros* (1997) ICJ, Rep.7, Judge C. Weeramantry, separate opinion.
26 Mowbray (2004), p158.
27 Judgment of the Grand Chamber in *Hatton and Others v. UK*, 37 EHRR 28 (2003) para. § 2, Joint Dissenting Opinion.
28 *Z. v. Finland*, 1997-I 323; 25 EHRR 371 (1998) Judge Meyer in his 'partly dissenting opinion'.
29 Taylor (1998), p309.
30 Breen (2002), pp2–7.
31 Mnookin (1985).
32 Mnookin (1985), pp16–24.
33 Mnookin (1985), p235.
34 Goldstein et al (1980), pp51–52.
35 Breen (2002), p49.
36 Dworkin (1971); Mill (1910)
37 Berlin (1969), p130.
38 Feinberg (1980), p11.
39 Feinberg (1980), p45.
40 Feinberg (1980).
41 *W. v. United Kingdom*, Judgment of 8 July 1987, Series A no.121, (1987).
42 *Olsson v. Sweden*, Judgment of 24 March 1988, Series A no.130, (1988).
43 *Rieme v. Sweden*, Judgment of 22 April 1992, Series A no.226 B, (1992).
44 Feinberg (1973), p94.
45 Beylesveld and Brownsword (2001), p165.
46 Berlin (1969).
47 Korten (1995).
48 Glasbeek and Rowland (1986); Westra (2004a).
49 Korten (1995).
50 Barlow and Clarke (2002).

51 Gilbert (1994).
52 Feinberg (1980).
53 Brown (2000).
54 Westra (2000b), pp465–476.
55 Fletcher (1971), pp401–437.
56 Westra (2004a).
57 Taylor, P. (1998).
58 Westra (2004a), Chapter 7.
59 *WHO Framework Convention on Tobacco Control*, WHA 56.1, 21 May, 2003; A56/INF.Doc./7.
60 Beaglehole and Bonita (2004), p270.
61 Fidler (2000), p122.
62 Fluss (1998).
63 Taylor, A. L. (1998).
64 Fidler (2000), p122.
65 Fidler (2000), p123.
66 *Agreement Establishing the World Trade Organization* (1994), 'Chapeau', and (b) and (g).
67 *Appellate Body Hormones Decision*, EC Measures Concerning Meat and Meat Products (Hormones), AB-1997-4, WT/DS 26/AB/R,WT/DS48/AB/R.
68 Howse (2000), p2330.
69 Howse (2000).
70 Shrader-Frechette (1991), pp46–50; Tickner (1999), pp162–186; Ashford (1999), pp198–206.
71 Barlow and Sullivan (1982), pA25; Clarkson (1993), pp3–20.
72 Laxer (1991), p209.
73 McBride and Shields (1993), pp162–164.
74 Wallach and Sforza (1999), Chapters 2 and 3.
75 EC Treaty, Part Three, Title 1, chapter 2.
76 De Burca and Craig (2003), p634.
77 *Officier van Justitie v. Sandoz*, 174/82, BV [1983] ECR 2445.
78 *Preussen–Elektra AG v. Schleswag AG*, Case c-379/98, [2001] ECR 1-2099.
79 De Burca and Craig (2003), pp633–634.
80 *Rewe-Zentrale AG v. Bundesmonopolverwaltung fur Brantwein*, Case 120/78.
81 Case 120/78 at para. ll.
82 *Simmenthal SpA v. Commission* (Case 92/78) [1979] ECR 777, [1980] 1 CMLR.
83 Howe of Aberavon (1996), pp190–193.
84 Tridimas (1996).
85 1983, 1 AllE. R. 1042, 1056.
86 *Appellate Body Hormones Decision*, EC Measures Concerning Meat and Meat Products (Hormones), Adopted Feb. 13, 1998, WTO Doc. WT/DS26/AR/R and WT/DS48/AD/U.
87 Fidler (2000), p233.
88 Fidler (2000), at para. 121.
89 Scott (2000), pp144–158.
90 Fidler (2001), p240.
91 Fidler (2001), pp245–247.
92 Epstein (1989).
93 Case C-149/96, (1999) ECR I-8395.
94 Case C-149/96, (1999) ECR I-8395 at para. 47.
95 A 56/INF.DOC./7.
96 Adv.Op., 1996 I.C.J. .66.
97 Kindred et al (2000), p363.
98 Falk (1998).

  99 Falk (1998).
 100 Falk (1998).
 101 Falk (1998), p174.
 102 Falk (1998), p175.
 103 Ragazzi (1997).

PART TWO

Ecojustice and Future Generations' Rights

CHAPTER 5

The Impact of Consumerism and Social Policy on the Health of the Child

A QUESTION OF PUBLIC POLICY

Now Europeans have a new dream, one more expansive than the one they left behind: to enjoy a quality of life, to respect one another's cultures, to create a sustainable relationship with the natural world, and to live in peace with their fellow human beings. Universal harm rights are the legal articulation of the new European Dream.[1]

Thus far, the research of this work has focused on an examination of various approaches to the protection of the life and the health of the child in law. But a consideration of both common law and civil law, as well as international law instruments, discloses that most applications of domestic, international and even supranational regulatory regimes eventually are decided according to an interpretation of the law that favours present social and public policy considerations. Cases do refer to precedent and to reasons why decisions have been taken in the past, as well as to the letter of the articles of various instruments. They use analogy sparingly, but appeal to public policy and social practices and beliefs on a regular basis, in fact, generally speaking, they do so more often than they refer to abstract arguments about justice or fairness.

Hence the vital importance of turning to a consideration of the institutionalized, political and even economic setting against which cases are adjudicated, laws are enacted and regulatory regimes implemented. In Chapter 4, the aims and goals of the WHO and the WTO were juxtaposed in order to show the vast difference between the consequences following upon the two disparate approaches to public policy. But even the WHO is not entirely the power for health and environmental protection it could be because of the economic power of the nations to which it is accountable, or rather the nations whose support it needs in order to function. This fact indicates that, contrary to the principles of justice and fairness (at least in the moral sense) even at the level of the highest defence of the human right to health (the WHO's mandate), too much of the economic motive is still present.

Today globalization is, for the most part, 'America's Quest for Global Dominance', as Noam Chomsky has it.[2] Chomsky traces the recent history of this approach, and he cites John Ikenberry, as describing:

> *a grand strategy [that] begins with a fundamental commitment to maintaining a uni-*
> *polar world in which the United States has no peer competitor. . . . [so] that no state or*
> *coalition could ever challenge the US as a global leader, protector and enforcer.*[3]

This strategy dismisses international law, its instruments and institutions, including the norms of just war and aggression, and especially self-defence, starting with Article 51 of the UN Charter.[4]

One may well ask how are these facts, even if obviously true, related to children's health and the environment. First, all approaches to children's health are embedded on globalized political regimes, dominated by the US and its neo-liberal mandate of aggressive, unprincipled individualism. Second, most of the world's countries need to ally themselves with the imperial power or submit to it, so that establishing contrasting, or 'deviant' institutions and instruments is, for the most part, not possible for any single country today, in the face of the overwhelming and ruthless power that operates on the 'idea' that was articulated repeatedly by the administration of George W. Bush, 'either you are with us, or you are against us'.

Hence the need to recognize and embrace the presence of innovation and advances in the new 'European Dream', a dream, and in some cases, as we saw, a reality that stands as a separate concept and at times in opposition to the US's hegemony.[5] The oppositions between the two systems are best understood when, 'the concept of globalization seems to be little more than a synonym for Westernization or Americanization'.[6] In addition, Marxist analysis of capitalism as a 'social order' with a 'pathological expansionist logic' needs to reach for a constantly growing field, as the whole world is viewed as 'markets' to be divided in ways that foster capitalist growth.

Indeed, 'International order is the order produced by the more powerful states',[7] at least for the most part. Hence, if our aim is to ensure that a specific sort of human rights be recognized and taken to be primary, over economic considerations or other 'freedom' issues, that is the right of the child to health and the environment, then it is important to understand these conflicting regimes, and to seek out the best 'power blocks' or jurisdictions within which our quest may come to fruition. The passage with which this chapter started points the way to what could be viewed as our best option in this quest, and we will return to it below. For now we should consider the role of consumerism and of the media, beyond state and global trade interests on a grand scale.

Capitalism and the pathological role of consumerism

In a recent paper, Robert Albritton argues that present Western national systems support and actively promote policies that have a grave effect on the health and the life of all human beings and the environment: more and more in the West, we are 'Eating the Future'.[8] His analysis of practices and conditions of life in the West today is based on and researched primarily from the viewpoint of everyday US activities, and the underlying beliefs that govern those activities. For the most part, the practices are those of legal persons, that is, individuals who can own property as well as buying and selling it. Their most basic value is 'freedom', to own, to move and to consume.[9] All of these 'freedoms' are based on a Hobbesian concept of an 'absence of external impediments to motion', and they foster the typical American 'dream' triad of car/home/television, perhaps the clearest example of these related freedom goals.[10] Home ownership is a suburb, the car to travel from this location to the work that enables the repayment of the long-term mortgage to which each individual family is committed, and the television that provides the basic entertainment, while it reinforces these same values, even as it promotes even more consumerism.

The parameters of one's personhood are circumscribed by what one owns and consumes. Albritton says:

> *Such externalized or hollow selves are lacking the qualitative materiality that goes into what we normally call 'character'. As legal persons they are caught in a world of economic calculation, where the direction that wills take are determined purely by short term quantitavitive forms of calculation.*[11]

Thus, if 'for legal subjects consumption is crucial to identity formation',[12] then even to suggest a communitarian agenda based on principles of respect for human rights, including the right to health, and 'ecological rights',[13] represents an attack on US/consumer identity.

The clearest conflict is perhaps between individualism and public interest, where the latter is properly understood to encompass the life and health of present and future generations. But the supposed 'conflict' is, in fact, nonexistent when the science that supports these paradigms is properly understood.[14] Even a wealthy, productive society is totally dependent on a healthy environment for its very existence, and this is true at a number of levels.

Human health, especially that of the most vulnerable – children – is acknowledged to be at risk from a wide variety of exposures, not only in occupational settings, but also in homes and elsewhere. Examples include routinely used household products such as solvents in all their applications;[15] pesticides including herbicides, and other substances whose effects are so varied, so terrible that not only the WHO devotes much of its research to these effects (Tamburlini et al, 2002), but they are even described as 'weapons of war', because they can be so used.[16]

Of course wars and armed conflicts provide an additional rich source of environ-mental health hazards, including the spraying of herbicides connected with the narcotics trade:

> *many Colombian farmers in sprayed areas report significant skin problems, headaches, vomiting, miscarriages and deaths of small children, effects they attribute to the spray-ing. Residents of the sprayed areas are not told when the spraying will occur for security reasons, so they cannot take any steps to protect themselves, their families, their crops or their livestock.*[17]

As most wars and armed conflicts are carried on for reasons where trade interests are prominently featured, this aspect on 'consumerism' is also relevant. In addition, industrial pollution is endemic to any war situation. In the 1991 Gulf War, more than 600 oil wells were set afire by Iraqi soldiers, and the toxic components of these oil fires 'include polycyclic aromatic hydrocarbons (PAHs), metals, sulphur and lead'.[18] The health effects of these exposures include 'cancer ... asthmas ... airway inflammation ...

and high blood pressure and kidney damage (from lead).[19] During the Kosovo offensive (1999), both NATO and US planes bombed industrial complexes, including those at Pancevo, near Belgrade, and the 'joint UNEP/UN Centre for Human Settlements Balkan Task Force,' 'found extreme pollution in the area, including ethylene dichloride and mercury, (causing neuro-logical and developmental damage), and large quantities of vinyl chloride monomer, dioxic, carbon monoxide and polycyclic aromatic hydro-carbons'.[20]

These effects are worsened by the fact that these conflicts do not occur in some pre-designated battlefield, but happen close to areas that include human habitation, industrial complexes and factories. Hence their effects can be compared to the 'ecoviolence' I described in situations where environmental racism is an issue. Although the latter occurs routinely in peacetime,[21,22] many of the same industrial substances affect not only people of colour in North America, or in the developing world, but they do so in ways that closely parallel the attacks on the 'enemy' of the West, from Iraq to Serbia. Thus my argument that the conditions that apply to just wars should, a fortiori apply to these attacks on peaceful citizens (non-combatants), whose only 'flaw' is to be poor, or to belong to an ethnic or racial minority that is more easily targeted by corporate 'free' enterprise.[23,24]

The research of the WHO, cited in Chapter 1, explains and documents the harm-ful role of pesticides, herbicides and fungicides in food production, distribution and storage. In addition, Albritton draws out the systemic similarities between food production, including its promotion, and consumerism in general:

> *Food production and consumption in the US has only gradually been transformed from petty commodity production to a highly concentrated form of capitalist industrial production. It is my belief that it is only in recent years after capitalism has almost totally subsumed food production and consumption, that we are learning the painful truth that the prominence of use-value considerations in the food industry make it ill adapted to capitalist production and consumption. It follows that my focus on the food system is meant to draw out some of the deep contradictions (serious degrading of human beings and the environment) of the current conjuncture of capitalism.*[25]

Much of my work and that of the Global Ecological Integrity Project has shown that human health and integrity are intimately connected and the WHO has confirmed the connection in 1999.[26] Albritton also connects 'human health and ecology'[27] Food is related to normal human function in many ways, ranging from malnutrition and starvation – which claims over 33,000 children's lives each year, according to Food and Agriculture Organization (FAO) statistics, with neither fanfare nor emphasis in the media[28] – to Western man's diseases, including overeating, obesity and their consequences, and we will return to these issues below, in relation to advertising and marketing.

It is noteworthy that many tobacco companies have turned from one highly lucrative addictive business to another: the food business, as fat is gradually replacing tobacco as the main killer in the North:

> *Corporate concentrations in the global food industry is increasing rapidly. Big Tobacco, traditionally one of the most profitable industries, has bought heavily into the food*

industry to protect themselves from tobacco liability suits. Now Philip Morris is among the top three food producers in the world, but alas obesity has now become a greater threat to health than tobacco, and they may in the future face obesity liability suits.[29]

Albritton's analysis helps to connect the many implications of the injustices perpetrated by the Northwestern ecological footprint.[30] It connects capitalist supported consumerism to the hazards of (a) the spread of capitalist supported practices and trade, including the trade of toxic waste; (b) the elimination of natural resources that provide 'nature's services',[31] and hence support health and normal function; (c) the regular transformation of health enhancing natural materials, into health-threatening wastes; and (d) the injustice of obesity and the consequent westerners' diseases (diabetes, heart conditions, many cancers), juxtaposed through the same industrial food production, to the diseases endemic to this form of industrial activity in developing countries (Bhopal comes to mind in this respect), and the accompanying hunger famines and lack of clean water suffered by these countries' populations.

ATTACKS ON THE HEALTH AND NORMAL FUNCTION OF THE CHILD: THE ROLE OF MARKETING AND THE MEDIA

Throughout the world cultural, social and economic transformation patterns are now driven by communication technology. Institutional restructuring responses occurring as a result, are dominated almost entirely by the dictates of the marketplace.[32]

There is a misguided vision that equates Western democracy with the primacy of liberty for all legal subjects, and it may be viewed as one of the sources of the hazards to human health and normal function to which children are exposed. But to view liberty as primary without considering the context of its exercise and the consequences that ensue may be wrong for those who can make decisions that affect society. The responsibility of that power is to consider and weigh the legitimate interests of those affected by their policy decisions.

Powerful private organizations such as chemical industries, for instance, do not have the explicit mandate to protect the citizens of their own and other countries, whereas domestic, international and supranational legal institutions do. The role of governments is to protect citizens (see Chapter 1). They also have the related task 'of supervising the activities of all persons and organizations within [their] jurisdiction and seeing to it that they all conform to certain appropriate standards of behaviour'.[33]

Hence the importance of turning to a consideration of political institutions and especially the use within these of the complex concept of freedom. Some have argued that not freedom, but the rights to which it is instrumental is most important.[34] When it is so understood, 'equality' has an important part to play in 'freedom', and so does the concept of a free market. If we accept the primacy of freedom as a simple concept, we may not see the role it plays in the promotion of certain policies and activities; as 'it does not tell us anything about which freedoms are important and which are not, and why'.[35]

It seems clear that 'there is no value-neutral definition of liberty; none that is, which is of any interest for moral and political thought'.[36] Thus the main flaw of the 'simple principle' of liberty, is at the heart of the problems inherent in present policies of neo-liberal Western states, and their support of the doctrine of 'limited government'. John Rawls' work on justice emphasizes procedural fairness at the expense of any substantive understanding of a common good, such that it might be used to qualify and specify which 'freedom' represents a desirable advance for a society, and which represents a regressive, harmful practice instead, even an attack on human rights.[37]

Neutrality in the face of human rights breaches is not desirable or even tolerable: it gives rise to such grave harms as the genocide in Rwanda, crimes against humanity in Serbia or Nazi Germany. It also promotes, as I have suggested, the rise of ecoviolence in the world: crimes committed through environmental conditions, affecting especially the most vulnerable, the poor, minorities, and our own subject, children. Viewing people as ends in themselves, as the Kantian imperative dictates, radically excludes the possibility of accepting the 'laissez faire' approach with regard to human rights, that is clearly present in Rawlsian neutrality.[38]

Nowhere is the deleterious effect of 'freedom' in its simplest sense and of neutrality more clear than in the role that media plays in children's health. Albritton noted the pivotal role of television in fostering the goals of capitalism, as part of the 'triad' including also 'house and automobile'. Its effect and those of other commercial exploitations of children such as video games and violent movies, are multiple and remarkable, as they range from promoting direct harms (advertising foods high in fats and sugars, at the expense of healthier food choices); advertising toys and computer games that may be chemically hazardous in their composition, but also intellectually hazardous and demeaning as they take time away from both physical exercise, and from reading and artistic creativity, on the other.[39] The prevalence of violence in all forms of so-called entertainment for children, both in video games and television, also has grave effects on the mind of children who become accustomed to senseless violence as 'normal' and acceptable, part of modern culture,[40] but, in addition, as they suffer physical reactions to the violence that are hazardous to their health.[41]

The addiction to unhealthy fast food starts early in life, as children's programmes depend on the marketing dollars of fast food producers, so that even older babies are able to identify certain foods, but also certain brands, advertisements or jingles. The logic of the market does not respect even the innocence and vulnerability of early childhood, as 'our economy became hooked on mass consumption'.

> *The logic is simple. As we become more and more productive, more and more things were produced. What is produced must be sold that is the essential requirement.*[42]

The requirements (a) to produce requires the further necessity, (b) to sell. This imperative respects nothing beyond the achievement of its goal, so that everyone becomes a fair target: children demand a certain product not because they are 'free' and make 'choices'. They do so because they have been manipulated to view the products offered as utterly desirable, even indispensable, and these beliefs are communicated to parents and other adults, who are equally victims of market strategies that exclude reflective, rational choices. Advertising admits its goal of 'conquering' to sell. Speaking of the Coca-Cola Company, Alan Durning relates:

> Adweek, *a trade journal, was so impressed with the brand's success that it praised Coke's mastery of global marketing with a two-page spread depicting Hitler, Lenin and Napoleon and a coke bottle. 'Only one' read the caption, 'launched a campaign that conquered the world'.*[43]

The 'freedom' of a corporate enterprise here is described as 'conquering' those who are persuaded to use their product, and are admittedly, as unfree as those who lived under the rule of tyrants.

Nor is corporate power daunted by the all-inclusive numbers of those who have been 'conquered': children are targeted as well as adults, and the same holds true for other unhealthy products beyond Coca-Cola, from McDonald's fast food empire, to highly sweetened cereals and candies. Hence the harm to children's health through consumerism goes beyond exposure to industrial and household chemicals (see Chapter 1) or even food products. As noted, exposure to violence through computer games or television programmes is also, largely, unchecked.

Harm to children through all the avenues to which we have alluded is part and parcel of a paradigm of consumerism, as the *sine qua non* of capitalism. Christine Harold, speaking of US capitalism, says:

> *At least since the 1920s, when Ford style assembly line manufacturing made it possible to mass produce consumer goods, armies of advertisers have been producing something more important than commodities, consumers. Consumers aren't born, they are made. And American culture is the Mercedes-Benz of consumer-makers.*[44]

Given that not only in the US, but also generally in North America, children are not protected from the barrage of 'over 3000 commercial messages a day'[45] through the media, representing unrelenting capitalist propaganda, it is important to consider whether there might be any other approach to public policy, more conducive to some measure of the protection children are entitled to receive.

In the previous chapters we noted the importance of public policy to society, even in case law and the related judiciary decisions. In the next section we will consider another approach: one that is not exclusively devoted to the pursuit and the support of consumerism. The European Union's policies, while not perfect, merit being seriously considered because of the difference between them and the entrenched policies of North America.

THE 'EUROPEAN DREAM' AND
THE IMPACT OF PUBLIC POLICY

The long paragraph at the start of the introductory section of this chapter shows the importance of the emerging supranational power of the European Union, and the presence there of a 'community public policy'.[46] *Ordre Public* is neither an obvious nor a simple concept, and it needs careful interpretation:

> *The problem of interpretation derives from the terminology. In Latin countries it is used to refer to a single notion,* ordre public, ordine pubblico, orden publico, *without distinguishing the possible nuances that a single term may incorporate. On the contrary, Saxon countries tend to differentiate between* ordre public, *and public policy, or* offentliche Ordnung, *according to the (private or public) legal sphere where it is involved.*[47]

Public order appears to have a more coercive, specific meaning than public policy, as it resonates, for instance in both Canadian and international law. In the case of forceful protests against G8/WTO meetings, from Seattle to Quebec City, from Geneva to Genova, riot policy or even the army may be called upon to maintain or restore the 'public order', without any explicit 'public policy' mandate, although that mandate may well be implicitly present. It is one of the themes of this work that characterizes that mandate: nothing must impede the unfolding of 'business as usual' and the march of Western hegemonic powerful institutions, not even the democratic expression of millions of citizens' 'anti-hegemonic' ideals.[48] In this sense it can be defined as a 'legal good directly protected by specific rules within a system, namely, public security, administrative rules and criminal law'.[49]

In contrast, 'public policy' entails an explicit mandate, clearly articulated in the instruments of a state, but also in those of supranational agencies such as the United Nations, the WHO and the European Union. Moral, economic and political values in the European Union:

> *are a reflection of the functions traditionally attributed to public policy, namely (1) the elimination of foreign law which offends 'natural' law, (2) the defence of the principles that are at the basis of a legal system and (3) the safeguarding of the legislative policies it pursues.*[50]

Public policy fulfils both a positive and a negative function: for the former, it is intended to inspire and direct the regulations of the system; for the latter, in the sense of exclusion, it helps to crystallize whatever might be foreign or incompatible with the vision it intends to implement. This is equally true of international law, and the values and principles it embraces:

> *The latter [international public policy] defines this public policy as a normative one, referring to the ideal system of values which inspires the whole legal order.*[51]

The importance of this distinction cannot be overemphasized: we noted in our analysis of cases that, not only regulatory regimes and instruments were cited, but that public policy was often an integral part of judicial decisions. Hence speaking of the community public policy in the European Community, Rodriguez-Pineau says:

> *The Rome Treaty made a reference to public policy in a specific Community sense, namely as an exception clause to Community freedoms, envisioned in Articles 36,*

48, 56 and 73 of the EC Treaty... Member States may invoke public policy in order to protect the interests of a democratic society[52] while they respect the principle of non-discrimination and the proportionality test.[53]

Thus, as the case law indicates, not only does the European Community benefit from an *acquis communautaire*, but it bases its jurisprudence on an *ordre public communautaire*, which imposes the limits required by the public interest to the exercise of fundamental rights.[54]

The direction each country's laws are taking and the accepted understanding of any European nation's public policy are limited and informed by the community's public policy mandates. Thus it is insufficient to look at the specifics of national/domestic legal instruments, unless the supranational directives are fully appreciated and acknowledged.

The impact of the general public policy climate everywhere interfaces in various ways with the possibility of establishing the rights of children to health and the environment, therefore, equally, the rights of future generations. If environmental health is a 'basic human right' as many have argued including the author,[55] then that right ought to be enshrined in all legal systems and in public policy, for children as well as adults.

If the health of the child is not only determined by conditions and exposures after birth, and by her genetic background, but also and most significantly by all her pre-birth exposures, then the protection of this basic human right should form an integral part of public policy. I have argued that ecoviolence represents a crime against humanity.[56] I have also proposed that, as Rifkin suggests in regard to the 'American Dream', the European dream, better understood as vision, or even public policy ideal, and which may well be the best hope for a blueprint for a world government that is capable of dealing appropriately with crimes against humanity.

Utilitarian Peter Singer reaches a similar conclusion as well. In a recent paper on 'How can we prevent crimes against humanity', he describes a 'distant vision' of a worthwhile world:

> *This world would be one in which the United Nations functions more like the way in which the European Union functions today, but with significant differences due to the fact that it is a global, not regional organization.[57]*

PUBLIC POLICY AND THE 'SOCIAL CONSTRUCT OF CHILDHOOD'

We have been considering the definition of the child, or what a child is understood to be, according to various legal systems and in the language of several judicial decisions. Perhaps we should have discussed this important question at the beginning of this work. But as we acknowledged that this understanding and even those definitions are heavily influenced by social policy, perhaps this is the appropriate time and place for this discussion.

Children are the living message we send to a time we will not see. From a biological point of view it is inconceivable that any culture will forget that it needs to reproduce itself. But it is quite possible for a culture to exist without a social idea of children.... childhood is a social artifact, not a biological category.[58]

This passage raises some serious questions and offers some answers to the problems we have encountered in this work. As the biological understanding of the child recedes, and is almost entirely taken over by the social 'artifact' definition, the vitally important differences between adult and child in the biological sense that the WHO has amply demonstrated (see Chapter 1) lose in significance and relevance.

Because neo-liberal social theory is intent upon disclaiming the traditional view of the child (as 'relational', or part of family, for instance), as it is contrasted instead with the existence of non-nuclear, non-traditional, or extended families,[59] its perspective lists other categories such as legitimate or illegitimate children or adopted, or fostered children, children viewed as 'legal subjects' as well as 'legal objects', in order to show how these categories, most of which seriously affect the life of children, are extraneous to what a child is, and simply reflect social conditions related to the adults with whom they interact.

Yet in their concern to free the child from these inappropriate and sometimes harmful categories, they ignore the most important aspect of childhood: the inherently unique biological existence of the child, and this neglect has grave implications for the protection of the health and normal function of the child, as we have shown. For instance, the 'social construct' theory is relevant for the 'end of childhood' aspect of the problem. Young women may be given the right to contraception and, failing that, to abortion at an increasingly early age. Their 'freedom' to pursue any course of action they prefer is also not to be restrained for any reason, including the possibility of serious harms to the unborn, including such practices as the use of tobacco and other drugs as well as alcohol.

Of course it is equally true that if childhood is a construct, then the routine affirmation that a child is not a 'human being' or a 'person' until after birth is also equally a construct, and it ought not to be affirmed as though it were an obvious, indisputable 'truth'. The emergence of concerns about the status of embryos and in general the unborn, in current technologically enhanced practices, is already debating these issues in the law.[60]

So far we have assumed and used a purely biological understanding of the child, based upon the research of the World Health Organization. Yet even the recognized presence of overwhelming scientific evidence about the continuity of development, hence of exposure to harm, from the preborn to the born child, has run aground when confronted with immovable social policy blocks, intent upon denying this continuity in order to protect the freedom of women, whether wanting to abort or to continue their preferred activities during pregnancy. It is noteworthy that the emphasis on freedom in the sense of negative rights to the lack of restraints, is equally applicable to corporate legal persons, as it permits them to continue their hazardous activities unabated. I am not suggesting that this might be an intentional alliance, but the thrust to individualism and the pursuit of private preferences without a countervailing consideration of either the public interest or moral principles, is equally present in both areas.

Of course the further question of the real meaning of 'public interest' is one of the problems we face, as it is often defined in purely in economic terms, especially in North America.[61,62] Appeals to the public interest become completely counter productive when so understood, because, as we noted, the thrust of the argument of this work shows that the public interest is, in fact, most often in conflict with economic considerations.

In contrast, in 'A lawman's view of the public interest', Julius Cohen argues that, in the law, the phrase has a dual sense, neither of which reflects economic considerations:

> *first, in a logical sense, i.e. to explicate the meaning of the established values of the community... Second, it is used in an instrumental sense, i.e. that a policy would be in the public interest if its consequences would implement one or more of the established basic values of the community.*[63]

Cohen's argument dismisses the sole reliance on economics as a measure of the public interest, as he states, 'Our values have a qualitative as well as quantitative dimension'.[64] He is speaking of such values as 'ideals of human well-being', and 'fundamental methods for achieving them',[65] hence we are once again in the realm of the sort of principled 'public policy' that we saw described, for instance, by Jeremy Rifkin, in relation to the European Union.

For children, public policy and – one hopes – the public interest in the non-economic sense were very much in the forefront when the *Convention on the Rights of the Child* (CRC) was drafted and ratified by most countries (with the notable exception of the US). Part I, Article 1, for instance, defines the end, but not the beginning of childhood, as a compromise between setting the beginning at conception, as the Holy See and other countries would have wanted, and the objection of many other states:

> *Article 1. For the purposes of the present Convention, a child means every human being below the age of eighteen years unless the law applicable to the child's majority is attained earlier.*

Part of the compromise was the suggestion by Sweden that the concern with pre-birth protection be placed, at least, in the Preamble:

> *Bearing in mind that, as indicated in the Declaration of the Rights of the Child, the child by reason of his physical and mental immaturity, needs special safeguards and care, including appropriate legal protection, before as well as after birth.*

Thus the same obstacles to the right of the child to health, normal function and the environment that was in evidence through the use of legal instruments in both civil and common law cases, that is, the 'public policy' concerns we have encountered throughout our research, are based in part on the 'social construction of childhood'.

It is not science, not biology, but neo-liberal social tenets that decree that a change of location is required for a child to acquire any rights, and even to be able to enjoy a possible inheritance or honorific rights that, though present after conception, become effective only after a live birth. Thus, although:

Every child has the right to grow in an environment which is supportive of their health and well-being this right is not stipulated in any specific provision of the Convention on the Rights of the Child, the most widely ratified human rights treaty, in fact such an explicit right is conspicuously absent.[66]

In contrast to this lack, Harry Post, after a detailed review of the right of the child to a clean environment in EU law, concludes that, as we have also argued, Europe seems to be a more fertile ground for appropriately protective child's rights than other countries and continents. He says that Europe is even superior in this regard to the regimes already present in international law. Other international regimes are not 'even remotely comparable to the EC in terms of effective rights of the child to a clean environment. These rights are to a great extent ready to be claimed'.[67]

THE *PARENS PATRIAE* DOCTRINE: A POSSIBLE JURIDICAL POLICY?

In the previous section, the role of social policy in the respective countries and legal systems were shown to be, on the whole, largely indifferent to the plight of the unborn and the possibility of ascribing any rights to her. Much of this indifference was ascribed to the individualism and consumerism endemic to the capitalist global enterprise: capitalism is inherently unsustainable as are its 'abstract calculations'. Richard Westra argues:

because value augmentation is an abstract quantitative goal, we can say that a most fundamental level capital, with its commodity economic material outcomes, is destined to conflict with concrete-qualitative human goals to the extent that the latter necessitate respect for the earth and the life-world within which a long-term human existence must be embedded.[68]

The argument of this work is that indifference to children's ecological human rights, rights to health and normal function, implies also indifference to the health (and survival) of future generations beyond the first. That is precisely the 'long-term human existence' referred to above. For the most part, governmental instruments that ought to protect children and prevent harm, do not do so, and we have speculated on the social convictions and public policy trends that prevent the development of more protective laws, such that would truly serve to protect the 'best interests of the child'.

In contrast, there is a history of protective jurisprudence, dating back as far as the Middle Ages. In its most recent instantiations, the *parens patriae* doctrine has been used to support judicial decisions that deal with the protection of those who cannot speak for themselves, especially in the case of health issues.[69]

The language of these judgements is extremely suggestive and well worthy of attentive study. But before turning to the cases, it might best to review briefly the history of the doctrine. The doctrine of *parens patriae*, despite its Roman name, is entirely a common law doctrine, and while the Canadian Supreme Court makes use of it, it does not exist in Quebec law.[70,71] It is perhaps an anomaly that a doctrine with a Roman name and origin is presently only found in the common law, as Morin indicates in his description of the doctrine's historical background.[72]

Until 1873 a fundamental dichotomy prevailed in Britain's legal system. From the Middle Ages, royal tribunals used the 'communeley', but the great majority of cases were heard by the lords and the local courts. Only rarely did the King, as 'fountain of justice' participate in decisions of the courts through the person of his Chancellor, who until the 16th century was, at the same time, the King's confessor, hence perhaps the use of the Latin phrase.[73]

The Chancellor's aim was the promotion and the triumph of equity principles, learned in his study of Roman law. The rules guiding these judgements and their results eventually became codified, hence 'precedent' was born.[74] The doctrine was used for custody and guardianship matters involving the relation between the lord and a minor, perhaps one whose father might have been a tenant of the lord before his death, so that guardianship was required until such time as the child could be recognized as a tenant in his stead, at age fourteen.

Eventually the 'Court of Wards and Liveries' was instituted by Parliament, after 1540,[75] and this court remained in operation for some time. The concept of royal protection was substituted in the 15th century by a Court of Chancery, which kept the concept of wardship alive, and was able to introduce a novel move by 1792, when it forbade a violent father to interrupt his son's schooling and continue with his guardianship.[76]

Although the Court of Wards was abolished, the concept of 'wardship' remained as an aspect of its *parens patriae* jurisdiction:

> *In time wardship became substantively and procedurally assimilated to the* parens patriae *jurisdiction, lost its connection with property, and became purely protective in nature.*[77]

The inception of the use of the doctrine thus explains both its Latin roots and its evolution from the protection of a minor's economic interests, to the protection of children's interests, simpliciter. Without any further effort to trace its antecedents, we will now turn to its development use, in order to see whether its development renders the doctrine applicable to the protection of children that we have been advocating in this work. The classic statement of the modern principles that govern state intervention in the best interests of the child, can be found in Rand, J's judgement:

> *The view of the child's welfare conceives it to lie, first, within the warmth and secur-ity of the home provided by his parents; when through a failure with or without parental fault, to furnish that protection, that welfare is threatened, the community, represented by the Sovereign, is, on the broadest social and national grounds justified in displacing the parents and assuming their duties. This in substance, is the rule of law established for centuries and in the light of which the common law Courts and the Court of Chancery, following their differing rules, dealt with custody.*[78]

La Forest, J. ties recent cases to their British background:

> *It will be obvious from these provisions that the Supreme Court of Prince Edward Island has the same* Parens Patriae *jurisdiction as was vested in the Lord Chancellor in England and exercised by the Court of Chancery there.*[79]

A further point worthy of note is the increasingly wide reach of the doctrine, giving the courts the ability to protect children from injury. In Re X (a minor),[80] Latey, J. cited,

> *a passage from Chambers on Infancy (1842), p.20 that indicates that protection may be accorded against prospective as well/as present harms.*[81]

With this statement we come a lot closer to the possibility of protecting children's health, in the sense we have been seeking to find explicitly, in legislation, without much success. If 'prospective harm' is explicitly a part of the *parens patriae* doctrine, then it is not only a juridical tool to be used after some crime has been committed or to prevent some obvious injustice. It could instead be especially powerful when there is an unconsented medical treatment at issue, as there it can be used 'to prevent ... damage being done'. A similar approach exists in the US.[82] In another American case, *Matter of Sallmeier*,[83] the Court said:

> *The jurisdiction of the Court in this proceeding arises not by statute, but from the common law jurisdiction of the Supreme Court to act as* parens patriae *with respect to* **incompetents**.[84] [emphasis added]

Essentially there are two possible approaches included in the doctrine the 'best interest' approach, and the 'substituted judgement' approach.[85] What is relevant from our point of view, is the fact that neither approach needs a 'person', in order to protect. In fact *parens patriae* only comes into effect when the rights of the individual needing to be protected are not those of a 'person', able to think and decide or even to protect her own interests. The classic locus for this approach is the case of the unborn[86] a case to which we alluded briefly in Chapter 3. It is worth revisiting the case, so that its policy position may best be appreciated at this time.

Winnipeg Child and Family Services (Northwest Area) v. D.F.G. [1997] 3 S.C.R. 925 – Revisited

> *Best Interests of the Child*
> *(3) Where a person is directed in this part to make an order or determination in the best interests of the child, this person shall take into consideration those of the following circumstances of the case that he or she considers relevant:*
>
> 1 *The child's physical and emotional needs, and the appropriate care or treatment to meet those needs.*
> 2 *The child's physical, mental and emotional level of development.*

3   *The child's cultural background.*

4   *The religious faith, if any, in which the child is being raised.*

5   *The importance for the child's development of a positive relationship with a parent and a secure place as a member of a family.*

6   *The child's relationship by blood or through an adoption order.*

7   *The importance of continuity in the child's care and the possible effect on the child of the disruption of that continuity.*

8   *The merits of a plan for the child's care proposed by a society, including a proposal that the child be placed for adoption or adopted, compared with the merits of the child remaining with or returning to a parent.*

9   *The child's views and wishes, if they can reasonably be ascertained.*

10   *The effects on the child of delay in the disposition of the case.*

11   *The risk that the child may suffer harm through being removed from, kept away from, returned to or allowed to remain in the care of a parent.*

12   *The degree of risk, if any, that justified the finding that the child is in need of protection.*

13   *Any other relevant circumstance.*[87]

Most of these points of consideration are psychological or social in tone, and perhaps these directives helped to influence social worker to leave children in physically hazardous circumstances, as we saw in recent cases in Canada. My emphasis, in contrast is on physical hazards and harms, as I believe that, on balance, these ought to be primary in any consideration of the rights of the child to protection and her best interests. Perhaps these thirteen points ought to be prioritized in some way, so that the child's continued existence and health is protected before cultural and social considerations enter the decision-making process.

At any rate, the case under consideration involved the possible forcible detention of a pregnant woman addicted to glue sniffing and unwilling to undergo an abortion. She was already the mother of two mentally challenged children, presently wards of family services (see Chapter 3). But, as McLachlin, J. affirmed:

> *Ultimately, however, as the Alberta Court of Appeal recently observed in* T. v. Alberta *(Director of Child Welfare) (2000), 188 D.L.R. (4th) 603, at para. 14), child legislation is about protecting children from harm; it is a child welfare statute and not a parents' rights statute.*[88]

The *Winnipeg v. D.F.G.* case, the topic of this section, has McLachlin, J. use, inter alia, a 'slippery slope' argument, citing Balcombe, LJ:

> *If a pregnant woman was to be subject to controls for the benefit of her unborn child, Parliament should so legislate, as it had in the case of mentally incompetent persons...(at para.53).*

Adding, 'taking it to the extreme were the Court to be faced with saving the baby's life or the mother's it would surely have to protect the baby's'.[89]

Her reasoning led McLachlin, J. to say (at para. 57), 'I conclude that the law of *parens patriae* does not support the order for the detention of the respondent.'

In contrast, Major, J. delivered the reasons for his and Sopinka's dissent, starting with highlighting the most important questions faced within this case:

> *There are three questions that arise in this appeal. What are the rights of the pregnant woman? Does the unborn fetus have independent rights? Does the State have a separate right to intervene to prescribe proper medical treatment in the hope of achieving the birth of a healthy child; as opposed to standing idly by and watching the birth of a permanently and seriously handicapped child who has no future other than as a permanent ward of the state? (at para.63).*

Major, J. also notes that:

> *Historically, it was thought that damage suffered by a fetus could only be assigned if the child was born alive... The logic for that rule has disappeared with modern medical progress. Today by the use of ultrasound and other advanced techniques, the sex and health of a fetus can be determined and monitored from a short time after conception. The sophisticated surgical procedures performed on the fetus before birth further belies the need for the 'born alive' principle (at para.67).*

We noted earlier (Chapters 2 and 3), that the 'born alive' rule is an anachronism, as it is 'a common law evidentiary presumption', rather than the statement presently taken as self-evident truth, that there is no one, before birth, who could be the subject of rights. Although the exercise of the *parens patriae* jurisdiction appears to be unlimited,[90] its use must be limited in some sense: it must only be exercised for the benefit of the 'person' involved.

But 'personhood' entails the presence of a complex number of characteristics, including the ability to think, entertain abstract concepts, to determine one's own course of action, to represent one's own interests. This is not a logical position: even the 'born alive' foetus will not possess these characteristics for some time. Some argue that the characteristics that denote personhood will not be acquired until at least age seven or even much later. In addition, most mentally challenged persons may never be able to meet that standard of mental competence.

Hence it appears that the application of the *parens patriae* doctrine excludes a priori its application to those who can be considered full persons. Thus, even to require that a foetus be born alive, does not guarantee that a 'person' will emerge, who therefore will have rights like other human persons. The 'born alive' rule should be eliminated from legal consideration. As Oliver Wendell Holmes has it:

> *It is revolting to have no better reason for a rule of law that that it was laid down in the time of Henry IV. It is still more revolting if the grounds upon which it was laid down have vanished long since, and the rule simply persists from blind imitation of the past.*[91]

Therefore, the *parens patriae* doctrine denotes a remarkably modern trend as a possible policy for the protection of children's life and health, for several reasons, despite the fact that no actual covenant exists to codify it into international law, nor does a domestic law act in common law support it explicitly. Its importance lies in its distrust of unproven and anachronistic historical standards, its wide range of applications and most important of all, its main focus is on those who cannot speak for themselves.

It would be highly desirable to empower a Law Commission to study the doctrine in all its possible policy applications and, in the next chapter, we might want to keep the doctrine in mind as we turn to a consideration of future generations' rights in the general sense of the concept, thus beyond the difficulties raised by the rights of the first generation discussed so far. In the next section a related issue will also be discussed: the transmission of HIV/AIDS.

PRENATAL TRANSFER OF HIV/AIDS: IS CRIMINALIZATION THE ANSWER?

In the previous section we focused on one aspect of a pregnant woman's possible responsibility for inflicting foetal harms, and we questioned the status of the preborn in that respect. The Winnipeg case discussed above was decided in favour of the free choice of the pregnant woman addicted to glue sniffing, who had already given birth to two children so damaged by her habit as to need permanent institutionalization. In that case, existing instruments and jurisprudence led McLachlin, J. to conclude 'that the law of *parens patriae* does not support the order for the detention of the respondent'.[92]

In contrast, those who knowingly but without the intent to cause the disease, transmit AIDS are, increasingly, not viewed in such a benign light by the courts. In 1987, ten years after the existence of HIV/AIDS made itself known, President Ronald Reagan of the US created 'The Presidential Commission on the Human Immunodeficiency Virus Epidemic'.[93] After one year and over 40 hearings, the Presidential Commission recommended that:

> *HIV infected individuals who knowingly conduct themselves in ways to pose significant risk of transmission to others, must be held accountable for their actions.*

By 1992, ten US States had enacted legislation 'criminalizing the transfer of AIDS or the HIV infection through sexual contact or the transfer of infected body fluids, blood or tissue'.[94] Children who are infected are totally vulnerable as they have no way of having information, protecting themselves or, obviously, consenting. In 1992 it was found that 87 per cent of such children are born to women infected with or at risk of HIV infection.[95]

> *Children so infected die within three to nine years of birth, ... and will be forced to endure extensive hospitalization during their brief lives.*[96]

In 1993, 87 per cent of HIV-infected children had the virus transmitted to them by their mother.[97] Today, with better blood transfusion controls, almost 100 per cent of HIV-positive children become ill in the same manner, because that is the most common form of transmission.[98]

Therefore, we must return to the difficult questions discussed in the first four chapters of this work: what, if any, are the rights of the unborn child. On this topic, as we saw, there are far more problems than solutions:

> *Recently courts and commentators have increasingly recognized the rights of the unborn child, limiting the liberty of the mother in order to safeguard the health of the child she carries. The New Jersey Supreme Court went so far as to declare that 'justice requires that the principle should be recognized that a child has a legal right to begin life with a sound mind and body'*[99]

But is tort law the appropriate remedy for an action the result of which is an incurable disease? Criminal law may provide a better fit, especially when, even lacking the requisite *mens rea*, it could be established that 'the mother knew with substantive certainty that her conduct would transfer the antibodies to her child'.[100]

However, this approach may fail when the mother is unaware of her disease at the time when she becomes pregnant. In contrast, any woman who has engaged in risky behaviour that may have resulted in her own infection, surely has at least the moral obligation to be tested before engaging in further activities that may lead to a pregnancy. Once she is aware of her own infectious status, then, although her behaviour may not bring her to the attention of the courts at the time, any act that results in a pregnancy should be treated in the same way as that of any other individual infecting other unsuspecting and unconsenting individuals.

As noted in *Roe v. Wade,*[101] and the highly liberal interpretation of that case that has broadened its reach over the years, the right to privacy of the woman supersedes any right of the foetus during the first trimester of pregnancy; for the second trimester individual states are allowed to make their own determinations 'to safeguard the health of the mother'. After viability, however, abortions should be permitted only 'to protect the mother's life'. The liberalization of this decision's laws has been adopted and repeated not only in US common law, but also in civil and international law.

The general trend in legislation has become, increasingly, that of not putting obstacles in the path of a woman's choice, rather than that of protecting life.[102] In contrast, in *Webster v. Reproductive Health Services,*[103] the Preamble to the Missouri Code[104] was used to regulate and specify the rights of unborn children, but only as applicable to tort and probate law:

> *the laws of this state shall be interpreted and construed to acknowledge on behalf of the unborn child at every stage of development, all the rights, privileges, and immunities available to other persons, citizens and residents of this state, subject only to the Constitution of the United States, and the decisional interpretations thereof by the United States Supreme Court ...*

But courts only have the say in specific cases, and after a specific event takes place, hence there is – admittedly – a need for criminal legislation to deter and clearly set limits to allowable conduct, even including the police power of the state.[105]

> *Traditional criminal law may prove to be an ineffective and inappropriate means of deterring the type of culpable conduct, responsible for transmission of the AIDS virus.*

> *Yet the aims and goals of HIV transmission legislation are arguably the same as the aims and goals of the more traditional criminal laws: to punish individuals who engage in prohibited behaviour; deter and prevent dangerous and risky behaviours; and provide social means of education regarding the norms of acceptable social behaviour.*[106]

The consequences of exposure constitute a clear danger to the public and an Indiana Statute[107] for instance, refers specifically to 'Transferring contaminated body fluids', as it provides that a woman who 'knowing or intentionally transfers such fluids (including blood), commits a Class C felony. If the child is then born and tests positive for HIV, the woman may be guilty of a Class A felony.[108] The transmission of infected fluids may be parental, that is, taking place during the pregnancy, as transmitted through the placenta, a thin organ capable of absorbing nutritive substances, but also harmful ones, such as viruses through the blood.[109]

Other states, such as Idaho,[110] and Arkansas[111] have similar provisions that criminalize the acts of the pregnant woman with regard to the developing foetus. In the next section we shall also note that parallel legal instruments and jurisprudence also apply to alcohol and drugs used by pregnant women.[112]

But there is a basic difference between enacting laws intended to restrain behaviour that will result in harm to a developing child, and proscribing, even criminalizing, behaviour leading to reproduction. The right to procreate is indeed a basic one, as the jurisprudence of several US cases have demonstrated. Even in the case of a statute intended to sterilize habitual criminals, the court noted that '[w]e are dealing here with legislation which involves one of the basic civil rights of man – marriage and procreation are fundamental to the very existence and survival of the race'.[113,114]

The question remains, however, whether the state's interest in preventing an incurable disease from spreading supersedes another fundamental right. In *Roe v. Wade* the state needs to 'demonstrate a rational basis between the regulation and a legitimate state interest'.[115,116] The presence of a compelling state interest in the prevention of the spread of AIDS is undeniable, and even *Roe v. Wade* noted that 'as long as at least potential life is involved, the state may assert interests beyond the protection of the pregnant woman alone'.[117]

There are several cases, however, that raise doubts about the correctness of the criminalization of the pregnant woman, and debate is still ongoing about the legitimacy of testing both the pregnant woman and the newborn.[118] In 1999 a panel of the Institute of Medicine recommended that routine prenatal care should include HIV testing,[119] and explained that such testing could take four different forms:

1   mandatory;
2   routine without notification;
3   routine with notification; and
4   voluntary.[120]

The report pointed out that women may be afraid of several adverse consequences of such testing, including possible domestic violence and other social harms, as well as changes in the treatment received from medical workers, and the spread of such information in the community. These are well-founded fears but none of these, or even all of the adverse effects taken together, can possibly compare with the fatal effect of non-testing, and hence no treatment, will entail for the infant.

In effect, all the negative effects listed above may be rectified, they do not represent either legal or morally right consequences that are guaranteed to occur, and – most of all – they are not irreversible.

In contrast, if untreated, the child exposed to HIV/AIDS is receiving an almost certain death sentence, a consequence that cannot be rectified, cannot be reversed as at least 70 per cent, and today probably even more, of exposed children will be affected. Therefore, leaving the testing optional, as a choice of pregnant women, is as dangerous as permitting hazardous corporate operations to start or continue, based upon their own self-assessment, or that of in-house testing. Of course it could be said that even a law requiring no sexual activity that might possibly result in pregnancy or requiring mandatory testing may not deter someone already suffering from a terminal disease. In addition, an infected woman who did use birth control that failed might be subject to prosecution for something over which she had only limited control (given the possibility of failure of any device). But these cases are not central to the issue; Wanamaker adds:

> *Nonetheless pregnancy results from the act of engaging in consensual sexual intercourse, conduct that is voluntary. Because the AIDS/HIV epidemic presents such a serious public threat, a state may be able to impose a duty on a woman to ascertain whether she has or could have AIDS before engaging in an act that may result in pregnancy, and rightly subject her to strict liability for her failure to do so.*[121]

Thus the application of criminal law restricting a woman's right to procreate in the public interest, may be possible and desirable, as even those whose religion forbids the use of condoms, could choose to abstain from marital intercourse.

The right to intercourse or to engage in sexual activity is not a guaranteed human right, it is not entrenched either in the Canadian Charter of Rights and Freedoms, or in the American Constitution, and even a right that is so entrenched, the right to religious freedom, 'ceases where it overlaps or transgresses the rights of others'.[122,123] This is true of all public health policies that restrict the guaranteed right to freedom of association or movement, by using quarantine for diseases such as measles or tuberculosis, as we saw in Chapter 3.

Public health approaches to foetal harms?

> *Governmental responses to prenatal drug exposure have proceeded under two venues: the criminal justice system and state legislatures. The purpose of the criminal justice system is to determine whether a crime has been committed and, if so, to punish the guilty parties – not to determine the most effective policy to combat a particular social ill.*[124]

It is important to note that the 'public health' approach is contrasted with the criminal law approach in the passage cited above. But there are two basic questions that must be answered, before attempting a comparison between different approaches to alcohol and abuse during pregnancy: (1) the status of the foetus; and (2) the import of *mens rea* considerations. From the standpoint of criminal law, if a woman were to be charged with child abuse, or child endangerment, or even with delivering drugs to a minor, the preborn must be viewed as possessing personhood, or at least, to be accepted as a 'child', something that, as we saw in earlier chapters, is hard to find either in civil or common law.

In the case of drugs, we noted the Canadian case discussed earlier in this chapter, where the decision went to protect the 'freedom' of the addicted mother, not the child. In the US, many high courts have recently ruled that the foetus was not a person.[125] A possible answer to this quandary would be to test the born child while still attached to the mother by her umbilical cord after delivery, then use the toxicology screen to show that the child has been receiving narcotics from her mother in that way.[126]

Of course, even if that prosecution were to succeed, the damage would already have been done at that point. In addition, there is always the possibility of legal challenges, even at the testing stage, that is, after the fact, as we noted for HIV/AIDS transmission. In addition, for the second question, that is that of *mens rea*, the requirements for a criminal conviction are also hard to establish in cases of this nature, although knowledge is far easier to establish than the intent to harm. For instance, both Wisconsin and South Carolina held that the foetus had a right to protective custody on the part of the state, in order to ensure that it would not suffer prenatal harm, although, contrary to the decision in the *Winnipeg v. D.F.G.* case, the protection entailed placing the pregnant woman in a treatment centre. That was the decision reached by the Wisconsin courts, while for South Carolina, the ruling was for an eight-year sentence for the mother of a cocaine addicted child.[127]

In these cases, questions emerge about the legality of unconsented testing, as they did for HIV/AIDS, as well as questions about possible social/racial inequalities, as most of the women so charged are poor and are African American, and these individuals are far more likely to use state rather than private hospitals where such testing may occur. As expected, another major hurdle lies in the interference with the 'reproductive freedom' of women.[128]

Returning now to our original question, that is, either a criminalizing, hence a punitive approach, or a public health oriented one; the way the contrast is viewed is instructive in itself:

> *The legislative responses to prenatal substance abuse can be divided into two basic categories, punitive and public health oriented approaches. Punitive approaches maintain that pregnant addicts must be coerced into behaving responsibly, while public health approaches emphasize education, medical treatment and the provision of social services to pregnant addicts.*[129]

The contrast between the two approaches is viewed as starkly divergent in the law, but this contrast is only valid if one (a) views these cases (of alcohol and drug abuse) specifically as 'women's issues'; and (b) totally ignores the regulatory regimes of public health already in place in most countries. Of course only a pregnant woman can transmit HIV/AIDS, drugs or alcohol to her foetus pre-birth, and in that sense, the issue is specifically a woman's issue.

But the language used of 'giving narcotics to a minor', or 'child abuse', or 'child neglect' is, not gender specific, so that even the possibility of involuntary commitment of the woman, is thus analogous to the expected treatment of someone of either gender, for those acts. In fact, when pregnancy is not the form of administering proscribed harmful substances, a man or woman will face prison terms, not commitment to a health facility for the remaining months of a pregnancy. In fact, by such commitment, pregnant women are helped to avoid criminal prosecution to the full extent of the law. For instance, over 18 states have laws that ensure commitment to appropriate facilities before birth, but would prosecute a woman if her baby were born addicted to 'hard drugs' such as cocaine or heroin, and at least 18 state laws contain some punitive component.[130]

Civil commitment laws may also include a pregnant woman who demonstrates a 'habitual lack of self-control in the use of alcoholic beverages, controlled substance or controlled substance analogs' as is the case in Wisconsin and South Dakota.[131] Thus, it can be argued against those who view all interference with women's rights to self-determination as improper and even illegal that civil commitment is a measure that helps women avoid committing a crime, a step that is unique to their situation, given that many states treat positive toxicology screens as avoidance of abuse, neglect, or their equivalent. These states include Minnesota, Florida, Nevada, Iowa, Indiana, Oklahoma, Missouri, Virginia, and California.[132]

For instance, Wisconsin terms prenatal drug exposure 'abuse', as it requires that,

> *Because of that compelling interest in the potential life of the fetus, the court may order protective custody of the child even though such custody requires custody of the mother as well.*[133]

In contrast, a public health orientation is said to use public education campaigns, do research and offer services for pregnant addicts (and 33 US states have taken this more cost-effective position): all these approaches view 'drug addition as a disease that is best treated as a medical and psychiatric condition'.[134]

But addiction, by its very nature entails that the practice does not represent a totally autonomous decision, so that it seems clear that while efforts to educate and help might eventually be at least as useful as they have been in anti-smoking campaigns, persuasion does not often seem to work. Young women are, for the most part among the most resistant to anti-smoking campaigns today, and – although persuasion and advertising campaigns have been used everywhere, there are also necessary punitive laws, such as those forbidding smoking in public places, and heavy fines, everywhere, in order to achieve some results.

Essentially, then, the problem is reduced primarily to a social one. Any state or nation has a strong interest in preventing the spread of HIV/AIDS, and the birth of drug-addicted children and babies with foetal alcohol syndrome. Not only is there the clear obligation to protect the first and future generations from harm, but there is also the question of the significant public expense needed by children who are mentally and physically challenged beyond the possibility of a cure, and the high medical costs involved.

Hence, I believe, we might want to consider using both approaches concurrently, rather than emphasizing either one or the other. There is no reason why one gender should not be accountable for the grievous harms their practices inflict on innocents, but also on society. In fact, reaching beyond strong criminal laws, and social assistance and education programmes, I propose to also take seriously the legal instruments presently available to public health regimes, discussed in Chapter 3, on the problem of the impossibility of permitting voluntary choices to avert public threats.

Contagious childhood diseases, from rubella (where a foetal harm is also at issue) to measles, to adult contagious diseases like tuberculosis, all involve medically mandated confinements or restraints that indicate their acceptance of all these events as diseases rather than crimes, but nevertheless allow no 'extenuating circumstances', such as childhood inability to consent perhaps, or poverty for homeless men (in regard to TB), to influence the necessity for immediate public force action. No need for excusing or justifying 'punitive' approaches, or to waste court time to seek *mens rea* conditions: none of the above are crimes, yet all are dealt with efficiently, expeditiously, for the public good.

Therefore, there seems to be far less contrast than previously indicated, between a criminal law and a public health approach. In fact, the latter is swifter and less nuanced than the former, and it does not 'discriminate' in favour of female risk imposers, as gender is not an issue, for the most part, in public health ordinances of this kind. Because the alcohol/drug abused child, even if it survives into adulthood, has a much stronger chance of continuing the cycle of abuse for her own offspring as we note later, in the section the on First Nation people of Canada, swift public health action is thus desirable not only for the immediate harm to children to be born now, but also for its far-reaching implications for the future.

NOTES

1   Rifkin (2004), p278.
2   Chomsky (2004).
3   Ikenberry (2002), cited in Chomsky (2004), p11.
4   See also Westra (2004a), Chapter 1.
5   Westra (2004a), Chapter 3.
6   Held and McGrew (2002), p3.
7   Held and McGrew (2002), p16.
8   Albritton (2004).
9   Albritton (2004), p11.
10   Albritton (2004).
11   Albritton (2004), p13.
12   Albritton (2004), p12.
13   Taylor, P. (1998).
14   McMichael (1995a, b, 2000); Tamburlini et al (2002); Westra (2004a), Chapter 2.
15   Taylor, P. (2004), pp956–961.
16   Schmidt (2004), ppA1000–1001.
17   Schmidt (2004), pA1001.
18   Schmidt (2004), pA1002.
19   Schmidt (2004).
20   Schmidt (2004).
21   Westra and Lawson (2001).

22 Bullard (1994).
23 Westra (2004a), Chapter 3.
24 Bullard (2001).
25 Albritton (2004), p25.
26 Soskolne and Bertollini, 1999; see also Pimentel et al (1998); Pimentel and Goodland (2000).
27 Pimentel and Goodland (2000).
28 Westra (2004a).
29 Albritton (2004), p27.
30 Rees (2000).
31 Daily (1997).
32 Dyson (2000), p142.
33 Raz (1986), p5.
34 Raz (1986), p6; Dworkin (1977).
35 Raz (1986), p11.
36 Raz (1986), p16.
37 Rawls (1971).
38 Raz (1986), pp145–146.
39 Linn (2004).
40 Dyson (2000).
41 Ruskin (1999).
42 Goodwin (2000), p248.
43 Durning (1992), p71.
44 Harold (2004), p1.
45 Harold (2004).
46 Rodriguez-Pineau (1993–94), pp43–85.
47 Rodriguez-Pineau (1993–94), p43.
48 De Souza Santos (2002).
49 Palaia (1974), p.115.
50 Rodriguez-Pineau (1994), pp52–53.
51 Palaia (1974), p115.
52 *Rutili* [1975]Case 36/75, ECR 1219 at p.32
53 Rodriguez-Pineau (1994), p46.
54 Simon (1976), p221.
55 Westra (2004a), Chapter 7; Taylor, D. (1998); Taylor (2004), pA1007.
56 Westra (2004), Chapter 7.
57 Singer (2003), p136; see also Westra (2004a), Chapter 8.
58 Postman (1994), pxi; Fionda (2001).
59 Kiralfy and Routledge (1980), p165.
60 Massager (1996); see also Chapter 2 of this book.
61 Barry (1966), pp191–204.
62 Braybrook (1966), pp129–154.
63 Cohen (1962), p156.
64 Cohen (1962), p157.
65 Cohen (1962), p156.
66 Jansen (2000), p210.
67 Post (2000), p102.
68 Westra (2006).
69 *E. (Mrs.) v. Eve,* [1986] 2 S.C.R. 388, [1986] S.C.J.No.60 (S.C.C.); *Winnipeg Child and Family Services (Northwest Area) v. D.G.F.*[1997] S.C.J. No. 96 (S.C.C.).
70 Morin (1990).

71   *Droit de la Famine*, 323, [1988] R.J.Q. 1542 (C.A.)
72   Morin(1990).
73   Morin (1990), p830; see also Baker (1979), p273.
74   Morin(1990).
75   Morin (1990), p32.
76   *Skinner v. Warner*, Dickens 799, 21 E.R. 473 (Ch.1792).
77   La Forest, J. in *E. (Mrs.) v. Eve*, [1986] 2 S.C.R. 388 and P.X.11. R. 273, 185 A.P.Q. 273 at para. 35.
78   *Hepton v. Maat* [1957] S.C.R. 606 (S.C.C., Rand, J. at 607–8).
79   La Forest, J. in *E. (Mrs.) v. Eve*, at 39.
80   [1975] 1 All E.R. 697, [1975] Fam.47.
81   Cited in *E. (Mrs.) v. Eve*, La Forest, J at para.44.
82   *Stump v. Sparkman*, 435 U.S. 349 (1978).
83   378 N.Y.S. 2d 989 (Sup.Ct.,1976), at para.991.
84   *Moore v. Flagg* 137 App. Div.338, 122 N.Y.S. 174; *Matter of Weberlist*, 79 Misc. 2d 753, 360 N.Y.S. 2d 783.
85   La Forest, J at para.64.
86   *Winnipeg Child and Family Services (Northwest Area) v. D.F.G.*, [1997] 3 S.C.R. 92.
87   R.S.O. 1990, c-11,s.37 (3),S.O. 1999,c.2,s.9
88   *Winnipeg Child and Family Services v. K.L.W.* [2000] 2 S.C.R. 519; [2000] S.C.J. No.48 at para. 80.
89   *Winnipeg Child and Family Services v. K.L.W.* [2000] 2 S.C.R. 519; [2000] S.C.J. No.48 at para. 80.
90   *Winnipeg Child and Family Services v. K.L.W.* [2000] 2 S.C.R. 519; [2000] S.C.J. No.48 at para. 100.
91   Holmes (1897), p469.
92   *Winnipeg Child and Family Services (Northwest Area) v. D.F.G.* [1997] 3 S.C.R. 925 at para. 57.
93   *Report of the Presidential Commission on the Human Immunodeficiency Virus Epidemic* at XVII (1987).
94   Wanamaker (1993), pp383–384.
95   Center for Disease Control (1992).
96   Center for Disease Control (1992), p12.
97   Wanamaker (1993), p97.
98   Dr S. Houston, Epidemiology, University of Alberta, personal communication, 2 May 2005.
99   Wanamaker (1993), p387, n.27; *Smith v. Brennan* 157 A.2d 497, 503 (1960).
100   Wanamaker (1993), p388.
101   410 U.S. 113(1973).
102   *Planned Parenthood v. Casey*, U.S. 112 S.Ct. 2791 (1992).
103   492 U.S. 490 (1989).
104   *Ann.Stat. Missouri* §1.205.2 (Vernon's 1992 Supp.).
105   Wanamaker (1993), p39.
106   Hermann (1990),p351–352.
107   *Indiana Statute*, Ind. Code Ann. §35-42-1-7 Burns 1992 Supp.
108   Wanamaker (1993), p395.
109   *Stedman's Medical Dictionary* (1990).
110   *Idaho Code* § 39-608 (1992 Supp.).
111   *Arkansas Code Ann.* § 5-14-123(b) (Michie 1991 Supp.).
112   Schroedel and Fiber (2004), 'p217.
113   *Skinner v. Oklahoma*, 316 U.S. 535 541 (1942).

114   *Carey v. Population Services Int'l*, 431 U.S. 678 (1977).

115   *Roe v. Wade*, 410 U.S. 155.

116   *Harvard Law Review* (1985).

117   410 U.S. at 150.

118   Wolf et al (2004), pp137–147.

119   Wolf et al (2004), p137.

120   Wolf et al (2004), p138.

121   Wanamaker (1993), p401–402.

122   Wanamaker (1993), p403.

123   *Cude v. State*, 377 S.W. 2d 816 (Ark.1964), 'finding a law requiring school children to be vaccinated to be within the police power of the State regardless of religious objections'.

124   Schroedel and Fiber (2004), p217.

125   Schroedel and Fiber (2004).

126   Schroedel and Fiber (2004).

127   Schroedel and Fiber (2004) p219; *State ex.rel. Angela M.W. v. Kruzinski*, 197 Wis. 2d 532; 541 N.W. 2d 482 (Wis. Ct. App. 1995), rev ed 209 Wis.2d 112; 561 N.W. 2d 729 (Wis. 1997); *Whitner*, 492 S.E. 2d 777; *Whitner v. South Carolina*, 523 U.S. 1145(1998).

128   Schroedel and Fiber (2004).

129   Schroedel and Fiber (2004), p220.

130   Schroedel and Fiber (2004), p221.

131   Schroedel and Fiber (2004), p221; Wis Stat § 48.193 (1999); S.D. Codified Laws § 34-20A - 70 (Michie, 1998).

132   Schroedel and Fiber (2004), pp222–223.

133   Wis.Stat. § 48.02 (2000).

134   Schroedel and Fiber (2004), p224; see also *International Classification of Diseases*, 1 TCD-9-CM 49-50 (5th ed., 9th rev., 1997).

CHAPTER 6

Future Generations' Rights: Linking Intergenerational and Intragenerational Rights in Ecojustice

INTRODUCTION

> *This case, however, has a special and novel element. Petitioners minors assert that they represent their generation as well as generations yet unborn. We find no difficulty in ruling that they can, for themselves for others of their generation and for succeeding generations, file a class suit. Their personality to sue on behalf of the succeeding generations can only be based on the concept of intergenerational responsibility insofar as the right to a balanced and healthful ecology is concerned.*[1]

This appears to be the only judgement that appeals specifically to intergenerational equity,[2] in international law. Barresi goes on to point to the significance of the case: 'it was decided by a national court on principles of intergenerational equity for future generations of nationals of that national state'.[3] This, I believe, is only partially correct: appeals to future generations for ecological purposes and to preserve 'environmental rights', a 'nebulous concept' according to Davide, J, have far wider implications than the protection of the area's citizens, present and future, as they affect a much larger proportion of the Earth, than appears, prima facie, to be the case.[4]

From our point of view what is particularly important is the appeal to *parens patriae* doctrine, as the minors request explicitly, 'protection by the State in its capacity as *parens patriae*'.[5] We concluded the first portion of this work, that is, the discussion of the rights to health and the environment of children and the preborn, by finding the *parens patriae* doctrine as the best approach to governmental/institutional responsibility for the rights of the first generation. We noted that the doctrine progressed from being used, initially, purely for economic/inheritance problems, to juridical use in cases that are exclusively medical and protective. Now we note that the same doctrine is used for the protection of life and health of children and future generations, by means of the preservation of naturally 'supportive' ecology. This case therefore explicitly links the two major areas of concern of this work: children's life and health and the environment.

Nevertheless, despite its explicit support of intergenerational equity and the novel use of *parens patriae*, subsequent cases did not follow in the footsteps of *Minors Oposa*. In 1997, the Courts in Bangladesh, in fact, took an opposite position.[6]

At any rate, the major work on intergenerational justice and the law is that of Edith Brown-Weiss.[7,8,9] Hence it might be best to approach the topic with a review of the 'Sustainable Development Symposium' where she revisits her 1990/1992 argument and responds to the critiques brought against it.

OBLIGATIONS TO FUTURE GENERATIONS IN THE LAW: THE PROPOSAL OF EDITH BROWN-WEISS

What is new is that now we have the power to change our global environment irreversibly, with profoundly damaging effects on the robustness and integrity of the planet and the heritage that we pass on to future generations.[10]

What are the main characteristics of Brown-Weiss's position? The first thing to note is that her proposal comprises both rights and duties, and that these include both 'intragenerational' and 'intergenerational' aspects.[11] Intergenerational duties include the obligation:

1 to pass on the Earth to the next generation in as good a condition as it was when that generation first received it;
2 a duty to repair any damage caused by any failure of previous generations to do the same.

Thus every generation has the right 'to inherit the Earth in a condition comparable to that enjoyed by previous generations'.[12] In addition, each generation has four duties:

1 conserve the diversity of the Earth's natural and cultural resource base;
2 conserve environmental quality so that the Earth may be passed on to the next generation in as good a condition as it was when it was received by the present generation;
3 provide all members with equitable access to the resource base inherited from past generations, and
4 conserve this equitable access for future generations.[13]

These duties impose non-derogable obligations especially on affluent Western developed countries, who are clearly in a position of power, as most of the degradation, disintegrity, elimination of biotic capital and other serious ecological ills proceed directly from the practices of the powerful West, to the vulnerable South. I have argued that these obligations should be viewed as *erga omnes*, and they should also be considered as founded on *jus cogens* norms, as the proliferation of harmful chemicals, the exploitation of natural areas, the many activities exacerbating global climate change represent a form of institutionalized ecological violence, or ecoviolence on vulnerable populations. As gross breaches of human rights, they should therefore be considered to be ecocrimes and treated accordingly.[14]

In contrast, some have argued that both limitations on economic expansion and commercial activities on one hand, and the demand for increased respect for the preservation of endangered areas and species only represent a Western, imperialistic conceit, one that flies in the face of the South's needs and cultural practices.[15] Guha and others contrast the Western concern with the environment as a source of leisure-time amenities, rather than understanding its role as foundational to survival, as has been demonstrated by many, including the WHO.[16,17,18,19,20]

This partial understanding allows Guha to make a specious distinction between humanity and their habitat, something that is biologically impossible.[21] The impossibility of separating human health and normal function from environmental conditions, and the consequences of human technological activities was also proven in regard to children and the preborn, as discussed in Chapter 1, on the basis of the WHO's research. Nevertheless it is obviously true that it is easier for developed countries to institute remedial regimes to correct and restore presently harmful environmental conditions, than it is for developing countries to do so.

Thus Brown-Weiss is quite correct as she links intergenerational obligations with intragenerational duties: rich countries and groups must discharge their duties inter-generationally in a direct form, but also by fulfilling their intragenerational obligations to developing countries and impoverished populations. The latter would not be able to fulfil their own obligations without help. But the rich countries' institutions can, and therefore must, ensure that the global communal obligations to future generations be met not only by them, but also by those who require their help in order to comply (this relation between the ability to help and the duty to do so can be found in the 'Kew Gardens principle').

The 'principle of equitable resource use' can therefore be understood in this way: rather than exacerbating a conflict between North–West preferences and South–East basic needs, as Guha proposed, if we combine the two under the Kew Gardens principle it ensures that both intergenerational and intragenerational basic rights are met and the correlative obligations are discharged. Paul Barresi lists Brown-Weiss's proposed rights and duties, and her strategies for the implementation of these duties. He acknowledges that her point is that these should be more than just moral obligations: they should be codified as law.[22] Strategies of implementation include establishing Planetary Rights Commissions, which might serve as a forum where indi-viduals and groups might bring complaints for the violations of these environmental rights.[23] Perhaps courts might be set up to complement the International Criminal Court (ICC) and other ad hoc tribunals, intended to bring to justice serious human rights violations.

I have argued that ecocrimes represent gross breaches of human rights and should be judged accordingly, and no less seriously than (a) attacks against the human person; (b) genocide; (c) breaches of global justice; and (d) crimes against humanity in general (Westra, 2004a). Appealing to international criminal law in this way might even eventually allow a Planetary Rights Commission to be part of the International Criminal Court. But far more important than thinking of the courts appropriate to try and convict those guilty of these crimes against future generations, is to prevent these irreversible harms from happening, by ensuring now that ecojustice should prevail by supporting it in both its aspects of intragenerational and intergenerational equity. Both these aspects should be codified in appropriate law regimes of course, and both should be enforced.

An aside on justice and ecojustice: Rationality in natural law

> *Il exist un droit universal et immuable, source de toutes les lois positive; il n'est que la raison naturelle, entant qu'elle gouverne tous les hommes.*[24]

Ross notes the existence of at least three traditions of justice, basic to understanding its full meaning: (a) the positivist doctrine, where each country's 'sovereign' expresses his will through the law, which therefore has an indisputable binding force; (b) the natural law theory, which views justice as an a priori rational principle. Ross adds that, therefore, the 'enacted law' in this case, possesses binding force only to the extent to which it is a realization or attempt at a realization, of the idea of law; and (c) 'the romantic or historical school of law', where law is custom, or 'the mirror of the popular mind'.[25]

The first alternative does not exist in today's legal regime, but both positive law and a principled approach may be found in common and civil law respectively, or they may both be present in some proportion, as they are for instance, where both 'general principles of law', including natural law, and customary law are explicitly considered as part of the sources of international law.

Justice may also be understood as the highest virtue, including in its reach both law and morality. Justice is a principle and a concept that permits us to assess the cogency and the thoroughness of laws and judicial decisions by how they compare to that standard:

> *As a principle of law, justice delimits and harmonises the conflicting desires, claims and interests in the social life of the people. . . Justice is equality.*[26]

Of course perfect equality is not a viable principle, nor well-founded, justice may take into consideration merit, or performance, or needs or ability.[27] We need not elaborate on issues that are very well discussed in the literature, and particularly by John Rawls.[28] What should be emphasized, however, is that certain human characteristics may never be taken in consideration if justice is to be served: these include race, gender, creed and social class. John Rawls's 'difference principle' captures well the need to ensure that the least advantaged be treated in a way that alleviates their disadvantage in some way, and that corrects, as does the law, the unfairness of their situation.[29]

The second approach to justice that Ross proposes, (b), that is natural law, is well adapted to provide the foundation for this understanding of justice, even if one prefers to purge it of its metaphysical underpinnings, as Hugo Grotius suggests, saying that, even if one assumed that God did not exist, 'the law of nature would still be valid'.[30,31,32] I have argued that, as natural law provides the basis for a just war theory, it is also foundational to the understanding of crimes against humanity, genocide and other breaches of basic human rights that singly and collectively represent aspects of what I have termed 'ecoviolence'.[33]

That said, just as certain characteristics of humankind such as colour, gender or creed should not be used to dictate a discriminatory treatment of certain humans, or the deprivation of their right to protection from harm, so too the geographical or temporal distance of humans from the actor or decision-maker, ought not to permit discriminatory treatment either. The argument in favour of rationality as foundational to justice even without the further inquiry about the origin of such rationality, can be found in Kantian doctrine, and it has been used to great advantage by such eminent Kantians as Onora O'Neill and Thomas Pogge, on the topic of global justice.[34]

The main theme of global justice in these thinkers is the continued presence of starvation and poverty globally, despite the rhetoric of providing aid, on the part of Western affluent countries. For instance the 1996 World Food Summit in Rome issued a pledge by the 186 participating governments that ends with the following words:

> *We consider it intolerable that more than 800 million people throughout the world, and particularly in developing countries, do not have enough food to meet their basic nutritional needs. This situation is unacceptable.*[35,36]

This situation is also exacerbated and fostered by global climate change and we have witnessed the lack of interest in signing the Kyoto Agreement by the countries who are among the worst polluters: the US and Australia. Yet the International Monetary Fund (IMF), the World Bank and the World Trade Organization (WTO), led by the US, 'had unprecedented power to shape the global economic order'.[37] Instead of reducing global poverty, the World Bank recognizes its increase and admits 'it will reach 1.9 billion by 2015'.[38]

Pogge discusses the failures of these institutions by showing 'three morally significant connections between us and the global poor'. In brief, these are (1) the causal/historical connections of a shared past where the presently wealthy imposed colonialism and slavery on the presently poor, so that the foundation of the former joint powers and affluence is suspect; (2) we all depend on a single 'resource basis', we share the Earth, but only in ways that benefit those who are currently better off and harm the others; and (3) the present 'global economic order', does not redress, but aggravates 'global economic inequalities'.[39]

The difficulty Pogge emphasizes through the example of global famine, supports Richard Falk's contention that the world as a whole has arrived at a 'Grotian moment',[40] but thus far we have been unable or unwilling to even attempt to reach across the 'normative abyss' that is before us: 'A neo-liberal world order based on the functional imperatives of the market is not likely to be a Grotian moment in the normative sense.'[41]

His main point coincides with the argument here presented: while Grotius was able to 'articulate a normative bridge between past and future' at a critical historical moment, the present world order is both unable and unwilling to do so.

Falk notes that the present world order 'reflects mainly economistic priorities,[42] and that the state system has lost much of its credibility in problem solving, in the face of 'the rise of market forces'. Falk adds:

> *We currently confront in this era of economic and cultural globalization a more profound normative vacuum: the dominating logic of the market in a world of greatly uneven social, economic, and political conditions and without any built-in reliable means to ensure that a continuing global economic growth does not at some point and in certain respects cause decisive ecological damage.*[43]

Neither Pogge nor Falk address intergenerational justice directly, and some who do so, like Hendrik Ph. Visser 't Hooft, find Rawls' work to be more helpful than I have found it to be. In sum, Rawls refuses to commit to a specific formulation of 'the good' as superior to other possible choices, as he allows perhaps too much power to the 'rational contractors' even when their formulation of just principles takes place 'behind a veil of ignorance'. In contrast, his 'difference principle' might be extended, as Visser 't Hooft would have it, to global society.[44]

In general, accepting the arguments for sustainability entails that moral judgements be used when scientific evidence is assessed and legal instruments are often designed to support such judgements:

> *Justice constitutes one segment of morality primarily concerned not with individual conduct but with the ways in which classes of individuals are treated. It is this which gives justice its special relevance in the criticism of law and other public or social institutions.*[45]

From the environmental point of view, intergenerational justice emerges in several conventions, such as the *Biodiversity Convention*, as 'biodiversity', for instance, is acknowledged to be a 'common concern of mankind', but it cannot be said that there are in any convention,

> *substantive provisions to treat living resources as 'common heritage' or give full effect to intergenerational rights as conceived by Brown-Weiss.*[46]

Some additional examples of this, somewhat limited 'concern', or of the presence of human interests, are left to the Preambles of international treaties. For instance, the Preamble to the *Whaling Convention* (1946) recognizes 'the interests of the actions of the world in safeguarding for future generations the great natural resources represented by whale stocks';[47] the 1968 *African Convention*, states that soil, water and fauna resources constitute 'a capital of vital importance for mankind'; the 1985 *ASEAN Agreement*, talks about 'the importance of natural resources for present and future generations'; the 1972 *World Heritage Convention* says that 'parts of the natural heritage are of outstanding interest and therefore need to be preserved as part of the world heritage of mankind as a whole'; finally the Preamble to the 1973 *Convention on International Trade in Endangered Species of Wild Flora and Fauna* (CITES) speaks of wild flora and fauna as 'an irreplaceable part of the natural systems of the earth which must be protected for this and future generations to come'.[48]

Even such a brief discussion indicates that Brown-Weiss's work is outstanding in that it considers both intergenerational and intragenerational equity, whereas most existing legal instruments do not. I have suggested that the integration of the two concepts represents true ecojustice, that is, justice that recognizes humans as embedded in their habitat, so that 'justice' that does not recognize this aspect of their humanity is – to say the least – incomplete. Other internationally used concepts, such as 'sustainable development' are mostly used as a device to attempt to 'green' an existing or projected policy or proposal that simply advances 'business as usual'. We will return to this problem in our discussion of Western ecological footprints[49] in the next chapter.

For now, it is clear that justice as a normative, rational principle is well-served by Brown-Weiss's doctrine because:

(a) it requires that present populations needing help to achieve appropriate environmental goals should receive such help from the affluent countries who, it must be noted, have more than a moral interest in ensuring the conservation of common resources;

(b) it escapes the critiques based on identifying specific individuals to ensure that we should understand fully what their needs (or preferences) might be in the future: it is not individual rights, but group/class rights that are at issue. All considerations of equity in regard to certain groups and classes look at the general characteristics of all, *not* at the individual preferences of any specific member of the group, as some have argued against the rights of future generations;[50,51,52,53]

(c) it defends implicitly the right of the present generation to protection that accrues from the present respect for 'nature's services',[54] thus, instead of showing an unfair bias toward the future, at the expense of the needs of the poor of the present generation, it mandates the preservation and the protective instruments that are needed for all present peoples, especially the most vulnerable, that is the poor, those in developing countries, and the children.

All these require sustainability in their habitat, which Visser 't Hooft terms:

> the ecological core of the concept, which after all is the historical prior one, and ... the judgments on quality of life called for by the conception of a future integrity of the environment.[55]

When so understood, Brown-Weiss's doctrine on intergenerational justice, not only reconciles inter- and intragenerational justice, but it also manifests the underlying integrity and unity of justice and ecojustice. Paul Wood argues in a similar vein by addressing the question of 'The connection between intergenerational equity and allocational equity'. He proposes designing specific regimes to meet the joint goals of developed and developing countries, especially those in deltaic regions or island countries: 'An equitable self-sustaining regime will meet intertemporal obligations by jointly benefiting present and future generations.'[56]

Visser 't Hooft also remarks that intergenerational justice involves classes of individuals, but in a very novel, original way. I believe he is mistaken on this point. Decisions proscribing apartheid, for instance, or discrimination against people of colour, once codified in law, are equally intended to cover unknown groups of individuals, included in an open-ended class of persons fitting, say, the definition of 'persons of colour'. Those legal instruments are based on principles equally 'processional and open-ended' as future generations are. He adds:

> Justice between generations forms a natural alliance with the search for transgenerationally valid criteria of environmental integrity, established by means offering the best chances for consensus and clear definition.[57]

In contrast, I have argued, following James Karr, Reed Noss and other biologists and ecologists, that ecological integrity needs a scientific understanding, and an index (the Index of Biotic Integrity, IBI) to allow the reconstruction of a baseline. Such a definition is certainly scientific and thorough, but it is not based on 'consensus'.[58] I also proposed that justice, both transgenerational and intergenerational would best be served by adherence to a 'principle of integrity' that would morally prohibit any activity or process that involved man-made products such as the ones that are putting at risk the most vulnerable among us, starting with the children of the first generation, but extending globally to the present poor and all future generations as well.[59]

Klaus Bosselmann on ecological justice

Klaus Bosselmann has noted that there is a dissonance between most environmental ethics theories, which do not really address social justice issues, and theories of social justice, that do not fully appreciate the impacts of ecological problems.[60] His analysis of the problem starts by noting that 'a theory of either environmental justice or eco-justice is lacking'.[61] He cites a definition of environmental justice that views it as 'equal justice and equal protection under the law without discrimination. . . .',[62] but he also points out that such a view ignores the intergenerational aspect of the concept.

This author's work on environmental racism, admittedly also focused primarily on 'Africana', that is, issues of concern to North America's African American, is therefore guilty of the same narrow scope, for the most part.[63] Some of the contributors to my work deal with issues of concern to African populations, which entail a more historical, less limited approach.[64]

Nevertheless, it is in the environmental ethics work that I have addressed future generations' rights, not the work on environmental justice. In the latter, it was important to note the impact of then President of the US, Bill Clinton's 'Executive Order' no. 12898 (Federal Actions to Address Environmental Justice in Minority Populations and Low-Income Populations, 11 February 1994), which ensured that the US Environmental Protection Agency (EPA) would be more available to redress environmental injustice and harms befalling the inhabitants of African-American neighbourhoods, than they had been before the introduction of the Executive Order. The grave concern for the life and health of presently affected populations had clear primacy over the possible rights of the future.

Yet, it must be admitted, a consideration of the latter would have eliminated the need for costly clean-up and remediation on behalf of the former. In addition, there is the problem I have alluded to in the previous section: minority groups and peoples from developing countries tend to perceive ecocentrism as a position in direct conflict with their own, justified, immediate needs and aspirations. Bosselmann acknowledges that this position portrays a false dichotomy: 'The concentric position is inclusive, as it merely extends intrinsic values of humans to non-humans rather than replacing one by the other.'[65]

I have argued in this way as well in defence of the 'Principle of Integrity', as the debate between anthropocentrism and eco/biocentric holism is based on misconceptions about the scientific underpinnings of the latter position, the holistic biocentrism I have defended.[66,67,68] The two positions are seldom, if ever, combined or even discussed together in the literature, although, as this work has indicated, they converge in the interface between health, normal function and ecological integrity.[69]

Bosselmann argues for an approach to 'eco-justice', based on Brenda Almond's proposal, involving:

- the relation between a modern liberal theory of justice and environmental ethics;
- the various forms of distributive justice with respect to the environment; and
- their application to environmental issues.[70]

This set of guidelines appears to be basically flawed. We noted in Chapter 5 the grave difficulties produced by relying on neo-liberal policies, and those arguments do not need to be repeated. Bosselmann himself sees the wrongheadedness of this approach:

> *But like the 'rights' issue, the liberal approach of justice tends to foster the very problems we are trying to overcome. Rather than fundamentally challenging the traditional idea of environmental management with its anthropocentric limitations, it would simply internalize the concept in the 'idea of environmental justice'.*[71]

Finally, invoking distributive justice leads to the problems on which Richard De George, for instance, bases his argument against future generations' rights,[72] as well as introducing the difficulties present in various forms of 'exponential discounting'.[73]

Bosselmann wants to link intra- and intergenerational justice, citing Brown-Weiss's own proposal (see previous section) and extending the meaning of 'future generations' to non-human animals. I have proposed going even beyond that, by including all life under the same protective umbrella, thus including the unborn, or first generation as well. By starting with the consideration of health and normal function, and thus relying not only on ecology but also on epidemiology and the work of the WHO, the form of ecojustice here proposed is indeed radical. But, by connecting existing regulatory regimes not only to their explicit environmental, even if non-anthropocentric thrust, but also to their implicit interface with all human health, I believe this proposal for ecojustice might be the most extensive one, best suited to inform supranational and international law regimes. In the next section the case of the First Nation Peoples of Canada will demonstrate the links between intergenerational and intragenerational harms, connected through health considerations.

INTERGENERATIONAL HARMS: THE CASE OF THE CANADIAN FIRST NATION'S CHILDREN

> *Chiefs must consider the impact of their decisions on the seventh generation* (paraphrase of precept of the Great Law of the Haundenosaunee (Six Nations Iroquois Confederacy); Seventh Generation Fund, P.O. Box 4569, Arcata, CA 95518)

In Chapters 3 and 5 we encountered cases describing grave threats to the health of aboriginal children, within their family unit, in Winnipeg, Manitoba. The case was only 'environmental' in an extended sense: the abuse of a common chemical compound, glue, by the expectant mother, against the background of the result of her previous similar choices to the irreversible detriment of her two previous children. Aside from the question of possible restraints of the addicted mother, there are two important issues that also emerge from the case, and that are particularly relevant in a discussion of group rights and transgenerational and intergenerational equity.

The first point of significance is the use, as noted in the previous chapter of the *parens patriae* doctrine, which, as we will see, is here also used for the protection of group rights. The second point relates directly to specific harms suffered by aboriginal peoples, especially the harmful legacy initiated by the policy of 'assimilation' of First Nation children. Social science research shows today a dismal picture of harm to these children, as the following statistics indicate:

> *Child functioning by Aboriginal and non-Aboriginal Children in Care*
> - *Substance Abuse Birth Defect: Aboriginal Children (7%), non-Aboriginal Children (4%); Other visible minority children (1%)*
> - *Behavioural Problems: Aboriginal Children (18%); non-Aboriginal Children (25%); Other Visible Minority Children (18%)*
> - *Irregular School Attendance: Aboriginal Children (15%); non-Aboriginal Children (10%); Other Visible Minority Children (6%).*[74]

These figures, coupled with what is presently known about pre-birth exposures,[75] indicates a persistent, ongoing, intergenerational form of injustice. Unchecked, this injustice leads routinely to harms to all First Nation's Peoples, as most of these children's problems arise because of exposures and circumstances beyond their control.

Many of the difficulties these children face are due to earlier Canadian and Provincial policies of 'assimilation', intended to eliminate all forms of cultural 'indianness' from children, by placing them in white institutional schools, removed from their parents and extended families except for two months each summer, forbidden to speak their native tongues, and forced to abandon all traditional practices of their bands.[76]

These practices, intended to educate Aboriginal children to 'the ways of the white man',[77] without any respect or appreciation for their own traditions and culture, placed a heavy burden on the children, and produced harms that cannot be righted, even with the best will, within one generation. The results of earlier Canadian policies continue to produce 'Intergenerational effects' today:[78]

> *Aboriginal communities have not yet recovered from the damage caused by the residential schools... For the first time in over 100 years, many families are experiencing a generation of children who live with their parents until their teens.*[79]

This is not the appropriate place for a lengthy historical discussion of the failures of the Canadian Government policies with regard to its Aboriginal Peoples. The main point is that this is another case where intergenerational justice should have been practised in several areas: (1) pre-birth protection, in order to prevent many of the childhood problems statistically prevalent in Aboriginal children, as noted above; (2) the proper implementation of *parens patriae* doctrine in the defence and protection of Aboriginal children with behavioural, emotional and neurological problems, arising (in part) from environmental or other substance exposure; and (3) the serious and informed consideration of intragenerational issues connected with the intergenerational ongoing harm inflicted upon these children.

Starting with the final point, (3), as the most obvious one, Canada's Aboriginal Action Plan addresses the question of 'intergenerational effects':

> *The intent of the residential school policy was to erase Aboriginal identity by separating generations of children from their families, suppressing their Aboriginal languages, and re-socializing them according to the norms of non-Aboriginal society.*

We noted in the discussion of Brown-Weiss's proposal, that one of the major objections to her position, was the open-endedness of the proposed obligation to the future. This is an example of harms to a whole class, present, future and – after the fact – even to the past generation; it is the reality of all social and legal changes imposed on Aboriginal children.

The first point, (1), is of greater importance to First Nation Children than to others, given the statistics exposing the grave problem disproportionately affecting them because of pre-birth drug and alcohol exposure.[80] These problems affect children immediately, but they also add to delinquency in older children and adults, thus representing another form of intergenerational injustice. Against this background, however, Canada's Child Welfare Statutes give primacy to the 'Best Interests of the Child'.[81,82]

Although these documents start with the 'Respect for family autonomy and support of families', and add 'Respect for cultural heritage especially for Aboriginal Children', they also include 'the paramountcy of the protection of children from harm'.[83,84,85] This has been the topic of the first chapter of this book: protection of children from harm should not only initiate after their birth, when the endangerment could happen long before it. Health Canada produced a study, the Canadian Incidence Study of Reported Abuse and Neglect.[86] Nicholas Bala writes:

> *Each child welfare statute has a definition of a 'child in need of protection' (or an 'endangered child'). This is a key legal concept as only children within this definition are subject to an involuntary state intervention under the legislation.*[87]

If the 'need of protection' arises long before social workers or the courts may be confronted with it, then it is worthy of serious consideration at the time of exposure, that is, at the time of the origin of the harm. In other words, it is worth ensuring that pre-birth child endangerment is viewed as impermissible and that legal and social measures are put in place before the harm occurs. Legal instruments are needed to prevent such harms before they affect both the child itself and society. Serving justice by preventing the harms would make both logical and economic sense a well. As a greater percentage of affected children is Aboriginal, it would seem that any instrument that does not consider the 'pre-conditions' of their humanity is flawed and incomplete.

Intergenerational and intragenerational justice would seem to require this additional protection, as mentioned in Chapter 1, additional protection seemed to be necessary, from the 'freedom' of chemical companies and other polluters to impose harm on the most vulnerable, based on the extensive research of the WHO.[88]

Finally the second point, (2), the implementation of the *parens patriae* doctrine, appears to be as justified to support the intervention required by the first point (1), as it is in the case where, for instance, a Jehovah's Witness parent refuses a blood transfusion to the serious detriment of the child.[89] As Justice MacLachlin said:

> *para. 76. Canadian Child protection Law has undergone a significant evolution over the past decades. This evolution reflects a variety of policy shifts and orientations, as society has sought the most appropriate means of protecting children from harm. Over the last 40 years or so, society has become much more aware of problems such as battered child syndrome and child sexual abuse, leading to a call for greater preventive intervention and protection. At the same time, Canadian law has increasingly emphasized individual rights to protection against state intervention.*

In addition to the Jehovah's Witness instance cited above, La Forest, J discusses the implications of that decision regarding s.7 of the Charter (citing Whealy Dist. CJ):

> *When an infant, totally incapable of making any decision, is in a life threatening situation and the appropriate treatment is denied or refused by its parents, it cannot be said that any potential protection as given under section 7 for the family unit can be invoked against the right of the infant to live. Section 7 addresses itself also to 'the principles of fundamental justice'. It can hardly be said that the principles of fundamental justice could be invoked to deny a child a chance to live.*
>
> *It is worth noting as well that the rights set out in section 7 are conditional and not absolute. The rights therein set out can be interfered with if done in accordance with the principles of fundamental justice. The scheme of the Child Welfare Act, in my view, meets all the tests of fundamental justice, including a fair hearing before an impartial judge (para. 54).*

It is important to note two major points here. The first is that the freedom of religion is here appealed to by the parents of Sheena B., the infant at risk, as they attempt to block the medically required blood transfusion. Freedom of religion is a very important principle, far superior, I believe, to the freedom of choice to engage in a lifestyle that includes the use of alcohol or drugs. Neither are protected by the Charter.

The second point is the appeal to 'principles of fundamental justice': if they could not be invoked 'to deny a child the chance to live', I believe they also could not be invoked to deny to a child the right to be well-born, that is to be born with normal physical and mental function.

THE RIGHTS OF THE FIRST GENERATION AND OF THE FUTURE: THE INTERFACE

> *by its very nature, law must play a protective role. If violence and dependency to strong men in a society is to be replaced by the rule of law, law fulfills a role according to its most fundamental principle, i.e. to protect the equal dignity of all men, in freedom and mutual responsibility.*[90]

Children are the world's citizens. But, for a long time, children cannot speak on their own behalf or represent themselves, and one cannot always guess exactly what their future choices and preferences might be. These are also the characteristics of future generations, in fact, the very characteristics that render future generations' rights hard to defend both in morality and in the law. I have argued that ecoviolence, an attack against the human person perpetrated through environmental means, is an accepted and institutionalized criminal activity against an 'other' we do not want to recognize as worthy of respect.[91] These 'others' could be citizens in developing countries, where the ecoviolence acquires a sinister racist perspective, as well as poor and 'different' citizens of the most developed countries. We also noted in the first four chapters that the 'other' may also be one of our own: the developing child of this population, that is, the first of future generations.

Similar thoughts and sentiments are found in an unexpected area of scholarship: in the reflections on the holocaust. Eva Hoffman says:

> *Systematic violence – especially what Primo Levi called '**unnecessary violence**' – that is the violence that does not serve the ends of battle or victory but is meant to humiliate and brutalize the victim, is the ultimate form of mis-recognition or deliberate non-recognition.* [92] [emphasis added]

The 'meaning', the 'intent', is absent from environmental harms, and it is also lacking in pre-birth and perhaps some other harms to children. But, as 'deliberate cruelty' is judged to be an attempt to discount, negate and ultimately destroy the identity, the subjectivity of its target,[93] perhaps we can also say that the converse is true. In other words, 'to discount, negate the subjectivity' of those who are harmed, even without the requisite *mens rea*, necessary for the commission of a crime is, ultimately, a form of destruction that manifests an unthinking but undeniable cruelty. The humanity of these 'others' is kept faceless, their identity denied.

Is this possible account of the converging plight of the first and future generations overdramatic? Perhaps. But if we cast our minds back, to consider the consequences of our refusal to recognize the mindless violence offered to future generations and to the unborn through environmental means, we will have to acknowledge that such wholesale harms are not compatible with respect for humanity.[94] Even within a war situation, where institutionalized violence is expected and accepted, it is not the case that any 'externality' (in capitalist/consumerist terms), or 'collateral damage' (in just war terms) is considered to be acceptable either morally or legally.[95]

In the ambit of just war, there are still *jus in bello* conditions to be met, even when the objective of winning a battle, or a just war itself, is at issue. Senseless cruelty or violence is not condoned, nor is any attack against medical personnel, prisoners of war, hospitals or the cultural or religious icons of a people. These restrictions apply even when the goal to be achieved is a legal one and – for the most part — morally just. Therefore, it seems fair to also ensure that both corporate profit-making enterprises, and the activities of common citizens, whose lifestyles may impose grave 'collateral damage' on those who are negligently or unintentionally harmed, be subject to similar stringent restrictions.

The freedom of persons, be they legal or biological, is not absolute and in earlier chapters, we noted the presence of many restrictions already in place: through public health (e.g. freedom of movement restrictions because of communicable diseases, from measles to TB; of smoking in public places; of having unprotected sex when HIV positive, as in the recent Canadian murder conviction); or through police powers (e.g. through restrictions of speed of movement on highways, or the very impermissibility of driving if intoxicated or under the influence of certain substances).

In these cases and many others, liberty is limited by our responsibility not to harm others, a responsibility that is not only moral, but also legal and enforced through public institutions and the courts. One may object that the harm imposed by drunk driving or second-hand smoke, or even TB exposure is clear and obvious. But, as we saw in the first chapter, the scientific research of the WHO and of many epidemiologists,[96,97,98,99] the results of unrestrained activities by industry or single individuals may be as well supported by research as the cases we now consider 'obvious'.

In some cases, these effects may not be immediately visible, but neither is the result of second-hand smoke, HIV exposure or even drunk driving. The latter, for instance, may continue for a period without accident; but the potential for accidents and grave harm increases exponentially, when the harmful preconditions persist.

Of course, neither the unborn's nor the next generation's harms may be immediately observable. But the scientific research today is clear and robust enough to prompt us to adopt laws that defend the rights of the future.

Edith Brown-Weiss and others on the protection of the future

> *Standards of Fairness*
> *Experts generally adopt one of two general approaches to fairness. One measure depends on a priori rules, or 'focal points' – cultural or ethical rules broadly perceived as measuring fairness, which derive authority from legal and cultural traditions. The second approach views fairness as the outcome of strategic bargaining emerging from the negotiating process instead of being pre-determined. Bargained for rules derive their legitimacy from the explicit consent of agreeing parties.*[100]

Given that the latter is usually subject to the will of Western power blocks as a main guiding principle, and that negotiated treaties are usually brought down to the lowest possible denominator,[101] I have argued that ethical norms, including natural law, represent a far better option to ensure that justice and fairness be served.[102] In fact, although *erga omnes* obligations do not explicitly include the rights of future generations, it seems that the right to survival and to – minimally – the health and normal function that will make such survival meaningful and reaffirm the 'basic rights'[103] of future people, are and should be at least as important as the right to escape racist or gender based harms.

Hence *jus cogens* norms, not politically motivated agreements should govern regulatory regimes to protect the survival of the future. Treaties support the obligations of signatories, that is of certain specific countries; but the harms of which we have been speaking are global in reach. Brown-Weiss speaks of the 'planetary legacy' that cannot be abused or consumed, as it presently is, through the 'produce of Western technologies and lifestyles'.[104] Wood suggests the creation of 'cooperative regimes' shifting 'the focus away from benefits, costs and targets', as in the present Climate Change Protocol.[105] He also proposes that Western developed countries should provide financial and technical assistance to developing countries, many of which are at least potentially, becoming major polluters, such as China, for instance.[106]

But Wood himself recognizes that, if standing for future interests is not universal, protection would be geographically as well as temporally incomplete.[107] In that case, relying on voluntary agreements and regimes would appear to be precarious at best, and to represent an approach that is doomed to failure. In contrast, Brown-Weiss views intergenerational obligations and the intragenerational duties that support them, as *erga omnes* in character.[108] This appears to be the best available option, as neither negotiated treaties, nor a 'world-based empathy for the environment',[109] could possibly be used to counteract the world hegemony of the US and the WTO, and their indisputable ability to dominate global policy decisions that they appear to view exclusively through an economic lens.[110]

Brown-Weiss's position is convincing instead: (a) the protection of future generations is specifically mentioned in various international instruments; and (b) in fact, 'the World Commission on Environment and Development (WCED), recommended the appointment of an ombudsman for future generations'.[111] In addition, (c) treating the 'Planetary Trust' appropriately means that, as is the case for all trusts, 'maintenance of the capital is an integral component of the investment'.[112] In general trusts require the long-term perspective demanded by the consideration of future generations. Finally, (d) the recognition of the rights of the future is but another aspect of a human right, not an anomaly, or a different issue altogether. The Preamble to the *Universal Declaration of Human Rights* begins as follows:

> *Whereas recognition of the inherent dignity and of the equal and inalienable rights of all members of the human family is the foundation of freedom, justice and peace in the world...*[113]

Considering the language of this declaration, Brown-Weiss concludes that:

> *the reference to all members of the human family has a temporal dimension which brings all generations within its scope. The reference to equal and inalienable rights, affirms the basic equality of such generations in the human family.*[114]

Both the UN Declaration and Brown-Weiss's interpretation support the understanding of the rights of the future, as imposing an *erga omnes* obligation on all presently existing members of the human family, in regard to the future. The non-derogability of this obligation shows that neither preferences nor negotiations may eliminate this grave duty. Therefore Wood's argument for viewing – for instance – the climate system as 'a common property resource', although well-intentioned, misses the full understanding of the situation. The 'commons' will be the topic of the next section.

THE INTERNATIONAL PROTECTION OF HUMAN RIGHTS AND THE PRINCIPLE OF THE COMMON HERITAGE OF MANKIND

> *In our search for an Ariadne's thread to lead us through the intricacies of international relatives we stumble upon a new concept creeping in and out of the intricacies of international reality: the 'common heritage of mankind'.*[115]

When we consider the historical development of international law, we note that the powerful Western countries have tended, as much as possible, to support the status quo in law, through the respect for the 'freewill of states' and the prevalence of custom and of positive law. In contrast, the developing countries and those in Eastern Europe, albeit for separate motives, supported the formation of principles and rules beyond those based on the agreement and cooperation of states. Cassese's insightful analysis shows that, while in earlier years a 'Hobbesian or realist tradition' prevailed, which saw each country's position as essentially self-defensive in regard to other states, a later Groatian or internationalist conception of state interaction emerged, emphasizing 'cooperation and regulated intercourse among sovereign States'.[116] Finally, the universalist, 'Kantian outlook' emerged: 'which sees at work in international politics a potential community of mankind, and lays stress on the element of "transnational solidarity"'.[117] The latter approach, together with a strong thrust toward the emergence of *jus cogens* norms and of obligations *erga omnes*, represent the preferred agents of change of developing countries, as they press 'for quick, far reaching and radical modifications'.[118]

In contrast, Eastern European countries, 'prefer to proceed gingerly, believing as they do, that legal change should be brought about gradually, as much as possible through mutual agreement'.[119]

Nevertheless, both Eastern European and developing countries joined in supporting Article 53 of the *Vienna Convention on the Law of Treaties* (1969). Cassese remarks:

> *To developing countries, the proclamation of* jus cogens *represented a further means of fighting against colonial or former colonial countries-as was made clear in 1968 at the Vienna Conference by the representative of Sierra Leone, who pointed out that the upholding of* jus cogens, *provided a golden opportunity to condemn imperialism, slavery, forced labour and all the practices that violated the principle of equality of all human beings and of the sovereign equality of all states.*[120]

For Eastern European states (such as Romania and Ukraine), *jus cogens* was viewed as 'means of crystallizing once and for all, peaceful coexistence between East and West'.[121]

Despite the support of both of these 'blocks', Western countries were initially 'on the defensive' before bowing to the inevitable will of the majority, and the need to espouse norms consistent with their own legal traditions.[122] It is instructive to consider that it is the weakest countries, those who felt most disempowered by Western alliances and treaties, who enthusiastically supported an approach that characterized the 'new' law (although the 'old' *Le Louis* case demonstrates a similar position). E. Jimenez de Arechaga (Uruguay) termed these developments 'a flagrant challenge to international conscience'.[123] I have argued that we are all disempowered in the face of mounting environmental threats to our health and survival, and the monolithic powers that support global trade and current economic policies instead of life. Perhaps that is why we see protesting groups joining forces not with those from developing countries, but also from Western environmental and animal defence groups. At any rate, Cassese summarizes the 'three principles that emerge and become codified' in the 1969 *Vienna Convention*:

> First, it introduces restrictions of the previously unfettered freedom of States;
> Second, there is a democratization of international legal relations;
> Third, the Convention enhances international values as opposed to national claims.[124]

A controversial principle is arising within the 'new law' paradigm, one that did not quite live up to its true potential, at least so far: the principle of the Common Heritage of Mankind. The concept appears prima facie to step forward, but this does not represent the whole picture. Birnie and Boyle say:

> An important factor contributing to the classification of living resources as common property is that they have generally been so plentiful that the cost of asserting and defending exclusive rights exceeds the advantages to be gained. A regime of open access in these circumstances has generally been to everyone's advantage. However, as Hardin has observed, the inherent logic of the commons, remorselessly generates tragedy, as the availability of a free resource leads to overexploitation and minimizes the interest of any individual state in conservation and restraint.[125]

The principle of the Common Heritage of Mankind

> Law does not spring anew, old concepts evolve and new ones emerge to fit new fields of human enterprise. In this manner, the unique historical developments manifesting themselves in the emergence of a North–South cleavage have been responsible for the introduction of a new international legal concept, the Common Heritage of Mankind (CHM) Principle.[126]

The new legal concept, CHM, can be defined as follows:

> (1) the area under consideration cannot be subject to appropriation; (2) all countries must share in the management of the region; (3) there must be an active sharing of the benefits reaped from the exploitation of the area's resources; and (4) the area must be dedicated to exclusively peaceful purpose.[127]

This appears, at least prima facie to be a wonderful addition to the small arsenal of ecologically constructive concepts. Nevertheless the language employed in that definition shows clearly its incompleteness and deficiencies. If an area is ecologically sensitive and, in that sense, important enough to fit the CHM concept, then both managing it and exploiting it may be contrary to the continued preservation of the area, a goal implicit in the CHM designation. All future generations comprising mankind would be deprived of any benefit whatever if the area were to be both managed and exploited.

That goal would be far better served if both present and future humankind were managed instead, so that their exploitive activities could be controlled and even excluded from the area to be designated as a common heritage: the area's existence and the natural services it may provide for all life both within and without its immediate confines, is what is primarily at stake.[128,129]

In essence, future generations or mankind can only benefit from non-exploitation which, in turn, is based on regulated restraint, or management of present human enterprise. Although the CHM principle is not yet established as either a treaty obligation or as an obligation *erga omnes*, and it remains a 'political principle' at this time,[130] it has emerged in international discourse because developing countries have been seeking a New International Economic Order (NIEO).

The developing nations, largely disempowered by free trade and the economically and politically powerful G-7, are attempting in this way to influence public policy opinion, at least in regard to areas 'outside the traditional jurisdiction of states: the deep seabed, outer space and, to a lesser degree, the Antarctic'.[131]

Our concern is with the natural systems of Earth, so that only the deep seabed and Antarctica are relevant to the argument of this work. The first point worthy of note in this regard is that this political principle is too accepting of the status quo, hence, it is not capable of protecting our common heritage as stated, because this natural patrimony of mankind does not only lie in areas that do not interest the North–West affluent states. Oceans, old forests, lakes, rivers, and all other areas where biodiversity still abounds are surely part of the global commons and should be protected urgently, before their tragic loss may deprive all life of the support they provide.[132,133,134,135]

Hence, the reference to the 'benefits' of exploitation is clearly an oxymoron, unless one interprets benefit in a purely economic and short-term sense that appears to be contrary to the letter and spirit of a principle aimed at benefiting mankind as a whole not only a rich and present minority.

Are we, for instance, to consider the global commons as *res nullius*, despite the tragic consequences that may follow the free and unrestricted appropriation of these areas by technologically advanced countries and other legal persons, bent on immediate economic exploitation? Or are we to consider it *res communis*, together with air and sunlight?[136] The 1974 separate opinion of Judge De Castro in regard to the *Fisheries Jurisdiction*,[137] clearly shows the fallacy of this approach, as he states that 'fish stocks in the sea are inexhaustible'.[138] But neither clean air nor safe sunlight are presently available to most people on Earth, and fish stocks themselves are often sadly depleted or have crashed into extinction.[139] The argument of this work implies that the Common Heritage of Mankind Principle should be applied as *territorium extra commercium* as Bin Cheng proposes, except that instead of 'management, exploitation and distribution', our concern should be with preservation, nonmanipulation, and respectful treatment, as these concepts, not the former, would ensure that mankind as such may enjoy the benefits of an unspoiled nature.

Here is Cheng's important passages discussing some of these concepts:

> *While* territorium extra commercium *and* Territorium commune humanitatis *(for CHM) shared the same characteristics that they cannot be territorially appropriated by any State, they differ, in that the former is essentially a negative concept, whereas the latter is a positive one. In the former, in time of peace, as long as a State respects the exclusive quasiterritorial jurisdiction of other states over their own ships, aircraft and spacecraft, general international law allows it to use the area or even abuse it more or less as it wishes, including the appropriation of its natural resources, closing large parts of such ports for weapon testing and military exercises and even using such areas as a cesspool for its municipal and industrial sewage. The emergent concept of the common heritage of mankind, on the other hand, while it still lacks precise definition, wishes basically to convey the idea that the management, exploitation and distribution of the natural resources of the area in question are matters to be decided by the international community (or simply the contracting parties, as in the Moon Treaty?) and are not to be left to the initiative and discretion of individual States and their nationals.*[140]

Larschan and Brennan, in contrast, are primarily concerned with distributive issues: they argue convincingly that even defining certain areas as protected under the CHM Principle, in practice only appears to protect the 'Group of 77', given that the 'one nation–one vote procedure of the Assembly is cosmetic'.[141] The Council empowered to make executive decisions is dominated by states 'on the basis of investments, social system, consumption, production, special interests and equitable geographical distribution'.[142]

Our concern, instead, is with long-term preservation, not with the present distribution of the economic benefits of the global commons. The distributive approach, as Cheng points out, permits the use of the patrimony of mankind as a 'cesspool', hardly appropriate to the Common Heritage of Mankind.[143] Even with its weaknesses, it would have been highly desirable to retain the use of the principle, beyond open space, the moon, and the deep seabed.[144] The Antarctic Treaty System (1991) protects the area and the related ecosystems 'in the interest of mankind as a whole' (1991 Protocol to the *Antarctic Treaty on Environmental Protection,* Preamble); and our most obvious common heritage, the air we breathe, has not been so designated; rather the 'global climate' has been referred to as a 'common concern'. In other environmentally related Preambles, the expression used is 'world heritage of mankind' (*Convention for the Protection of World Cultural and Natural Heritage,* 1972).[145]

In contrast, referring to any aspect of the commons as a 'property resource' eliminates the requirement of respect and preservation and substitutes an approach that only requires 'fairness of allocation procedures'. The latter will not support ecojustice as the combination of intragenerational and intergenerational justice, and replaces it with an approach that retains an economic/procedural flavour, as 'maintaining quality, allocating capacity, and controlling access'.[146] I have argued that we are facing the 'final enclosure movement', as the tragedy of the commons reaches its final stage.[147]

To propose, as Wood does, 'stable institutions [that] include equitable arrangements, efficiency, assumed expectations through compliance monitoring and graduated sanctions',[148] misunderstands both the nature and the gravity of the situation. It is not only a matter of slowing down the inevitable elimination of the resource base by procedural fairness and 'assurance games'.[149] It is rather a question of viewing the Earth not only as property to be divided and exploited, even when fairness is employed , but to consider it as comprised of natural systems whose integrity and support is essential to our survival present and future.[150]

The protection of ecosystemic function supports our own natural function as the WHO has indicated[151] both in the present and in the future, starting with the first generation.[152]

INTRAGENERATIONAL AND INTERGENERATIONAL EQUITY: ECOJUSTICE FOR THE FIRST AND DISTANT GENERATIONS

This we know: the earth does not belong to man: man belongs to the earth... Whatever befalls the earth, befalls the sons of the earth. Man did not weave the web of life: he is merely a strand in it. Whatever he does to the web, he does to himself (Chief Seattle, patriarch of The Duwamish and Squamish Indians of Puget Sound, to US President Franklin Pierce, 1855)

This is indeed the position of today's ecology, and of biocentric and ecocentric environmental ethics, from Aldo Leopold on.[153] There are both scientific and moral reasons to support the need for ecojustice, or equity that respects the present as well as the future. From the scientific point of view, the unpredictability of future events, based on recent chaos theory research, ensures that any prediction that makes claims to certainty and accuracy, is most likely incoherent and false.[154] Scientific uncertainty is an accepted paradigm today, but even the use of the precautionary principle is, in some sense, insufficient, as it promotes the idea that we are not sure whether ecological or biological harm will follow certain practices or activities. In contrast, what might be uncertain or imprecise, might be the specific form the expected harm will have, not its occurrence. In this sense, it might be like saying that the recent outcry for devices capable of predicting the occurrence of a tsunami (such as the one that devastated Indonesia, Sri Lanka and Thailand on 26 December 2004), should not be put in place, because such devices cannot predict exactly the number of victims for each affected country, or the precise amount of economic damage we can expect.

The precautionary principle proposes that we should err on the side of caution, because we are not sure. But many of the harms resulting from ecological/biological disintegrity are well, if not precisely, known and expected.[155] The problem is not lack of knowledge, but a combination of inevitable partiality for short-term gain, and for visible immediate advantages, particularly economic ones, over both precaution and long-term safety; and the consumerist/capitalist thrust of corporate activities, protected as they are by the possession of unreasonable 'rights' and 'freedoms' against the undefended rights of vulnerable peoples and populations to survive unharmed.

That is why such soft law instruments as the *Earth Charter* are widely praised and welcomed in the developing worlds, but they are viewed with suspicion and distrust by wealthy, affluent countries, although the latter are the ones most in need of its principles of respect for all generations, and for the integrity of the Earth. Morally speaking, Brown-Weiss is certainly correct as she affirms:

> *As part of the natural system, we have no right to destroy its integrity; nor is it in our interest to do so. Rather, as the most sentient of living creatures, we have a special responsibility to care for the planet.*[156]

The combination of up-to-date science and moral belief, culminates in some of the legal instruments we have cited earlier. The 'right' sentiments are often expressed in Preambles and such, but the quest for true equity escapes: economic interests, noted in the previous chapter, tend to block normative considerations. Thus harmful exposures destroy the lives and decimate the healthy functioning of the first generation, while the harmful substances continue to accumulate to wreak a worse havoc on the future.

A link between first and future generations can also be found in the economic concerns found in most families.[157] At least two common approaches found in families favour the future: first, the accumulation of wealth on the part of many parents in consideration of future needs of their children, is useful, 'Both as insurance for the parents, and an inheritance for the children'; second, the motive to secure a better future for the children, prompts parents to reduce spending in favour of saving: 'the bequest motive thus tends to defer consumption and promote investment'.[158]

This example illustrates some of the consequences of the serious concern for the future we may find in parents, but it is probably not readily present in the general population in relation to our own collective future offspring. Both the desire not to waste, but to respect (ecological) wealth, and to curb consumption of (natural) resources, would provide an excellent basis for the intergenerational equity we are seeking to promote. The aspect of respect is certainly present in the beliefs and attitudes of aboriginal peoples, including the First Nation peoples of Canada, and most African peoples.[159,160]

Respect, in turn, may well breed concern and even distaste for overconsumption, when the consequences that will surely follow are clearly understood. But neither respect nor restraint may be left to spring up naturally in the heart and the thoughts of all people, although both are natural and expected when our own future (first) generation is under consideration. That benevolence must be legislated and enforced, if we ourselves and our future are to be protected and if equity is to be required.

CONCLUSION

In his important 'Dissenting Opinion', Judge Christopher Weeramantry discusses equity in detail.[161] Perhaps most important in the long and thorough analysis provided in 'Opinion', Weeramantry says: 'in the context of sharing of natural resources … equity is playing an increasingly important international role'.[162] Equity, as Weeramantry explains it, is far more than procedural fairness It may be used by the courts as 'rationale' to reach a decision when faced by facts that may not have been considered before in the Court's jurisprudence;[163] but equity, as Judge Jimenez de Arechaga affirms, cannot be used to reach a 'capricious' decision, but must exhibit 'reasonableness' in the light of individual circumstances';[164] it can be used in the sense of 'applying distributive justice and redistribution of wealth';[165] equity considerations permit, and in fact mandate, the consideration of the ensuing results of a judicial decision. Finally, it is intended:

> *to render justice through the rigid application of general rules and principles of formal legal concepts, but though an adaptation and adjustment of such principles, rules and concepts to the facts, realities and circumstances of each case'*[166]

Thus the arguments purporting to prove that no full knowledge or precision is available to direct and inform our thinking when seeking a just approach to all future generations, fail. Equity itself may be brought in as the necessary corrective, through its role in 'tempering the application of strict rules'.[167] Weeramantry cites Aristotle in the Nichomachean Ethics in support of his position:

> *The reason for this is that law is always a general statement, yet there are cases which it is not possible to cover in a general statement.... This is the essential nature of the equitable: it is the rectification of law where law is defective because of its generality.*[168]

But the judicial leeway and flexibility here indicated show that judicial discretion (c) can only be applied 'through the choice of an equitable principle'.[169]

We noted that not only some of the causes of the harms to which all future generations are exposed, from the first one onward, are similar, but also that the reasons why these exposures are not yet clearly proscribed in the law have similar roots. They include the belief in absolute freedom as paramount for both individuals and legal persons, and the pre-eminence of the economic motive, the so-called 'sovereignty' of the consumer.

It is hard, in fact almost impossible, to restrain freedom and preference satisfaction even in the name of intragenerational equity; it is much harder to do so for inter-generational motives. Nevertheless it should be possible to do so, as Weeramantry's 'dissent' suggests, because many 'principles of equity' are already embedded in the law:

> *Many principles of equity such an unjust enrichment, good faith, contractual fairness and the use of one's property so as not to cause damage to others are already embedded in positive law. In the field of international law, the position is the same.*[170]

The appropriate use of equity, in fact, starts with assessing which facts and circumstances must be considered.[171] The existence of the harms befalling the future from present practices, it seems clear, cannot and should not be excluded from any consideration used to reach an equitable position regarding those practices.

In the next chapter, some of these practices will be examined through a discussion of cases of corporate criminality that easily demonstrate the extent, the reach and the basic injustice of ecofootprint harm.

NOTES

1   *Minors Oposa v. Secretary of the Department of Environment and Rural Resources*, 33 I.L.M. 173 (1994), Davide, J. R.J., p200.
2   Barresi (1997), p10.
3   Barresi (1997).
4   Wackernagel and Rees (1996).
5   33 I.L.M. 173 (1994).
6   *Farooque v. Government of Bangladesh* (1997) 49 DLR (AD) 1.
7   Brown-Weiss (1990), p199.
8   Brown-Weiss (1992).
9   D'Amato (1990), p190.
10 Brown-Weiss (1990), p198.
11 Brown-Weiss (1993), p333.
12 Barresi (1997), p2.
13 Barresi (1997), p2.
14 Westra (2004a), chapter 7.
15 Guha (1989), pp312–319.
16 McMichael (1995a).
17 McMichael (2000).
18 Karr and Chu (1995), pp34–48.
19 Westra (1998).
20 Soskolne and Bertollini (1999).
21 Westra (1998, 2004a).
22 Barresi (1997), p3.
23 Barresi (1997), p3.
24 *Code Napoleon*, cited in Ross (1958), p246.
25 Ross (1958), 106–107.
26 Ross (1958), p268.
27 Velasquez (2000), chapter 2.
28 Rawls (1971).
29 Rawls (1971).
30 Grotius (1625).
31 Cited in Ross (1958), p246.
32 Westra (2004a), chapter 1.
33 Westra (2004a), chapter 1.
34 O'Neill (1996); Pogge (2001a).
35 *Rome Declaration on World Food Security*, www.fao.org/wts/policy/english/96-eng.html
36 *Rome Declaration on World Food Security*, at p10.
37 *Rome Declaration on World Food Security*, at p11.
38 World Bank (1999), p25.
39 Pogge (2001a), p14.
40 Falk (1998), p4.
41 Falk (1998), p14.
42 Falk (1998), p28.
43 Falk (1998), p26.
44 Visser 't Hooft (1999), pp55–56.
45 Visser 't Hooft (1999), p54; Hart (1961).
46 Birnie and Boyle (2002), p604.
47 Birnie and Boyle (2002), p604.

48   Birnie and Boyle (2002), p605.
49   Rees (2000), pp139–156.
50   De George (1981).
51   Partridge (1990), pp40–66.
52   Westra (1998).
53   Parfit (1984).
54   Daily (1997) pp3–4.
55   Visser 't Hooft (1999), p17.
56   Wood (1996), pp293–307.
57   Visser 't Hooft (1999), p54.
58   Pimentel et al (2000).
59   Westra (1994, 1998).
60   Bosselmann (1999), p30.
61   Bosselmann (1999), p31.
62   Bosselmann (1999), p31.
63   Westra and Lawson (2001).
64   Gbadegesin (2001), pp187–202.
65   Bosselmann (1999), p34.
66   Westra (1994).
67   Westra (1998).
68   Norton (1995).
69   Soskolne and Bertollini (1999).
70   Bosselmann (1999), p37; citing Brenda Almond.
71   Bosselmann (1999), p39.
72   De George (1981).
73   Farber (2003), p289; Farber suggests that discounting is unavoidable, but he proposes 'the perpetuation value of environmental resources and the use of Hyperbolic discounting where the discount rate itself declines over time'.
74   Blackstock and Trocme (2004), Table 4.
75   Tamburlini et al (2002).
76   Sinclair et al (2004), chapter 7.
77   Sinclair et al (2004), p202.
78   *Report of the Aboriginal Justice Inquiry of Manitoba: The Justice System and Aboriginal People*, 1991, Province of Manitoba, Winnipeg.
79   *Report of the Aboriginal Justice Inquiry of Manitoba.*
80   Blackstock and Trocme (2004).
81   Human Resources Development, Canada, *Child Welfare in Canada* – 2000.
82   Ottawa (2002) www.hrdc.gc.ca/sp-ps/socialp-psociale/cfs/rpt2000/rpt 2000e_toc.shmtl
83   Bala (2004), p17.
84   *Child and Family Services Act*, s.1(a), as amended S.O. 1999, c.6.
85   *Child, Family and Community Services Act*, R.S.B.C. 1996, c.46, s.2(a) and 4(1).
86   Ottawa (2002).
87   Bala et al (2004), p18.
88   Tamburlini et al (2002).
89   *R.B. v. Children's Aid Society of Metro Toronto* [1995] 1 S.C.R. 315.
90   Hirsch (1999), p7.
91   Westra (2004a).
92   Hoffman (2003), p280.
93   Hoffman (2003), p280.
94   Westra (2004a), chapter 7.
95   Westra (2004b), chapter 1.

 96 Aron and Patz (2001).
 97 Soskolne and Bertollini (1999).
 98 McMichael (1995a).
 99 McMichael (2000).
100 Wood (1996), p305.
101 Koskenniemi (1992), pp123–128.
102 Westra (2004a), chapter 7.
103 Shue (1996a).
104 Brown-Weiss, as cited in Barresi (1997), p64.
105 *Protocol to the Framework Convention on Climate Change (Kyoto)*, 37 I.L.M. (1998), 22.
106 Wood (1996), pp296–297.
107 Wood (1996), p303.
108 Brown-Weiss (1988), pp540–544.
109 D'Amato (1990), p198.
110 As Brown-Weiss remarks (1992, p25), 'Future generations are not effectively represented in the marketplace today'.
111 Brown-Weiss (1992), p25.
112 Brown-Weiss (1992), p26.
113 *Universal Declaration of Human Rights*, pmbl., G.A. Res. 217, U.N.GAOR, 3d Sess., at 71, U.N.Doc. A/810 (1948).
114 Brown-Weiss (1992), p21.
115 Cassese (1996), p376.
116 Cassese (1996), p31.
117 Cassese (1996), p31.
118 Cassese (1996), p123.
119 Cassese (1996), p123.
120 Cassese (1996), p176.
121 Cassese (1996), p176
122 Cassese (1996), p177.
123 Cassese (1996), p178; Vienna Conference, Official Records, para.48.
124 Cassese (1996), p189.
125 Birnie and Boyle (1992), p118; see also Birnie and Boyle (2002), pp97–100.
126 Larschan and Brennan (1983), pp305–337.
127 Goedhuis (1981), pp218–219.
128 Daily (1997).
129 Westra et al (2000), chapter 1.
130 Larschan and Brennan (1983), p306.
131 Larschan and Brennan (1983), p310.
132 Noss (1992).
133 Westra (1994).
134 Ulanowicz (1995).
135 Daily (1997).
136 *Black's Law Dictionary* (1979), p1173.
137 *UK v. Iceland*, 1973 I.C.J. Rep. 3.
138 *UK v. Iceland*, p97.
139 Westra (1998).
140 Cheng (1980), p337.
141 Larschan and Brennan (1983), p323.
142 Larschan and Brennan (1983), p322.
143 Cheng (1980), p337.
144 Birnie and Boyle (2002), pp97–100.

145 Birnie and Boyle (2002), pp97–100.

146 Wood (1996), p307.

147 Westra (2004a), pp107–120.

148 Wood (1996), p311.

149 Wood (1996), pp312–313.

150 Westra (1998); see also Rockefeller (2002), ppx–xiv.

151 Soskolne and Bertollini (1999).

152 Tamburlini et al (2002).

153 Leopold (1949); Westra (1994, 1998); Sterba (1998); Ulanowicz (1995, 2000); Noss (1992).

154 Goerner (1994).

155 See for instance the research of the WHO in Tamburlini et al (2002), and in Soskolne and Bertollini (1999).

156 Brown-Weiss (1990), pp198, 199.

157 Epstein (1989), p1465.

158 Epstein (1989), pp1472–73.

159 Adams (1995), p181.

160 Oke (2005).

161 *Maritime Delimitation in the Area Between Greenland and Jan Mayer* (Denmark v. Norway) 1993 I.C.J. 38.

162 *Gabcikovo-Nagymaros* (1997) ICJ, Rep.7, Judge C. Weeramantry, separate opinion, p118(d).

163 *Gabcikovo-Nagymaros* (1997) (see note 169), p114.

164 *Gabcikovo-Nagymaros* (1997) (see note 169), p115.

165 *Gabcikovo-Nagymaros* (1997) (see note 169), p121.

166 *Gabcikovo-Nagymaros* (1997) (see note 169), p124, citing Judge Jimenez de Arechaga, paras.71 and 107.

167 *Gabcikovo-Nagymaros* (1997) (see note 169),(c).

168 *Gabcikovo-Nagymaros* (1997) (see note 169), p133.

169 *Gabcikovo-Nagymaros* (1997) (see note 169), p135(d).

170 *Gabcikovo-Nagymaros* (1997) (see note 169), (h) C 115.

171 *Gabcikovo-Nagymaros* (1997) (see note 169), (c) C 151.

CHAPTER 7

Ecojustice and Consideration for the Future: The Persistence of Ecofootprint Disasters

INTRODUCTION

In the last chapter we showed the connection between intra- and intergenerational justice, culminating in the concept of ecojustice. Ecojustice joins first generations with the remote future. Ajar Malhotra also argues, as this work does, for the unavoidable interface between the rights of the child and those of the future, as he outlines three major points, two of which are cited here below:

> *Firstly, many legal systems on the material plane do provide for laws of inheritance that accept persons not yet born as being beneficiaries. Secondly, while the similarity between future generations, which do not yet exist, with those existing but legally incompetent is certainly arguable, legal systems do confer rights on human beings who are incapable of regarding themselves as bearers of rights, for instance infants and those severely mentally disabled.*[1,2]

The third point refers to the language of the *UN Convention on the Rights of the Child*, as he comments on the setting of an upper limit to the definition of the child, while the convention 'deliberately avoids setting a floor'[3] as was noted above as well.

There is no question that 'future generations' are also never clearly or precisely defined, thus allowing the connecting inclusivity here proposed between the first generation and the future. If this inclusion is basic to true ecojustice, then we need to view all possible obstacles under this joint perspective. Obstacles to the rights to health and environment of the child, such as the ones we observed through the scientific research, both medical and epidemiological, are not only similar to the obstacles to future rights: the obstacles to the safety and security of both classes appears to be very close, and based on the same issues in many cases.

Identifying joint obstacles, or at least similar foundations for the difficulties in both cases, represents a first step before possible remedies might be identified. In the next section we will return once again to consumerism, to try to elucidate these connected obstacles in the path of protecting whole classes of endangered humanity.

CONSUMERISM AND THE RIGHTS OF THE FUTURE: THE CASE OF THE 'VULNERABLE CONSUMER'

An environmental justice critique of trade liberalization also suggests that it is import-
ant to focus on local environmental struggles in order to understand the precise social
and economic forces that promote environmental degradation and social injustice
and to develop effective policy responses. Top-down solutions driven by the North's
environmental and economic agenda exacerbate environmental injustice by reinforcing
Northern economic and political dominance, and by failing to take into account the
needs and priorities of those most affected by environmental degradation.[4]

In Chapter 5 we noted the powerful role of neo-liberalism with regard to rights and responsibilities; we even saw that influence on the social considerations that inform decisions in the jurisprudence and case law both civil and common.

Neo-liberalism views all people as individuals intent upon satisfying their preferences and asserting their interests, hence being primarily consumers rather than citizens of a country.[5] By collapsing two distinct and often contradictory aspects of human life with all its aspirations, into one single aspect based on economic characteristics, this approach reduces human life to the pursuit of the one activity that serves to support corporate profit-making, whether domestic or transnational.

But transnational capitalism is the basis of neo-liberal globalization. In turn, as we noted, it depends on consumers to keep on buying the array of products and services that are marketed to ensure economic growth, without any consideration of its extensive negative impacts.

The main tool of a capitalism economy is advertising. Marketing strategies are carefully researched, not only to inform but, and primarily, to influence, persuade and manipulate. There are some groups for whom the barrage of advertising to which the media exposes all of us, is particularly deleterious. Michael Schudson explains, as he outlines:

> *five groups whose situational or structural ignorance makes them unusually vulnerable*
> *to advertising: highly mobile people, immobile people, children, the poor, and many of*
> *the relatively poor and poorly educated people in the Third World.*[6]

Among these most vulnerable groups, the present poor and the people of the developing world represent the intragenerational aspect of vulnerability based on 'situations' that prevent a critical appreciation of marketing. Poverty and the lack of education combine to ensure their lack of mobility, and render diminished or absent their ability to make informed, rational choices.

In addition, the poor in developed and developing countries tend to see their aspirations embodied in the least desirable Western icons, such as cola drinks, or Macmeals, for instance. These are choices that do not nourish, hence they do not represent rational choices especially for those whose resources are severely limited.

The intergenerational aspect of vulnerability is present in the children, born and unborn, who are 'structurally' ignorant, and unable to reason about possible choices, express their wishes, or otherwise represent their interests. Their 'structural' and 'situational' position is even worse during the most vulnerable period of their development, in the early part of pregnancies. At that time, they are totally unprotected and exposed to the effects of both advertising and marketing on their 'habitat' thus on the choices, informed or not, by the person most intimately responsible for their health, their mother.

Poor mothers in developing countries are among the most vulnerable and the best known example of that vulnerability, in the case of Nestlé's infant formula. Third World mothers were convinced by various means, by both advertising and marketing ploys, including the hiring of 'milk nurses' who served in Third World hospitals and clinics as well as maternity centres.[7] The 'nurses' role was to convince mothers to try the 'better', Western way: feeding babies formula that (a) they could not afford to use at full strength, for optimal nutrition; and (b) had to be mixed with water that was, for most part, unsafe for consumption. The result of these circumstances was death by malnutrition or infection of a great number of babies.

The basic cause of these deaths was the corporate motive and the marketing techniques employed. We can therefore conclude that the vulnerability of the groups named, especially those exposed to activities contrary to intragenerational and inter-generational justice, must be recognized in law, perhaps through the presence of an ombudsman or a guardian *ad litem*, and we will return to this proposal below.

That said, advertising and marketing are products of the general obsessive consumerism that characterizes present Western lifestyles, and we will return to that topic in the next section.

Consumerism, public health and public policy

> *Consumption-induced environmental damage remains pervasive, and we are in the midst of widespread failures of public provisions.*[8]

In Chapter 5 we noted the particular relation between US values and beliefs and consumerism, a relation that far exceeds similar relations in other Western countries. From the 1960s and 1970s and from the time of the critique of John Kenneth Galbraith, the American 'consumer culture' has been critiqued by many:

> *They argued that Americans had been manipulated into participating in a dumbed-down artificial consumer culture, which yielded few true human satisfactions.*[9]

But the whole social environment has changed dramatically since those times, and not for the better. The idea of 'neighbourhood' and the standards that underscored the earlier concept of 'keeping up with the Jones', were based then on the ideal present in an almost homogenous group. Within this group, some effort was made to 'belong', even to exceed social standards, perhaps, but these efforts were always kept within specific limits.

Now, in contrast, few if any limits are accepted. The new concept that prevails is that of 'competitive consumption', starting with the 'redefinition of reference groups'. Constant mobility, lack of neighbourhood roots and so on, while media representations of the 'good life' foster an endless desire for ongoing 'betterment', are also promoted by media and various marketing techniques. They have promoted a form of consumerism that is essentially new. The 'social context of consumption' entails that now, more than ever, you are what you consume. Unlike the standard provided by the mythical 'Jones', however, the goal is now intrinsically elusive, a constantly 'moving target', as 'income adequacy' becomes a social construct rather than a reality, as those earning around $100,000 believe, just like those with half that income, that they cannot afford to buy all they need:

> *But 85% of the population cannot earn the six figure incomes necessary to support upper middle class aspirations. The result is a growing aspirational gap: with desires persistently outrunning incomes, many consumers find themselves frustrated.*[10]

Thus 'competitive consumption', the need to 'keep up' through conspicuous status goods, is a new and highly dangerous aspect of consumerism, as 'luxury rather than mere comfort, is a wide-spread aspiration' today.[11]

The neo-liberal political climate in Western countries fosters and promotes these self-defeating aspirations. More and more work is also needed to support more and more spending, allowing less and less time for living in the style to which one is aspiring. The promotion and marketing of shopping itself as a desirable leisure-time activity, supports the goals of capitalism and the aims of the wealthiest corporate individuals, but frustrates the aims of the average persons who are, essentially, more than just 'consumers'.[12]

Not only are North American goals self-defeating, however, they are basically immoral, as the mantra of 'more' in the West, is juxtaposed to the reality of poverty for the great majority of their own citizens and the starvation and disease fostered by poverty, and prevalent in the South-East. These goals are self-defeating in the most basic way, as a lifestyle devoted to the accumulation of 'stuff' is as void of real satisfaction as it is unhealthy. It parallels the fast food industry's larger and larger portions, leading to a host of Western men's diseases, starting with obesity, an epidemic as Albritton rightly saw.[13] In addition, the ongoing quest to 'acquire' indicates the presence of constant tension and malaise, thus aggravating the spread of disease.

Finally, and most importantly from our point of view, the protection of 'public goods', such as the environment, are neglected in favour of the ongoing need for more and more growth of 'private goods', that is, the growth of the income and profits of the corporate elites. Such ongoing institutionalized harms as the exploitation of workers (including children) in developing countries, the deliberate neglect of serious measures to halt and reverse climate change, and the continued promotion of chemicals, pesticides and all manner of hazardous substances, represent some of the gravest aspects of today's consumerism. The foundations of all these practices and activities is the neo-liberal belief in the primacy of freedom over any other rights, as we saw earlier in the discussion of Raz's work (see Chapter 5) in the context of the right of the child to health.

Like the rights of the future, the rights of the first generation are deeply and inescapably embedded in ensuring that clear limits are enacted to the proliferation of consumerism. Schor herself proposes the need for a collective response, in addition to the numerous individual responses on the part of those who are rebelling against the prevailing consumerist trend. No doubt, such limits would not be welcomed either by corporate supported politicians, or by those who – predictably – continue to respond to the 'cultural environment' in which they are embedded, by embracing wholeheartedly the unattainable quest for the 'good life' of competitive consumerism.[14]

The need for radical changes is clear. Whether anyone might be ready to join in a collective acceptance of our responsibility for an irrational present and a blighted future, is in doubt at this time. The story of the frog, eventually boiling to her death, because of her lack of reaction to earlier lukewarm to warm conditions, appears to be particularly appropriate. We have passed 'lukewarm' conditions a long time ago, and are reaching closer and closer to the boiling point. But those who have the power to make changes, also possess the means to mitigate the harsh effects unavoidable by those who are not protected by their wealth. It is undeniable that action must be taken in the quest for ecojustice. I have argued that criminalizing some of these activities might be helpful,[15] and in the next section we will consider some of the most glaring environmental cases.

ECOLOGICAL FOOTPRINT AND ECOCRIME: THE INTERFACE

It is the overconsumption of the North that poses the greatest threat to the global environment, while the environmental costs go to the South. Environmental law has traditionally emphasized pollution control and protection of national resources while ignoring the ultimate cause of pollution and resource degradation: the problem of overconsumption and a remarkable dearth of legal scholarship on the issue.[16]

The connection between present and future people, and between neo-liberal globalization with its emphasis on trade and consumerism, and public health, is here made explicit, and the work of William Rees[17] and others, as well as my own work, emphasizes the same point.[18]

It took several acknowledged disasters, from Bhopal, India, to Seveso, Italy, and many others, to prompt the emergence of laws that mandate practices that protect exposed populations, rather than corporate practices: the best known of these regulatory instruments in the *Seveso II Directive*.[19] Of course not all disasters based on ecofootprint come to the courts and are acknowledged as 'cases', at least as torts, if not crimes. The ecodisaster in Ogoniland, Nigeria, for instance, is only recently getting a proper hearing in the New York Courts,[20,21,22] and the disaster at Walkerton, Ontario, Canada, has been treated as a failure of administrative law, at best. We can return to these cases below. For now, it might be best to start by considering the Seveso case. The case is based on an accident that occurred at a Hoffman-LaRoche plant, 'which led to a large release of dioxin, that contaminated surrounding areas and caused substantial alarm over future health consequences of exposed persons'.[23]

We will return to the details of the *Seveso Directive* in the next section. The main point here is that, even in the face of terrible multi-generational health damages, as we shall see, chemical companies' 'trade secrets' are still protected and they continue to rank above the citizens' right to know, but also, above the right to life and health. Nor was the Seveso disaster the only one of its kind. On 2 December 1984, 'A toxic gas called methyl isocynate escaped from an underground storage tank of a fertilizer plant ... in the city of Bhopal, India'. This plant was owned and operated by Union Carbide India, Ltd., a subsidiary of Union Carbide Corporation of the United States. The gas quickly spread over an area of 25 square miles, resulting in 1800 deaths and affecting over 200,000 more people. The latest death total has been calculated at 4200 people.[24]

The substantive scholarly literature available on the Bhopal tragedy, pinpoints the importance of the connection between transfers of technology and, in general, trade, and the harm perpetrated upon developing countries on one hand, and the lack of corporate restraints, on the other.[25,26] Sudhir Chopra emphasizes the role of transnational corporations (TNCs), the 'true culprit of the cost/benefit approach', who are willing to export cheaper technology especially when it is no longer allowed in the home country. Of course the complicity of the accepting governments is also required for these transfers to happen, and it is most often present, because of the desirability of importing cheaper technologies and to provide new jobs.[27] The imposition of unacceptable harms is the main component of the oppression that characterizes the ecofootprint of the North–West.

Appeals to the Code of Conduct for TNCs are insufficient for several reasons.[28,29] First is the problem of an international law that does not always supersede municipal or domestic instruments, hence a gap exists even today that has not been bridged in the intervening years. Second, there is no 'enforceable legal framework' to deal with the transfer of harms arising from Western ecological footprint practices. Finally:

> *A binding dispute settlement mechanism is also needed either in the form of a 'Court of Arbitration', or a more innovative 'international corporate dispute settlement court'. Another option would be to change the current structure and jurisdiction of the International Court of Justice so that it could rule on the cases involving transnational business activity.*[30]

I have proposed a similar approach in my recent work,[31] as I have argued there is little difference in the results of political conflicts resulting in genocide and crimes against humanity, and the corresponding results of corporate crime, absent perhaps the political motivation, while the basic economic intent remains present as it often is, in both cases. Another possibility, though equally remote at this time, would be to modify the 'structure and jurisdiction' of the International Criminal Court, for similar reasons.

Nor is the Bhopal case unique, or the only location where similar circumstances have existed, although in some cases state responsibility plays a determinant role, and in others, it is the TNCs that bear most of the responsibility for the disasters that occurred. In the following sections we will examine some of these examples of the imposing of harms, coupled with almost total disregard for ecojustice.

Ecofootprint crimes: Seveso and the *Seveso Directive*

> *While Chernobyl and Sandoz are textbook examples of State responsibility cases, Bhopal and Seveso are not. In the latter cases, new laws were created judicially or*

legislatively to address the problem. However these laws are very limited in scope. They neither address the causes of such accidents, nor satisfy the aspirations and desires of the victims.[32]

Chopra is absolutely correct: in no case are the causes we have discussed, as producing the resulting present and future harms, addressed in these regulations. We pointed to globalization, the primacy of trade over human rights, the capitalist-driven neo-liberal agenda, and the rampant consumerism engendered by it, as giving rise to the policies and practices that show no respect or consideration for present or future justice. A brief look at these cases will help to emphasize the role played by the policies we believe are causative of these disasters. The cases and the related regulatory regimes will emphasize how limited and incomplete are the policies intended to eliminate these disasters.

The first of the major known disasters is precisely the one in Seveso/Meda, in North Italy, near Milan, at a Giveaudan Corporation subsidiary of Swiss Hoffman-LaRoche. The accident was caused by malfunctioning safety equipment, which released dioxin, a toxic gas. It caused ecological damage that spread well beyond the immediate surroundings of the plant and, although the legal literature simply reports that 'no death occurred',[33] the intergenerational harms continued long after the time of exposure, as women who were pregnant at the time of the spill, or who became subsequently pregnant while living in the area, gave birth to severely deformed or handicapped children with malformations ranging from having only one eye, to a body so contorted that their normal motion and function would never be restored.

The first thing to note is that there are a number of organizations and institutions responsible for the safe production, use and transport as well as disposal of hazardous substances produced by industrial activities. In addition:

> *For some product risks, government may be culpable because it reviewed the hazardous product but allowed it to be sold without adequate warnings or for inappropriate uses. Government may also be culpable if it required the product to be used, as in the case of asbestos insulation installed in ships and public buildings.*[34]

Baran also notes that the whole life cycle of many of these substances is hazardous, hence not only 'primary producers (and importers); [but] intermediate producers, end-user firms, transporters of substances and associated wastes, and waste-disposal firms' and, last but not least 'individual consumers' might be held responsible.[35,36]

But, although Seveso II (1996), or the latest iteration of the *Seveso Directive* attempts to strengthen measures intended to better prepare for all industrial health/ environment related accidents, even the present measures are insufficient, although they are intended to be harmonized with individual States' regulatory instruments. There have been advances in protection, as at this time all forms of mining-related activity and the industrial use of potassium nitrate are included in the directive to prevent industrial accidents such as Seveso, and some subsequent ones, for instance Baia Mare, Toulouse and Asnacollar, from ever happening again.[37]

Not only are specific problems of industrial activities still not addressed but, from our point of view, the major difficulty is not even discussed: the very existence of these substances. A dog may bite once or twice at the most, but then, despite the fact that both bites could be considered accidents, not deliberately imposed harms, the dog is ordered to be killed. How many 'bites' is the chemical industry permitted, before if not its existence, at least its production is designated as illegal? It is instructive to consider the language of the *Seveso II Directive*:

> *Definitions*
> *Article 3.4. 'dangerous substance' shall mean a substance, mixture or preparation listed in Annex 1, Part 1, or fulfilling the criteria laid down in Annex 1, Part 2 ...*
> *Article 3.6. 'hazard' shall mean the intrinsic property of a dangerous substance or physical situation with a potential for creating damage to human health and/or the environment.*

The question that arises is why these 'substances', intrinsically hazardous though they are, are not prohibited, and why corporations are not required to research safe substitutes instead.

The increasing strictness with which the directive treats these hazards, indicates that the risk of harm they impose goes well beyond the possibility of a disastrous accident. In fact, the directive's 'Aim' should be amended accordingly:

> *Article 1*
> *Aim*
> *The directive is aimed at the prevention of major accidents which involve dangerous substances and the limitation of their consequences for man and the environment, with a view to ensuring high levels of protection through the Community in a consistent and effective manner.*

Noteworthy is the expression 'limitation of their consequences', thus the implicit acceptance of the presence of some consequences despite the presence of the directive. This is the pernicious connection between the ecofootprint of the industrial West, and the affected populations, present and future, given that these substances' consequences for health and the environment are not limited, either geographically or temporally. Moreover, even the original aim here presented, that is the prevention of future industrial disasters, was clearly not achieved, although most countries either 'harmonized' their laws with *Seveso II Directive*, or at least used it to frame their own regulatory regimes. Baran, however, states:

> *The Seveso Directive requirements are being implemented most smoothly in countries that already have relatively well-developed public rights of access to environmental information, such as West Germany and the Netherlands.*[38]

France, the UK and other countries take a stronger view on the protection of trade secrets and other pertinent information regarding these substances, their manufacture, production and their related processing in industrial operations.[39] The insufficiency of the Seveso approach will be demonstrated by the other well-known disasters that followed, despite the clear alarm provided by the Seveso disaster.

Ecofootprint crimes: Bhopal and Chernobyl

The tragedy of Bhopal is long gone from the minds of the Western public. The commercial charisma that the news carried for some time is all but dead. However the victims of this accident continue to suffer and will endure further suffering for decades to come.[40]

Bhopal, unlike Seveso, demonstrates the absolute injustice of TNC operations in developing countries, where even the weak regulatory instruments that protect citizens from industrial harms in the West, are not in place. (See note 24, for a repeat of the well-known facts.) But what is less commonly known is that in India, at the time of Bhopal, the courts did not even apply strict liability rules, but preferred to apply negligence theory instead.[41] In addition, the court's efforts to ensure that the US should be made responsible for the damages appear to be motivated more by the desire to shield Indian Government-owned insurers from harm, than by the duty to protect the victims.[42]

Eventually, the cooperation of two countries, India and the US, combined to acknowledge the harms that had been perpetrated on a vulnerable population, and the torts were 'compensated'. This approach, however, excludes (a) the consideration of the criminality of Union Carbide's actions and – particularly, of its omissions such as the lack of information given to workers and their families, and the lack of safety measures; and (b) the institution of serious limits to what can legally be produced and marketed.

The aggravating circumstances are based on the political implications of 'eco-imperialism' of a hegemonic power that simply does not consider human rights to be primary. Like all environmental disasters, the harms that follow are not limited in either time or space. Also, like all environmental disasters, its roots lie in the policies that privilege trade over life and health, and the 'rights' and 'freedoms' of natural and corporate individuals over the common interest and the public good.

In this case, unlike Seveso, the issue of 'eco-imperialism' is strongly in evidence.[43] Chopra proposes a 'grotioan innovationism' to replace the present piecemeal 'grooming' of existing laws that are, at this time, incapable of restraining the inequality between industrial advances and social progress.[44,45]

In contrast, the Chernobyl accident (26 April 1986) involves quite different factual components. For instance, no multinational corporate actor was involved in this case. Yet, the Chernobyl accident 'was the worst nuclear chemical explosion resulting from meltdown of one of the four reactors in the nuclear plant, killing thirty-one workers and causing acute radiation problems for several hundreds more'.[46] In this case, however, as in Seveso, the resulting harms are not limited in either time or space, although most of the existing literature on the topic emphasizes the geographical spread of the hazards, not their intergenerational aspects.[47]

Aside from Internal Corporate Responsibility for the management of the facility, the 'long-term radiation pollution' was responsible for health effects long after the accident. These effects included harms to women, unborn children and infants, as well as severe damage to the ecology. Undeniably, it was a case of failure to protect on the part of the state. The classic Trail Smelter Arbitration[48,49] demonstrates how transboundary harms should be handled.[50]

Yet, despite its obvious responsibility (then) Soviet Russia refused to offer compensation for the extensive crop damage that occurred almost everywhere in Europe, and did not offer redress even to those facing health damages. The very notion of transferring the burden of proof to those affected presently, and to those in the future, including first generation individuals, is inherently unjust. Similar intragenerational injustices are present in racist practices in North America, especially in the US, as Robert Bullard has suggested.[51] Similarly, the practice of expecting the victims to mount their own defence, and demonstrate the harms they have suffered in a court of law, is one of the greatest obstacles to environmental justice in domestic law.[52]

This difficulty becomes even more acute when the victims of hazardous activities are infants, children or even the unborn at the time when the damaging exposure occurred, or women, who would experience reproductive harms in the future, or men, whose sperm count would be negatively affected. All these harms are so serious that preventive regulatory regimes should have been employed, although the powerful nuclear and chemical industries' presence at international conferences and pressures at the level of government regulatory activities, have made such advances impossible so far.

Ecofootprint crime: Sandoz-Basel, Switzerland

The Sandoz case is, in many ways, quite different from either Bhopal or Chernobyl, as it involves only developed countries within Europe; it also manifests an approach to 'fairness' and a compensation situation quite different from the one obtaining in the Chernobyl case, as we shall see. Finally, it is less a case of state responsibility than one involving irresponsible TNCs. The accident happened several months after Chernobyl, on 1 November 1986, and it started with a fire lasting five hours, in the Sandoz agrochemical warehouse in Muttenz, Schweizerhalle, near Basel, Switzerland.[53]

It was viewed as 'Western Europe's worst environmental disaster in decades', as the spill of toxic chemicals in the Rhine River, 'formed a red toxic trail 70 Km. long moving downstream through four countries into the North Sea'.[54] Boos-Hersberger states that the Sandoz spill's major proportions can best be understood when viewed in conjunction with the other spills into the Rhine during the same period:

A total of fifteen accidental releases of significant amounts of toxic substances into the Rhine were recorded at Swiss and West German chemical plants between June and December 1986:

- *In mid-October 1986 the Bayer Works at Leverkusen leaked 10 metric tons of a benzene compound into the Rhine.*
- *The night before the Sandoz fire, Ciba-Geigy, Switzerland's largest chemical company and Sandoz's neighbour at Schweizerhalle, illegally released approximately 400 kilograms of the herbicide Atrazine into the Rhine. The discharge was discovered only when the river was tested for pollution from the Sandoz accident. Ciba-Geigy did not report the discharge until days later.*

- *In another accident on 2 December 1986, 2.7 metric tons of polyvinyl chloride leaked into the Rhine from the Lonza chemical factory in Waldshut, West Germany, when an employee accidentally left a valve open.*

The ecological results of these spills were grave indeed, as the entire fish population of the Rhine was eliminated and the river's ecology was gravely affected. Amazingly, however, 'bacterial self-purification' enabled the river to regenerate itself.[55] However, this astonishing result was not paralleled by similar successes either on terrestrial ecosystems or by the results of human health.[56]

Criminal proceedings were initiated on several grounds:

qualified negligence on causing a fire, negligent exposure to hazardous gases, negligent pollution of drinking water, negligent violations of environmental protection, animal protection and water pollution legislation, as well as manslaughter and negligent bodily harm.[57]

Nevertheless the Basel-Land authorities found a 'lack of sufficient proof of the cause of the fire and of the blame attaching to the accused under criminal law'.[58]

Eventually, even the tort cases that came to court were not treated seriously enough, as the fines imposed were drastically reduced for various reasons. In contrast, Sandoz itself settled over 1100 claims for damages from most of Europe, including Switzerland, France, Germany and The Netherlands.[59] Despite the private settlements that occurred in this case, the 1976 *Rhine Convention*[60] is one of the few Western European treaties that permits any party to refer to 'binding arbitration' any dispute concerning 'interpretation or application' of the convention.[61]

Following the Sandoz disaster, the *Rhine Convention* requires 'notification to other states and relevant international organizations in case of accidental discharge of toxic or seriously polluting substances likely to affect other states',[62] because Switzerland had not offered timely warnings of the Sandoz disaster to other, potentially affected parties.

Thus the provisions of the 1976 *Rhine Convention*, as well as the 1976 *Rhine Chloride Convention*,[63] jointly supports sustainability of the Rhine ecosystem, beyond the pre-existing pollution control requirements: 'The parties are to be guided by the precautionary and preventive principle, the "polluter pays" principle, and sustainable development.'[64]

The requirements of the Rhine Commission (especially after the 1999 Convention), manifest more stringent requirements than the *Seveso II*, as, for instance, NGOs must be consulted in all its decisions, and may be invited to Commission meetings. In addition, NGOs input must be publicized in the Commission's reports.[65] When the 1999 Convention will be ratified, it will become the most powerful and transparent environmental convention in Europe and, possibly, in the world.

Yet, until the spill occurred, the Rhine Treaty Regime was not successful in preventing the ongoing pollution, described above, any more than other such regimes, including the Canada/US joint Commission.[66] The Swiss authorities were also negligent, as the warehouse where the chemicals had been stored had been built in 1968 to house machinery, but in 1979 its use as a chemical storage warehouse was approved instead, and the danger posed by its closeness to the Rhine was not acknowledged, despite the presence of a 'Risk Report' that had been prepared by a Swiss Insurance Company to discourage the change in warehouse use, in 1981.[67] In addition, Switzerland was in breach of several Articles of the Convention (especially Articles 7 and 11); but the Sandoz disaster served as a 'wake-up' call to move Switzerland to reconsider adopting the *Seveso Directive* that it had so far refused to accept.

The cases we have considered are well-known and their ecological impact has been acknowledged. They are cited in international and supranational law jurisprudence and literature, and they have influenced these legal regimes and the way ecological disasters are viewed. They are not unique: many others have occurred but have not captured the public opinion and the attention of the media in the same way. What they all share, however, is the clear willingness of the involved TNCs to expect at least some level of 'collateral damage', to use the term used for civilian casualties in armed conflict, and for the involved governments and political regimes to be complicit in the ecocrimes that ensue. Their role would be to curtail if not proscribe hazardous corporate activities, and we will return to that topic below, and the problem of state responsibility, through a Canadian case.[68]

Another aspect of the problem, the North–South conflict, is in evidence in Bhopal. But it is vital to acknowledge that it is not only the spills and accidents that impose grave harms to human and ecological health, but also the practices that accompany 'business as usual', especially when the North–West ecofootprint extends, as it invariably does, to the vulnerable peoples in the South. Gonzales notes:

> *like the environmental justice movement in the United States, Southern environ-mentalism is inextricably intertwined with the struggle for social and economic justice.*[69]

One of the clearest examples of the North–South injustice, fostered by the North's endless appetite for oil to sustain an unsustainable lifestyle, is that of Royal Dutch Shell Oil and their interaction with the Sani Abacha military regime in Nigeria.

'DEVELOPMENT' AND ENVIRONMENTAL RACISM: THE CASE OF KEN SARO-WIWA AND THE OGONI

> *The environment is man's first right*
> *We should not allow it to suffer blight*
> *The air we breathe we must not poison*
> *They who do should be sent to prison*
> *Our streams must remain clean all season*
> *Polluting them is clearly treason*
> *The land is life for man and flora,*
> *Fauna and all: should wear that aura,*
> *Protected from the greed and folly*
> *Of man and companies unholy.*

Ken Saro-Wiwa, 'A Walk in the Prison Yard,' 1994

Playwright George Seremba writes:

> *Last Monday I got news of the five attempts it took before they finally hanged him. In the Wild West they would let you walk at the failure of the first attempt. I will remember the words 'Why are you doing this?' I also heard that he said, before they were all martyred: 'Lord take my soul, but the struggle continues.'*[70]

Seremba is speaking of the murder of Ken Saro-Wiwa on 10 November 1995, an unspeakable crime committed by General Abacha and his military tribunal, with the complicity of Nigeria's powerful elites, but also with the tacit support of Royal Dutch Shell Oil, and of all of us who overconsume and overuse, in affluent North–West countries. For the most part, our silent complicity and our responsibility goes unnoticed and unacknowledged. Therefore, after briefly detailing a chronology of Nigeria's history from June 1993 to February 1995,[71] and presenting Ken Saro-Wiwa's case,[72] I will argue for the need for a new approach to personal morality and public policy that includes an *environmental* assessment of all technological projects. I will also argue that a holistic assessment of all developmental issues is the only approach capable of imposing respect for all life support systems, hence for all human and non-human life.

Nigeria under the dictatorship of Sani Abacha: Ken Saro-Wiwa and the Ogoni people

The events of 1995 and the killing of Ken Saro-Wiwa may be seen as the culmination of two separate but intertwined historical lines, one tracing the political developments in Nigeria, the other, that country's economic interaction with oil companies, primarily Royal Dutch Shell Oil and Exxon.

Political Developments

In June 1993, General Babangida sanctioned presidential elections in Nigeria: Chief M.K.O. Abiola was the clear winner, but Babangida cancelled the elections after the fact, claiming that fraud had been committed. The international community reacted by cancelling all but humanitarian aid, suspending military cooperation and restricting visas to Nigeria. Wole Soyinka describes what happened:

> *On June 23, 1993, the day of the annulment of the presidential election, the military committed the most treasonable act of larceny of all time: it violently robbed the Nigerian people of their nationhood.*[73]

Through the summer, July and August, the country was plagued by demonstrations and several hundreds were killed in clashes. The government in power detained human rights workers and charged them with 'sedition', 'unlawful assembly' and other 'crimes'. At this time, both Babangida and Shonekan, his intended successor, were ousted by General Sani Abacha.

In November 1993, Abacha disbanded all elected bodies, such as the state legislature, 30 houses of state assemblies, all local councils and banned all political activity. He also suspended the 1979 Constitution, including all provisions for human rights carried by that document. In April 1994, a Civil Disturbance Tribunal was established with the power to impose the death penalty: capital offences now included 'unrest crimes' and 'attempted murder'. By May 1994, four Ogoni leaders had been murdered and several hundred people, supporters of the Movement for Survival of the Ogoni People (MOSOP) were arrested, including Ken Saro-Wiwa.

The documents of Amnesty International relate that 'he was severely beaten, his legs chained'.[74] Former senators, governors and members of the House of Representatives were also detained without charge. From June to September, a major Gas and Oil Union went on strike, causing riots and protests, and President Clinton sent Jesse Jackson as a special envoy, to attempt mediation. This effort was not successful; and the whole Nigerian Labour Congress, representing 40 unions and 3.5 million workers, joined the strike. This prompted the authorities to dissolve all unions and to replace their leaders with government-appointed officials. In September, the strike collapsed, and General Abacha issued a series of decrees, retroactive to mid-August, allowing 'administrative detention laws, for up to three months, renewable', and specifying further that this particular law could not be challenged in court.

Abacha also fired the Attorney General, Olu Onagoruwa, and arrested union officials and leaders. In 1995, a ban on all political activities was executed; still, no time was set for the present regime's departure. In Ogoniland hundreds of villages were destroyed and hundreds killed, while Saro-Wiwa was still detained, suffering ongoing inhuman treatment and often tortured: he was expected to be tried by the 'Civil Disturbances Tribunal' for the murder of four officials in Ogoniland.

Economic and Technological Developments

In 1958, Shell discovered oil in Ogoniland, 404 square miles of largely wild, fertile land, home to a variety of flowers, plants and animals, both terrestrial and marine, beyond its coast, and to 500,000 Ogoni people.[75] Chevron moved its oil exploration to Ogoniland in 1977, and both companies, jointly, have extracted an estimated US$30 billion worth of oil from Ogoniland. Saro-Wiwa adds:

> *In return for this we have received nothing but a highly polluted land where associated gas burns twenty-four hours a day, belching carbon monoxide, carbon dioxide, methane and soot into the air; and oil spillage and blow-outs devastate much needed farmland, threatening human existence.*
>
> *Flora and fauna are all but dead, marine life is destroyed, the ecosystem is fast-changing. Ogoni is a wasteland.*[76]

However, Nigeria's military dictatorship was geographically removed from this devastation, and enjoyed a mutually supportive relationship with the oil companies, as they depended on the wealth the oil companies provided. In turn, the oil companies depended on the dictatorship to ignore the environmental disasters they continued to create, without imposing restraints or demanding remediation or compensation for the land and people affected. Throughout this increasingly distressing state of affairs, Saro-Wiwa maintained that 'the environment is man's first right. Without a safe environment, man cannot live to claim other rights'.[77] He also steadfastly opposed the devastation of Ogoniland, demanding remediation of environmental problems and royalties to assist his people. The Ogoni desperately needed help, as the families could no longer depend on the land and the sea, but had to have financial help and medical aid to mitigate the many ills besetting them and destroying not only their livelihood, but also their health, as they were now living in 'absolute poverty'.[78] They had no access to safe water, to electricity, telephones, or any educational or health facilities.[79]

Examples of the harms inflicted on the Ogoni people from Shell's economic exploitation abound. In one case, Grace Zorbidon was walking near her mud hut one night in January 1994, 'carrying a kerosene lantern to light her way'. She did not see 'the oil slick oozing from a rupture in a pipeline that runs hard up against her tiny village'.[80] When she put down her lantern, she was engulfed by flames and, in May 1994, was still lying on the floor of a healer's hut, in terrible pain, and treated only with traditional potions made from leaves. Shell neither enquired after her, nor saw to her treatment or to the fate of the eight children of this 'subsistence farmer'. Their excuse? Shell said they were 'hazy' on the accident, and could not substantiate Zorbidon's report because of the 'tensions in the area'. Shell was much quicker to react to protests and demonstrations that had forced it to close its operations in early 1994. Shell's reaction was to 'ask for assistance' from the military authorities, who responded with swift and brutal retribution against the protesters.

The Nigerian government was not prepared to tolerate any interference with its business relations with Shell: neither human rights, nor environmental concerns could be allowed to interfere. The *Wall Street Journal* reports:

> *Nigeria's government depends on oil for 80% of its income, and sees any threat to the industry as imperiling its shaky hold on power. Oil produced by Shell accounts for about half of these revenues.*[81]

Nigeria's military dictatorship and Shell operate as a 'joint venture' in which Shell holds a 30 per cent interest, the Nigerian government holds 55 per cent, Elf Aquitaine of France, 10 per cent, and Agip Francaise, 5 per cent. Furthermore, the US was also benefiting from the arrangement: they imported 36 per cent of Nigeria's oil production in 1993, which accounted for about 11 per cent of all US oil imports.

In all these large business transactions, what, if any, are the benefits the Ogoni have reaped from their land's exploitation? When large multinationals interact with impoverished developing countries, the benefit accrues primarily to their constituents in the affluent North–West. The usual 'tradeoffs' offered in those cases are (a) employment; (b) 'improvements' such as roads, hospitals and schools; and (c) remediation of environmental impacts. Shell's record appears to be dismal on all counts. 'Of Shell's 5000 employees in Nigeria, only 85 are Ogoni';[82] there are '96 oil wells, two refineries, a petrochemical complex and a fertilizer plant' in Ogoniland, but the only available hospital is described as an 'unfinished husk', and the promised schools are seldom open, 'because there is no money available for teachers' salaries'.[83]

In addition, Shell's spokesman, Mr Nickson, claimed that Shell 'deplored' the military's 'heavy-handed clampdowns and the pain and loss suffered by local communities'. However, there is no record of Shell initiating any policy to ameliorate the Ogoni's lot, or to mitigate the damage they had perpetrated. Given the strength of their economic interests in Shell's operations, the military continued to organize raids to 'punish' the

Ogoni for obstructing Shell, and responded to protests by 'shooting into the crowd', killing and maiming civilians, using any pretext to lay 'entire villages to waste'. The raids were often conducted by a Mobile Police Unit, 'nicknamed 'Kill and Go'. On Easter Sunday, 1994, villagers who had fled the raids were felled by random shooting. 'One ten-year old girl says she was gang-raped. Three days later, the whites of her eyes were bloodshot, the flesh around them purple and swollen'; she explained that the soldiers attempted to gouge her eyes out, 'so that she would not be able to identify them'.[84] Health facilities, says a European nurse, are minimal, and Shell refused to even pave the roads to prevent patients having to walk through the mud to reach the clinic.

What of the 'economic benefits'? In response to increasing protests from the Ogoni, the government ostensibly offered 3 per cent of its oil revenues to them. In practice, these percentages never reached the Ogoni, as the money was spent in the tribal lands of the ruling majority instead, or vanished 'in corrupt deals'.[85] As far as remediation is concerned, one example will suffice. More than 20 years ago, there was a spill near the village of Ebubu that has not been cleaned to date; today, in 'an area the size of four football fields, cauliflower shaped extrusions of moist black tar cover the ground to a depth of about three feet'.[86] Shell claims that while unrest continues, they are not prepared to do any cleanup work: it is worth noting that the spill occurred in the late 1960s.

As an additional corollary to the government's role in the economic development by the oil companies, foreign observers are denied access, and even a fact-finding mission from The Netherlands was denied permission to visit, and 'checkpoints' were set up instead in order 'to monitor Western travellers'. The *Wall Street Journal* reporter who compiled most of the data summarized in this section, concludes by relating her own experience:

> When I approached an army officer to ask for the military's account of a violent incident, I was handed over to the secret police, held and interrogated for two days, and then deported 'for security reasons'.[87]

Although the US Government commissioned a 'Human Rights Report' on the Ogoni in 1993, the report only admitted 'some merit' to the Ogoni's claims, but refused to accept the definition of 'genocide' urged by Saro-Wiwa, as appropriate to describe the Ogoni's plight. Saro-Wiwa remarked that 'one thousand dead Ogonis out of five hundred thousand', is comparable to half a million dead US citizens, and that situation, had it occurred, would surely have been termed a case of 'genocide'.

In essence, the perversion of human rights and the clear presence of racism (or even of attempts at 'ethnic cleansing') that was manifested by the oil companies with the support of the military dictatorship of Nigeria, was more than a particularly lethal case of environmental racism (Westra and Wenz, 1995): it was and is no less than an 'ecological war' that was being waged (and still persists), it is 'omnicide', Saro-Wiwa says. He adds:

> men, women and children die unnoticed, flora and fauna are threatened, the air is poisoned, waters are polluted, and, finally, the land itself dies.[88]

Again, a question of responsibility

So far we have pointed to joint activities by the military regime under Sani Abacha and by Shell Oil as the primary source of the crimes committed against the Ogoni and against their land. But are they the sole culprits? We can learn a lot from Shell's public relations response to Saro-Wiwa's murder, and the international revulsion and anger that followed upon it. After all, Saro-Wiwa was well-known as the recipient of several prizes and grants (The Goldman Environmental Prize (1995); the Right Livelihood Award (1994); and the Bruno Kreisky Human Rights Award (1995), one of which, the Goldman Environmental Prize, was deliberately given to him in advance, in the hope of drawing international attention to him, as he had already been declared a Prisoner of Conscience by Amnesty International). A well-known writer and activist, his death made an impact that Shell attempted to offset by buying prime space in international newspapers, in the effort to shift blame for their actions and omissions, as they disclaimed any responsibility for either the environmental devastation or the murder.

In a carefully worded newspaper advertisement[89] entitled 'Clear Thinking in Troubled Times', Shell explicitly allied itself with 'clear thinking', and patronizingly dismissed a 'great wave of understandable emotion over the death of Ken Saro-Wiwa', together with the anger and disapprobation it faced from all nations. 'The public have been manipulated and misled' was one of its statements, as they attempted to whitewash themselves because they had spent millions on 'environmentally related projects'. The environmental problems were due, they claimed, to 'over-farming'(!), soil erosion, deforestation and population growth, in areas where only the most meagre subsistence farming existed: Geraldine Brooks of the *Wall Street Journal,* describes it as 'pulling tubers from the earth with sticks'.[90] Shell further appealed to a 'World Bank Survey' to support their position, but the World Bank was one of the few major 'powers' who, together with the Royal Geographical Society, withdrew all their support from Nigeria, in protest, and categorically denied Shell's allegations.

Shell also remarked that, after all, they were not the only ones at fault, as all humanitarian protests and even international sanctions could not (and in fact did not) succeed. One can speculate that no other 'sanctions' could prevail, as they would not carry the same clout for a money-hungry military clique, as would the continued cash-producing presence of Shell and other oil companies.

Finally Shell raised a question and veiled threat common to all industries that are the target of environmental protests, worldwide. The ad continues, 'What if we were to withdraw from the project' and with it, withdraw all employment the project entails? 'The oil extraction would continue,' they say, 'and it might not be done any better.' One could respond that other companies elsewhere *have* in fact done much better. For instance, Conoco DuPont drilled a well in Gabon between 1989 and 1992:

> *it flew in much of its equipment to avoid pushing a major road through the rain forest. When trees had to be felled, the company hired scientists to cultivate cuttings so that sites could be replanted with exactly the same species that had been removed.*[91]

Hence a technology assessment based on a holistic management perspective would have made a large difference *at the outset* rather than demand remediation after the fact, a largely useless procedure from the environmental standpoint, and – as we saw – based on total disrespect for human rights as well.

Even more appalling from the moral standpoint, was the final paragraph of Shell's page-long ad:

> *Some campaigning groups say we should intervene in the political process in Nigeria. But even if we could, we must never do so. Politics is the business of governments and politicians. The world where companies use their economic influence to prop up or bring down governments would be a frightening and bleak one indeed.*[92]

It is both 'frightening' and 'bleak' to read such vicious travesty of the facts: Shell is a partner in the 'joint venture' with Nigeria's ruthless and inhumane military regime, and knew full well the impact its financial support had on the latter's existence. Further, when negotiations and consent *both* are conducted and originate from non-elected, non-representative authorities, one is clearly already 'meddling' in the politics of the country with which one deals.

Environmental ethics and responsibility

Nevertheless, even ascribing responsibility for the gross miscarriage of justice and the environmental devastation of Ogoni and to Shell and the military regime of Nigeria, is necessary, but not sufficient for a serious ethical evaluation of the situation. Shell and others like them could quickly point out that they only have a profitable market for their operations because we, the North–West affluent consumers, are hungry for abundant, low-cost oil and gasoline products. Hence, it is not enough to point the finger at Shell and other corporate exploiters. It is also necessary to confront the morality of our lifestyle and of our policy choices.

This is the raw, evil side of technological progress. It is ecoviolence perpetrated against the most vulnerable people: it shows the worst face of 'environmental racism' in a most deadly form. Retaliation against pro-environmental protest ended in a murder, orchestrated by a kangaroo court: Ken Saro-Wiwa was murdered by hanging, in Nigeria, on 10 November 1995, at 11:30 a.m. The dictatorial regime that plotted and executed his murder on a trumped-up charge was heavily dependent on the oil revenues generated by Shell's operations. The question now is, how should that technology have been evaluated before its impact on Nigeria was felt?

Traditional moral theories could and should indict the gross abuse of human rights that took place when Saro-Wiwa was murdered; they could decry the lack of justice and due process in his trial and sentencing and appeal to Rawlsian principles in defence of all the Ogoni people; finally, they could appeal to Bullard's 'five principles of environmental justice' to combat environmental racism.[93] But all these arguments are end-of-pipe attempts at mitigation, after the fact. The fundamental question remains: how should the introduction of a large technological system like oil extraction, have been evaluated in that particular part of the world, and in that geographical area? From the ecocentric point of view, the environmental impact should have been anticipated, if not precisely, at least with enough accuracy to discourage Shell unless an impartial international commission, including both appropriate scientists and environmental ethicists, could be put in place to oversee, with veto powers, all Shell's plans and activities.

In contrast, if we would counsel a purely anthropocentric position for our starting point, we might still be able to put in place some restraints, based on risk assessments of the situation. But, without knowing the actual results of Shell's operations, it would have been extremely difficult to stop them or establish tight limits to their activities, *before the fact.*

Hence, if we simply appealed to traditional moral principles, we might not have been able to stop the violence that followed. It also would have rendered us guilty of 'complicity', as would have our isolating ourselves from the information, and simply turning our eyes while availing ourselves of these products' easy availability.[94] The question is one of moral responsibility, one that Hans Jonas, for instance, viewed as the most important question to be asked in regard to technology: for him responsibility was the 'keyword' for the ethics of human conduct in dealing with technology.[95] Jonas argued that 'the new kinds and dimensions of action require a commensurate ethics of foresight and responsibility, which is as novel as the eventualities which it must meet'. And when 'foresight' is difficult because of science's lack of predictive capacities, since 'care for the future' is the 'overruling duty', we must face the fact that the only possible moral choices might be the careful application of the precautionary principle, or even abstention from certain non-basic lifestyle and technological choices.

One wonders whether an appeal to traditional, anthropocentric moral doctrines is sufficient not only to address, but also to prevent such problems from developing, in the face of increasing environmental disintegration and degradation, and mounting scarcity of 'resources' as populations increase. Many have addressed the need to ensure that cost/benefit analyses and economic evaluations of technology are made to focus prominently on ethical considerations beyond aggregate utilities and majority preferences.[96] I believe that the anthropocentric/nonanthropocentric distinction presents a false dichotomy in several senses, and that it is no more than a red herring, advanced by those concerned with defending the present status quo. Accordingly, they are led to propose a somewhat modified, 'greened' revamping of the same hazardous, uncritically accepted practices to which all life on Earth has been subjected.

Utilities and preferences are normally understood (in philosophical and political theory) as reflecting the wishes, and maybe the (descriptively) perceived 'good' of a society, as do appeals to rights, justice, fairness, and due process. The question, however, is whether ethical considerations based on moral doctrines designed primarily for intraspecific interaction – that is, designed to guide our interpersonal behaviour – are in fact sufficient, as well as being clearly necessary to ensure that our activities conform to an inclusive and enlightened morality. Recent global change affecting our resource base everywhere *proves* the inadequacy of calculations that depend solely on economics, so that evaluations founded on moral doctrines and upholding both 'natural' and 'civil' rights, appear indeed mandatory.

Would this approach have been sufficient to redress the terrible ills done to the Ogoni people and their land? In other words, had a democracy been in place, and had the citizens of Ogoniland been polled about their wishes in regard to the projects of Shell and other corporations, would that have been enough to save the environment on which they depend? One problem is that even if a technology impact assessment had been required and openly publicized, it is unlikely that a community of subsistence farmers would have been well-informed enough to foresee the irreversible ecological damage that would have been their lot eventually, even if they would have received a fair percentage of the oil royalties, and roads, schools and clinics might have been built for their use. Saro-Wiwa would have known, but it is at least an open question whether he would have been listened to, before the fact.

This remains a routine problem whenever hazardous operations move into minority or economically depressed areas in their home countries, although perhaps both education and standards of living might be higher, comparatively, than those of the Ogoni.[97] Hence, I suggest that even in an ideal situation, where legal restraints on environmental hazards are in place and where democratic institutions prevail, the environmental and health protection of all are by no means guaranteed.

The basic problem, for us anywhere, is sustainability. William Rees, for instance, proposes adopting an 'ecological worldview', in contrast with the prevailing established 'expansionist worldview', which represents 'the dominant social paradigm'.[98] As Leopold did before him, Rees recognizes that we are not independent of, and separate from, an 'environment', but ecological sustainability is foundational, so that it makes perfectly good sense to abandon our present unsustainable and indefensible worldview. Wackernagel and Rees (1996) say, 'By contrast, an ecological economic perspective would see the human economy as an inextricably integrated, completely contained, and wholly dependent sub-system of the ecosphere.'

This position is supported by Rees's research in the Vancouver–Lower Fraser Valley region of British Columbia, Canada, but can be easily generalized for all urban, affluent Northwest centres. His findings show that, 'assuming an average Canadian diet and current management practices', the local 'regional population support(s) its consumers' lifestyles' by importing 'the productive capacity of at least 22 times as much land as it occupies'. To put this in a more general way, 'the ecological footprints of individual regions are much larger than the land areas they physically occupy'.[99]

When we continue to import others' carrying capacity, we are 'running an unaccounted ecological deficit', and 'our populations are appropriating carrying capacity from elsewhere or from future generations'.[100] The same can be said about 'sinks' for our wastes: for both resource appropriation and waste disposal, our North–West approach has been one of neo-colonialism in regard to less developed countries, and one of ruthless exploitation (through 'environmental racism') toward minorities and the disempowered in our own countries.[101]

Thus, although it is both easy and even necessary to indict: (1) the military rule and the despotism that was instrumental in the killing of Ken Saro-Wiwa and the devastation of his land; and (2) the large corporations that wreaked havoc on the environment, leading to the Ogoni's protests and resistance, and these enterprises' callous and unjust exploitation of a vulnerable people for purely financial reasons, this is not enough.

On 13 November 1995, the *Wall Street Journal* reports that, although they issued 'sanction threats', and they cut military aid (US), and although the UK banned arms sales and the European Union recalled its ambassadors and suspended all aid, *no nation* had 'halted purchases of Nigerian oil or sales of drilling equipment, as a result of the hangings'.[102] Halting the oil trade would bring Nigeria to its knees, as oil represents 90 per cent of its exports, and 80 per cent of its revenue; but the US would *also* be hard hit, as it imports 40 per cent of Nigeria's oil. Hence, the US recalled its ambassador, but did not make the principled stand made by the World Bank. The International Finance Corporation (Private Sector Lending for the World Bank) withdrew its support in the form of a US$100,000 loan to Nigeria, from a liquefied natural gas project.[103]

The problem is that, as long as we elect leaders and governments on the basis of promises of 'low taxes' and 'low prices', as well as the 'right' to development, without any consideration of the *size* of our 'ecological footprint', let alone its *location* (that is to say, without considering who is to pay for our choices), we cannot claim to be free from responsibility. Each one of us is, to some extent, an accomplice and a contributor to the evil deeds perpetrated in Nigeria.

It is both what we *do* and what we *fail to do* that is at stake. In essence, we cannot continue to consume and to waste as though we had the *right* to take from the poor and the vulnerable, just because we can afford it. We must reconsider our political choices, when these are explicitly insular, isolationist and segregationist in intent, and when they are both supported by and supportive of big business, such as oil companies, tobacco producers, manufacturers of chemicals or transgenics, all of which (in their present forms) often spell death for our environment, and ensure severe threats to our health and to the persistence of our species on earth. Thus the problem is a question of personal as well as ecological integrity: it is a moral problem to which no facile solutions exist at this time. In some sense, Ken Saro-Wiwa died because of our moral failures, our negligence and our lack of commitment to justice and a moral ideal.

This, however, is one case where the law is moving slowly to attempt to redress some of the unspeakable harms that occurred. In New York, the son of Ken Saro-Wiwa, initiated an action under the Alien Torts Claims Act.

ECOJUSTICE AND INDUSTRIAL OPERATIONS: AN IRRECONCILABLE CONFLICT?

The previous sections reviewed some of the so-called 'accidents' in both the developed and the developing world. I am referring to them as 'accidents' not because I have any indication, or belief that there was any criminal intent, or *mens rea* involved, but it seems clear that, even in technologically advanced countries, a certain amount of technical failures and/or human error must be expected. Bluntly, the operation of chemical industries and related corporate activities, even in the most advanced countries and under the optimal circumstances found in affluent Western countries, is not safe for all stakeholders, even when all possible precautions, legislated by the regulatory regimes of North–West nations, are implemented.

Most of all, these operations are unsafe for the ecosystems that are affected by their products, even under 'ideal' conditions. But this is by no means their only effect. Any pesticide leaves residues not only in the fields, but also in all foods that are not organically grown. The increasing rates of diseases such as cancers in the developing world, attest to the accuracy of medical research[104] and most of all that of the WHO, as was noted in the first chapter of this book. There the effects of routinely used chemicals on the most vulnerable of human beings, the children, were discussed. Hence, it must be acknowledged, industries that have produced some comforts and advantages for mankind in general, and huge profits to many, have also been a dangerous, and insidiously harmful presence in the lives of almost everyone.

Chemical companies' immense profits are the result of their worldwide marketing drives. But the 'side-effects' of these operations affect the life and health of too many to be simply dismissed as 'externalities' or the cost of doing business. The cost of doing business by Royal Dutch Shell Oil included genocide, crimes against humanity, multiple rapes and assaults, but their ecocrimes are not even factored in the Alien Torts Claims Act (ATCA) indictments, or mentioned, as we saw.

Yet the destroyed environment also destroyed a people's way of life, their present and future health. Thus Royal Dutch Shell participated in the crimes against humanity that were committed there with the complicity of the local military government.

In this regard, it might be instructive to consider the *Statute of the International Criminal Court*,[105] which, unlike the Nuremberg Charter, envisions the possibility of internal crimes against humanity, committed by individuals, not states (Article 7), although the environment as such is only spoken of in connection with situations of armed conflict. Article 7(h) refers, for instance, to 'the crime of apartheid', a crime that may be politically motivated but that is not exclusively, or even primarily a 'war crime'.

I have argued that even negligent harms of the magnitude of these industrial disasters should be included as 'crimes against humanity'.[106] I am well aware, however, that we are considering *lex ferenda*, at best. Perhaps the best hope to see these crimes indicted and properly categorized may eventually be found in the definition of Article 5(d), in 'the crime of aggression' (under the provisions of Articles 121 and 123), as its full extent is, as yet, undefined. Similarly, it is not too far-fetched, I believe, to acknowledge with the language of the 'Preamble', the presence of *erga omnes* obligations, based on *jus cogens* norms, as applicable to all peoples, as they are in the worst crimes:

> *Recognizing that such grave crimes threaten the peace, security and well-being of the world. Affirming that the most serious crimes of concern to the international community as a whole must not go unpunished and that their effective prosecution must be ensured by taking measures at the national level and by enhancing international cooperation.*

When one considers the seriousness and the pervasiveness of the harms produced by the combination of corporate 'freedom' to pursue its goals with few restraints, on one hand, and the primacy of trade 'efficiency',[107] on the other we discover that all human rights are at stake. Even, as Jennifer Downs argues, 'first generation rights',[108] which are codified in the *International Covenant on Civil and Political Rights*,[109] while second generation's rights – refer to the *International Covenant on Economic, Social and Cultural Rights*[110] – are under fire. Neither first nor *second* generation rights ever mention health, either human or ecological. Yet the 'Preamble' of the latter refers to:

> *The ideal of free human beings enjoying freedom from fear and want can only be achieved if conditions are created whereby everyone may enjoy his economic, social and cultural rights as well as his civil and political rights.*

Freedom from 'fear and want' should include conditions of life that start with the 'basic rights' to 'subsistence and security' as Shue describes them,[111] that must include health and normal function, as well as a safe habitat able to support both. We will return to the possibility of establishing in law, third generation rights, or 'solidarity rights',[112] below.

But the argument here proposed is clearly supported by the Ogoni case, the case in Bhopal and in some measure, the other cases addressed in this chapter.

Yet some might argue that perhaps industrial activities in general are exclusively hazardous in circumstances of under development in the South or the East. That, however, is not a defensible position. The next topic will be the case of Walkerton, Ontario, as similar hazardous industrial activities, and similar failed regulative regimes produced a case that resulted in at least eight deaths and over 3000 serious illnesses in Canada's richest Province, Ontario, and within 150 km of the Province's capital, Toronto.

THE MANY FACES OF ECOFOOTPRINT CRIME

Before leaving the topic of ecofootprint crime, we need to move beyond examples, in order to better understand its meaning and the different aspects under which it manifests itself. These various 'faces' are really masks, often bland and even benign manifestations, representing jobs, economic possibilities and even progress. We have seen the effect of 'disasters' and later will also discuss the effects of 'business as usual', and the regular operations and activities that result in harm.

To understand it better, the first thing to note is that the harmful/criminal aspects of ecofootprints can be both direct and indirect. For instance, in the last example, Ogoniland, there are direct physical harms arising from the oil extraction operations, and we noted the direct impact on the health and the life of the local communities. But there are also at least two kinds of indirect impacts, no less heinous: (1) the impact on the community's habitat, the land and water upon which they had depended for generations for their subsistence and survival; and (2) the impact of the complicity between Royal Dutch Shell Oil and the Sani Abacha military dictatorship, with the subsequent suppression of protests, rapes, murders and other attacks upon the populations.

The direct effects of the North–West ecofootprint, therefore, do not only result in direct physical harms, but also, by their presence, produce indirect harms, beyond the easily observed material harms and damages to local environment and public health. Indirect harms may be far more subtle: they include supporting racism; engaging in illegal business practices; supporting industrial activities through the silencing of protests and other human rights violations.

The cases we have been considering include both direct and indirect material harms. The activities of Royal Dutch Shell Oil were directly harmful to the health of the inhabitants, and they also eliminated the basis for the population's survival as they made it impossible for the Ogoni to continue in their traditional lifestyles. Eventually, the strongest representatives of the protests, Ken Saro-Wiwa and the rest of the Ogoni 9, were indicted and murdered precisely for speaking out against the operations of Shell.

But a glance at the recent jurisprudence under ATCA[113] indicates that intimidation, attacks, even murders occur even when the corporate entity responsible and intent on promoting and protecting the efficient operations of its business is not intrinsically harmful in its products or processes, as in the *Sinaltral v. Coca Cola* case.[114] Most of these ecofootprint harms are inflicted by a North–West corporate organization, on a vulnerable population in the South–East, where regulatory regimes protecting human rights are not well-entrenched, and impoverished governments are greedy for the economic benefits these organizations will bring. Hence, it is systematic exploitation of those who cannot defend themselves that characterizes the criminality of the harms imposed.

Ecofootprint harms and institutionalized violence: The interface

In general, cases covered by litigation under ATCA are only the ones where the crimes committed are obvious, and the perpetrators are easily identifiable, although their legal responsibility may not be so easy to prove, and this was the case for the murder of the Ogoni 9 as well.[115] But there is a major problem that escapes this scenario altogether: the problem of institutionalized harms, or 'ecoviolence' as I have termed it.[116] For instance, the grievous harms imposed on the most vulnerable populations, arising from the effects of climate change through the intensification of both droughts and arid spells, as well as the melting of glaciers, fit under this category. They cause the destruction of the agricultural basis needed for the survival of peoples in developing countries, especially those living in coastal areas and islands, but not these exclusively, witness the conditions in sub-Saharan Africa in general. The resulting famines, starvations, and the intensification of the disease burden of the population, especially that of children, will be discussed in Chapter 9.

These harms are both direct and indirect: direct, as when climate change engenders stronger and more frequent storms, hurricanes and tsunamis that destroy both people and their ways of life. Indirect, as when the drought eliminates their food sources and water, with the disastrous conditions that ensue (see Chapter 9).

The language of the *Convention against Genocide*, envisions various forms of eliminating populations, including, under Article 2, (b) causing serious bodily or mental harm to members of the group; and (c) deliberately inflicting on the group conditions of life calculated to bring about its physical destruction in whole or in part.[117] In the far North, the Inuit's way of life is under immediate threat, as is the life of the fauna upon which their existence is predicated, and that of the ecosystem that is the habitat of both. On 7 December 2005, at the 11th Convention of the Parties (COP-11), in Montreal, Canada, a side event took place, entitled, 'Is there a right to be cold?', organized by Canadian Inuits.

What is at issue is not just the comfort or the continuity of familiar temperatures appropriate to the area, but their very survival. What are the Inuit or other First Nations (Canada) or other indigenous populations to do, when their living conditions are no longer as they have been in the past. Where will they go and how will they survive?

Similar questions may be asked about the inhabitants of the Caribbean, the Maldives, and other island and coastal nations, whose homes and lifestyles are washed away by rising seas and violent ocean perturbations. It is likely that a whole new category of 'environmental refugees' will need to be created, as the traditional reasons for attaining refugee status do not apply to such populations, although their plight is no less terrible than that of those who are exposed to more traditional forms of violence.

Refugees normally flee from genocide, torture and so on. *The Convention on the Prevention and Punishment of the Crime of Genocide* has 130 parties as of March 2000, and its addresses the question of personal responsibility as it specifies what the treaty parties undertake to prevent and punish. As we noted above, Article 2(b) and 2(c) are quite close to describing the conditions imposed by climate change on the South as well as the far North, where Inuit and Canadian First Nations peoples are losing the basis of their traditional lifestyles, hence the security of their survival.

Some, however, may argue that the aspect of 'intent' is absent from these crimes. Whatever the motivations of governments and corporate actives, the specific intent to eliminate a particular population is hard to prove. I have argued that at least knowledge of the consequences is clearly present and perhaps only what the Canadian criminal code defines as 'willful blindness' may prevent a government institution or a corporation from admitting to that knowledge.[118]

For the purpose of this argument (1) *mens rea* and (2) deterrence are the most important questions. Starting briefly with the latter, it is worth noting that some regional EPA offices, such as California and Ohio, have created specific task forces that target such areas as the 'mishandling of pesticides, failure to report leaking underground storage tanks, falsification of environmental documents' as well as whole 'critical geographical areas' such as the US/Mexican border.[119] The Ohio EPA has also shifted from prosecuting 'midnight dumpers', to established businesses intent on improving their profits and competitive advantages: 'Such companies may simply regard civil penalties as a cost of doing business, and can be brought into compliance only through the individual deterrent of criminal prosecution.'[120]

Corporate interests find it too easy to reduce all values to economic ones, so that the difference between (1) harms to human life and health, and even human rights, and (2) possible harms to corporate economic goals, are perceived as different in degree, rather than in kind. The shock of a criminal prosecution, as argued by Cooney et al, may possibly bring home the vast gulf present between harm (1) and harm (2), and thus to emphasize the grave responsibility borne by corporate offenders for harm (1), and the latter's incommensurability with harm (2).

Turning now to the knowledge element in US law, regarding environmental crimes, we need to consider several aspects of that question. First, environmental crimes are viewed as general intent offences; where knowing violations are not truly defined, allowing instead the courts to give meaning to the term 'on a case-by-case basis'.[121] The concept is often understood to mean that the defendant had 'mere consciousness' of an act or omission,[122] which amounts to a 'violation of law, regulation or permit', without demanding proof 'that the defendant had knowledge of the relevant statutory provision'.[123]

Second, the 'Public Welfare Offense Doctrine' applies 'when the substance involved is so inherently dangerous that the defendant's knowledge of the legal issues can be presumed'.[124] Third, the 'Crime of Knowing Endangerment', created by Congress 'to deal with particularly offensive conduct that directly threatens human life' with graver penalties, is an important tool to approach these crimes. All that is required other than the presence of graver consequences, is general intent, which is shown when evidence demonstrates that the 'discharger knew it was dealing with a material that could harm humans or the environment'.[125] Examples include discharge of 'dioxin from paper mills, arsenic from metal operations, vinyl chloride from other industrial operations' and so on. Cases that involve less lethal materials or compounds are misdemeanors and, for those cases, 'negligently violating a permit' represents sufficient knowledge. In contrast, aggravated felonies require a knowing violation and proof that the defendant 'knows at the time that he thereby places another person in imminent danger'.[126]

Individuals may be charged with environmental crimes on the basis of '(1) direct evidence, (2) willful blindness/conscious avoidance, (3) circumstantial evidence, and (4) the responsible corporate officer doctrine'.[127] The last of these requirements is particularly relevant in cases where it is hard to show knowledge through other means. Under this doctrine, criminal liability can be imposed on:

1   a corporate officer,
2   who is directly responsible within management for the conduct in question,
3   who knew that they type of improper activity allegedly committed by his or her subordinates was occurring.[128]

The doctrine permits imposing liability on officers at corporate headquarters, who have no direct responsibility for the operation of the offending facility,[129] when this facility is not located nearby. Liability is imposed solely by virtue of the position of responsibility of the corporate officer in question. The strongest support for this doctrine can be found in Britain,[130] where a city's public utilities' director was charged with allowing the discharge of pollutants into a local creek, in a case reminiscent of Walkerton (see Chapter 8). If US laws had been applied in Walkerton, as environmental crimes are subject to a *de minimis* knowledge requirement, it would have been easy to argue that, whatever his educational failings, a public utilities employee, such as Koebel, who knew enough to falsify reports to the ministry, would be aware of the dangerousness of the presence of E. coli bacteria in the water supply, and would certainly meet the *de minimis* requirement, as above.

Similarly, the Ontario Premier who initiated the deregulation, and monitoring cuts spiral, eventually leading to the documented deaths, could not avoid criminal prosecution, but would be charged under the corporate officer doctrine. One wonders why some of these approaches to environmental crime have not long since been introduced in Canada and internationally, and whether perhaps there might still be time for an interpretive appeal to the US approach for the Canadian case, as no criminal prosecutions have been initiated to date. In contrast, Lazarus argues that even in the US, present Supreme Court decisions are viewing the precedents upon which many environmental felony prosecutions have relied, as becoming increasingly unstable,[131] thus possibly leading to a regression away from environmental protection.

In this book I have emphasized the North–South dimensions of ecocrimes, hence the discussion of genocide appeared to be the most appropriate to the topic of first and future generations' harms. Yet, as we saw , the problem of the absence of *mens rea*, or mental element, is present for genocide, while crimes against humanity or against the human person do not appear to be defined by a specific intent to achieve a certain result. William Schabas says: 'But in cases that cannot be described as purely accidental, the accused's mental state may be far from totally innocent'.[132]

The *Rome Statute of the International Criminal Court* (1998) Article 30, declares that 'mens rea or mental element of genocide has two components', that is 'knowledge and intent'.[133] Thus awareness of the consequences that will follow upon the adoption of certain practices and policies can be objectively determined.[134] This form of 'know-ledge' or awareness has several aspects, such as constructive liability, recklessness, wilful blindness, and objective dangerousness.[135]

All the injuries are imposed as the result of inappropriate mental attitudes, but Edgerton says:

> Negligence neither is nor involves ('presupposes') either indifference or inadvertence, or any other mental characteristic, quality, state or process. Negligence is unreasonably dangerous conduct – i.e. conduct abnormally likely to cause harm.[136]

This is not the appropriate time for a detailed discussion of *mens rea* and of the mental element of ecocrime because, for the most part, it is extremely difficult to establish the direct, proximate causality required to identify one or more perpetrators. In addition, when none of the latter are natural persons, but are legal persons instead, the question of intent becomes even more complex and difficult to assess.[137]

In contrast, ATCA deals with torts, so it may be best to turn to a review of some of the cases litigated under ATCA, after a brief discussion of the interface between the criminality of some of these cases, and the treatment of such ecofootprint crimes in those cases.

Environmental harms and human rights: A question of jurisdiction?

> On February 28, 2002 ... Judge Wood's opinion found that plaintiffs' allegations met the requirements for claims under the Alien Torts Claim Act, in that the actions of Royal Dutch Shell and Anderson constituted participation in crimes against humanity, torture, summary execution, arbitrary detention, cruel, inhuman and degrading treatment and other violations of international law.[138]

Environmental harms/human rights violations are hard to place and prosecute from the standpoint of jurisdiction: are we to consider the nationality of all those affected? Or are we to consider all those who contribute to the harms, including both 'complicit' states and corporate bodies and including diversely incorporated companies, within a multinational corporate empire? And how is a diffuse harm, originating from multiple actors, to be analysed in terms of the three aspects of jurisdiction: (a) jurisdiction to prescribe; (b) jurisdiction to adjudicate; and (c) jurisdiction to enforce?[139]

The first aspect, (a), raises the question of which Court, hence which State may have the authority 'to prescribe rules that impact the conduct and behavior of individuals' outside its own national borders. The second, (b), addresses the most obvious aspect of the problem: which state has the right to rule on a matter in a specific dispute that might have taken place outside its borders, and might not have caused harm to its own citizens. The third aspect, (c), raises an even harder question (in practice): even winning a case and receiving a favourable judgement leaves unanswered the question of how to enforce a court's decree.[140] The problem is exacerbated because following the changes in human rights, international humanitarian and economic law, international organizations and even individuals (both biological and juridical) 'have attained some measure of international legal personality'.[141] Bederman analyses these aspects of 'jurisdictional problems', from the starting point of the 'Lotus Presumption' (that is, allowing States 'to assert jurisdiction to the maximum limits allowed'),[142] in the light of US law, especially the 1987 *Restatement (Third) of the Foreign Relations Law of the United States*, section 403. The paramount role of several standards emerges from the criteria listed, that is, the need to use what is 'most reasonable', (only with respect to (b)), 'comity', and the balancing of interests, before applying the doctrine of *forum non conveniens*.[143] One of the most recent and important examples of unclear and conflicted jurisdiction is apparently being addressed and is on the way to being 'resolved' in the US, in the case cited at the beginning of this section.

In the Opinion and Order,[144] Judge Kimba Wood addresses the question of jurisdiction and gives the disposition of the case:

> *Plaintiffs filed the first action against the corporate defendants on November 6, 1996 and filed an amended complaint on April 29, 1997. By order dated September 25, 1998 ['1998 Order'], the Court found that the corporate defendents were subject to personal jurisdiction in New York [2], but dismissed plaintiffs' amended complaint on* forum non conveniens *grounds. On appeal, the second Circuit Court affirmed that the corporate defendants were subject to personal jurisdiction, but reversed the Court's* forum non conveniens *dismissal and remanded the action for further proceedings. See Wiwa v. Royal Dutch Petroleum Company et al., 226H.3d 88 (2d Cir.2000). Plaintiffs filed a new action against Brian Anderson on March 5, 2001.*
>
> *Presently before the Court are: (1) defendant's motion to dismiss the actions for lack of subject matter jurisdiction; (2) defendant's motion to dismiss claims for failure to state a claim for which relief may be granted; (3) defendant's motion to abstain on the basis of act of state doctrine; and (4) defendant Anderson's motion to dismiss on the grounds of* forum non conveniens. *For the reasons stated below, the Court grants defendant's motion to dismiss pursuant to Fed.R.Civ.P.12(b)(6) with respect to two claims only: Owens Wiwa's Alien Torts Claim Act claims, 18 U.S.C.§1350[ACTA], founded on an alleged violation of his right to life, liberty and security of person, and his ACTA [3] claim for arbitrary arrest and detention. Plaintiffrs are given thirty days from the date of this Order to replead those claims. Defendant's motion to dismiss is denied in all other respects.*

There are both positive and negative aspects to dealing with this case under ATCA. It is indeed highly desirable to make Oil Corporations accountable for the havoc they wreak,[145] and we will return to this point below. But it is insufficient to highlight the most obvious and serious aspect of the tragedy in Ogoniland, while ignoring the *causal nexus* between environmental crimes, the citizens' resistance, and the state/corporate terrorist activities that ensued. The fact that no International Environmental Tribunal exists today that might have brought to justice the ecocrimes that gave rise to all ensuing cascading effects supports Judge Postiglione's pleas for the necessity of such a tribunal.[146]

In essence, Nigerian citizens in the area had no resource when their lands and waters were degraded and, with them, their only food supply. Had the ecocrimes been brought to an appropriate forum, perhaps the gross human rights violations that are now in the Court, might not have occurred.

After the murder of Ken Saro-Wiwa in November 1995,[147] I prepared a case study with the help of documents provided by Amnesty International, the Goldman Prize Organization and Dr Owens Wiwa, brother of the deceased. The case is one that includes both 'genocide' and 'ecocide' as Saro-Wiwa himself describes it.[148] After the continuing and unrelenting practice of gross abuses of human rights, ranging from the suppression of peaceful protests for the irreversible damages to the land and waters of the Ogoni people, to rapes, organized military raids and slayings, culminating with the murder of the Ogoni 9, including Ken Saro-Wiwa, no international body brought the perpetrators to justice.[149]

The main point is that 'any company that profits from crimes against humanity should be brought to justice wherever they are', and the most appropriate forum for such a legal exercise should be the one best able to mount a successful prosecution.[150] What is at stake is the defence of the most basic human rights, but also, at the same time in this case, the defence of our common environment/habitat, and this issue is not even mentioned.

In the 'Discussion' of the case, Judge Wood clarifies the reach of ACTA and of Torture Victim Protection Act (TVPA) with respect to the case:

> A. ATCA and TVPA
>
> Plaintiffs premise jurisdiction over their international law claims on the ATCA, 28 USC§1350, and general federal question jurisdiction, 28 U.S.C. §1331 (1993). The ATCA provides that 'the district courts shall have original jurisdiction of any civil action by any alien for a tort only, committed in violation of the laws of nations or a treaty of the United States.' 28 U.S.C.§1350. Section 1350 was enacted in 1789, but was rarely invoked until the Second Circuit's 1980 decision in Filartiga v. Pena-Irala, 630 F.2d 876 (2d Cir.1980). In Filartiga, the Second Circuit 'recognized the important principle' that ATCA 'validly creates federal court jurisdiction for suits alleging torts committed anywhere in the world against aliens in violation of the law of nations.' Kadic v. Karadzic, 70 F.3d 232,236 (2d Cir.1995) ['Kadic I'].

This paragraph brings out clearly the requirement for an international crime in violation of 'laws of nations', hence for violations encompassing breaches of *erga omnes* obligations. In some sense, it is insufficient to view these crimes as torts, but the presence of universal, non-derogable obligations breached in the cases ATCA considers, paves the way for further criminal prosecution, especially given the coming into force of the International Criminal Court in July 2002.

In a much simpler and lower profile case, a similar principle is upheld in the Supreme Court of Canada decision in *Ward v. Canada* (March, 2002). This was a sealing case, where Ford Ward was charged with using his fishing licence to kill certain seals and sell their pelts, against Federal Laws enacted in the common interest for the protection of these marine mammals and their habitat. Although he justly claimed he had a valid licence to pursue his chosen occupation, the Supreme Court of Canada argued that Section 27 of the *Marine Mammals Regulations*, prohibits the sale, trade or barter of young harp seals, and that it falls under the federal powers over fisheries, 'which is not confined to conserving fish stocks, but extends more broadly to maintenance and preservation of the fishery as a whole, including its economic value'.[151]

Notably, the latter is clearly not the primary consideration in the case; rather, the main concern is the 'management of fisheries as a public resource'. It may seem strange to return to a case such as *Ward v. Canada*, where no human rights violations were at issue, in order to compare it with the murder, destruction and torture present in the Ken Saro-Wiwa case. What they have in common is, primarily, (a) the choice of jurisdiction and of law instrument based on whatever best supports the common interest; and (b) an environmental issue that is much more in evidence in the Royal Dutch Shell Case, but is not mentioned in the ATCA analysis of the case. Yet the facts show that ecological concern was indeed the starting point and foundation of the Ogoni protest, on behalf of their 'basic rights'.[152]

Ward is a case where a Court upholds Federal prescriptive jurisdiction, while Royal Shell is about interpretive adjudicative jurisdiction; in addition, the common interest institutional function for one state (Canada) is quite different from the actual scope of the ATCA. Nevertheless, it can be argued that the appeal to the 'common interest' is the key that links the two apparently disparate cases. Even the Canadian case, ostensibly about the Canadian common interest, has several features that might bring Ward closer, in principle, to the *erga omnes* requirements of ATCA. These are: consideration of European negative assessment of seal hunting practices, the consideration, through that issue, of animal rights (a universal issue), even if it is primarily its Canadian economic aspect that emerges.

In conclusion, although the *mens rea* issue is not easily resolved in the presence of such diffuse and complex crimes, the knowledge element appears to contribute significantly to a possible resolution. The treatment of ecofootprint crimes under ATCA remains useful because it clarifies the factual elements and brings the perpetrators, at least initially and in principle, before a court of law. In addition, I suggest it may well be a first step to the possible indictment of ecocriminals by the International Criminal Court.

ATCA jurisprudence: Direct and indirect ecofootprint harms

In the US, the *Alien Torts Claims Act* of 1789 was instituted originally with exceedingly laudable aims and purposes, primarily, to further Congress' intent that 'the new nation take its place among the civilized nations of the world'.[153] Harms caused by climate change, and other conditions engendered by institutionalized and accepted forms of violence, must be assessed from a different point of view.[154] But all the ATCA litigation involves human rights as well, from torture and war crimes.[155] For the former categories, the Court recognized all these as violations of international law, specifically, 'genocide, war crimes, torture and summary execution'.[156] Hence only some of these cases can be classed as ecofootprint crimes. In some of the cases most of the aspects listed are combined, as in the Wiwa case. For the most part, however, the activities of transnational enterprises are the most prominent, and they do so in a surprising number of ways. The harms reach beyond direct impacts on the environment or on public health.

The first ecocrime (1) is thus the imposition of extreme environmental degradation (a direct harm), but also (2) direct, environmentally related harms to person and peoples. Other right-related harms include (3) labour-related human rights violations (as in the Coca-Cola case; or *Doe v. Unocal Corp.*, 110 F.Supp.2d 1294 C.D.Cal.2000

(Burma)), or (4) non-labour-related human rights violations (*Abdullah v. Pfizer, Inc.*, No.01 Civ.8118, 2002 U.S.Dist.LEXIS 17436 (S.D.N.Y. Sept.16, 2002)). Also, *Restatement (Third) of the Foreign Relations Law of the United States* 404 (1987), Section 702 provides that:

> *A state violates international law if, as a matter of state policy, it practices, encourages or condones:*
>
> (a) *genocide;*
> (b) *slavery or slave trade;*
> (c) *the murder or causing the disappearance of individuals;*
> (d) *torture or other cruel, inhuman or degrading treatment or punishment;*
> (e) *prolonged arbitrary detention;*
> (f) *systematic racial discrimination;*
> (g) *a consistent pattern of gross violations of internationally recognized human rights.*

Abdullah v. Pfizer concerned the liability of Pfizer, a pharmaceutical company, hence an activity that was not harmful to environments or person as such. But Pfizer:

> *administered Trovan to children from one to thirteen years, after obtaining the approval of the Nigerian government to conduct testing in response to epidemics of bacterial meningitis, measles, and cholera in Kano.*[157]

The corporation did not obtain parental consent, and did not explain the risks associated with that medication. As a result, several children died, and others 'suffered paralysis, deafness, and blindness'.[158]

Even the briefest review of the sort of harms imposed by the footprint of transnational corporate activities demonstrates the criminal aspects of these operations, even when their products or processes are not environmentally hazardous. The Coca-Cola case, for instance, represents a case of indirect harm. In order to promote its activities and its profits, the Florida owners of the Colombian operation hired a local man to discourage the forming of unions and to squash labour protests or workers' demands. With the aid of local paramilitary groups, Isidro Gil, a union representative was murdered as he entered the plant one morning. After that, loud speakers informed all workers that they had better sign documents immediately signifying their intention to disband the union, or risk a similar fate.

In this case then, it was not the product or process that was harmful, but the determination to push economic advantage at all costs, without any consideration of human rights violations, or any concern for labour laws. Therefore, when we consider the reach of ecofootprint harms, we must be prepared to go beyond an examination of its direct harms, and to acknowledge the various aspects of its indirect harms, most of which manifest clear criminal components.

The presence of these criminal relations demands both a review of present international law and the introduction of strong compliance and enforcement mechanisms. Benedict Kingsbury argues that, for the most part, today's international law is based on '(1) the Anglo-French focus on dispute settlement and litigation, and (2) the US focus on managerial problem solving'.[159] Both approaches exclude a priori the possibility of a strong normativity of moral principles providing the main focus.

But in cases involving the responsibility of the whole international community, human rights and moral obligations are primary as they determine the necessity for intervention:

> *International Law scholarship has been a vehicle of an internationalist morality, expressing ideas of shared responsibility for human rights, for basic human needs, and for the realization of environmental values.*[160]

Hence it is vital to demonstrate that ecofootprint activities are for the most part, lacking any 'internationalist morality'. Their effects are viewed – at best – as possible torts, but not as contrary to *erga omnes* obligations, despite the clear components we noted of accepted international crimes such as genocide or attacks against the human person.

We are facing a 'normative abyss',[161] and we need to appeal to Grotian 'rationality',[162] or, as I believe, to Kantian cosmopolitanism, where respect for every individual and for his or her rights is primary.[163] The latter would permit not only the primacy of moral ideals, beyond the accommodations and compromises present when states are viewed as the sole authority, but also steps toward the ideal 'universal state' Kant envisioned. This ideal could be embodied in a stronger UN, less dependent on the interests of powerful groups, therefore acting more as a true 'actor', than as a 'stage' where others act out their preferences.

NOTES

1   Malhotra (1988), pp41–42.
2   See also Timoshenko (1994), pp209–215.
3   Malhotra (1988), p42.
4   Gonzales (2001), p1016.
5   Sagoff (1988) .
6   Schudson (1984), p117.
7   Schudson (1984), p124.
8   Schor (1999), p436.
9   Schor (1999), p436.
10 Schor (1999) p438; I am indebted for much of the previous discussion to Schor's work as well.
11 Schor (1999), p438.
12 Sagoff (1988).
13 Albritton (2004), chapter 5.
14 Schor (1999), pp441–443.
15 Westra (2004a).
16 Gonzales (2001), p1010.
17 Wackernagel and Rees (1996).
18 Westra (2004a); Rees and Westra (2003), pp99–124.
19 *Council of Europe Communities Directive on Major Accident Hazards of Certain Industrial Activities* (82/501/EEC, 24 June 1982; as amended by 87/216/EEC, 19 March 1987; and 88/8610/EEC, 24 November 1988; hereinafter *Seveso Directive*).

20   Under *Aliens Torts Claims Act.*
21   Westra (2004a).
22   Westra (1998).
23   Baram (1989), p128.
24   Majupuria (1993). See generally *Business India* (1985); *India Today* (1984); Hazarika (1984); Diamond (1985); Nanda and Bailey (1988); and *Implications of the Industrial Disaster in Bhopal, India: Hearing before the Subcomm. on Asia and Pacific Affairs of the House Comm. on Foreign Affairs,* 98th Con. 2d Sess. 3, 6, 28 (1984) (statements of Robert A. Peck, Deputy Assistant Secretary for Near Eastern and South Asian Affairs, Department of State, and Ronald Wishart, Vice President for Government Relations, Union Carbide Corporation).
25   Ugelow (1982), p167.
26   Lutz et al (1985), p303.
27   Chopra (1994), p238.
28   *UN Declaration on the Establishment of a New Economic International Order,* May 9, 1974, G.A. Res.3201, 29 U.N.Gaor Supp. (No.31) C 50, U.N.Doc.A/9631 (1975).
29   *UN Conference on Trade and Development Draft International Code of Conduct on the Transfer of Technology,* May 6,1980, rep. 19 Int'l Legal Mat. 773 (1980).
30   Chopra (1994), pp239–240.
31   Westra (2004a), chapter 7.
32   Chopra (1994), p246.
33   Baram (1989), p128.
34   Baram (1989), p88.
35   Baram (1989), p89.
36   Draper (1991).
37   Lisi (2003).
38   Baram (1989) p133.
39   Kafka (1984).
40   Chopra (1994), p236.
41   Chopra (1994), p248.
42   Chopra (1994), p248.
43   Gonzales (2001).
44   Chopra (1994), pp240–241.
45   Falk (1998).
46   Chopra (1994), pp244–245.
47   Chopra (1994); increased radiation levels were found in Scandinavia, Poland, France, UK, Finland, Ireland and West Germany; see 'Government withholds information/then says radiation levels not serious', 9 *International Environmental Report* (BNAI) 188, 11 June 1986; 'EEC lift ban on East European food imports, substitutes U.S. limits on radiation levels', 9 *International Environmental Report* (BNA) 442, 11 June 1986: 'Radiation levels from Chernobyl prompts limits on livestock slaughter', 10 *International Environmental Report* (B1A) 442 9 Sept. 1987; 'Effects of Chernobyl in Finland', 9 *International Environmental Report* (BNA) 420 12 Nov 1986.
48   *US v. Canada,* 3 I.A.A. 1911 (1941).
49   *Corfu Channel Case, UK v. Albania,* 1949 I.C.J., Rep.4.
50   Malone (1987), p203.
51   Bullard (1994).
52   Bullard (2001), pp3–28.
53   Boos-Hersberger (1997), pp103–105.
54   Boos-Hersberger (1997), pp103–105.
55   Boos-Hersberger (1997), pp106–107.
56   Sandoz (1996), p8.

57   Sandoz (1996) pp10–11.
58   Boos-Hersberger (1997), p108.
59   Sandoz (1996), p14.
60   *Convention on the Protection of the Rhine Against Chemical Pollution* (Bonn), 1124 UNTS 375; 16 ILM (1977), 243. In force 1 February 1973.
61   Birnie and Boyle (2002), p206.
62   Birnie and Boyle (2002), p322.
63   *Convention on the Protection of the Rhine from Pollution by Chlorides* (Bonn), 16 ILM (1997), 265. In force 5 July 1985; Amended by the 1991 Protocol; note also the *1999 Convention for the Protection of the Rhine from Chemical Pollution*, not in force, as not yet ratified by all Rhine States.
64   Birnie and Boyle (2002), pp324–325.
65   Birnie and Boyle (2002), p324–325.
66   Brunnee and Toope (1997), p26.
67   Boos-Hersberger (1997), p118.
68   Westra (2004a), chapter 4.
69   Gonzales (2001), n. 20.
70   Seremba (1995), p.H3.
71   Amnesty International (1995).
72   *Goldman Environmental Prize*, Goldman Environmental Foundation Documents package on Ken Saro-Wiwa, San Francisco, CA, 1995; see also Silverstein (1995).
73   Soyinka (1994).
74   Amnesty International (1995).
75   Saro-Wiwa (1994b).
76   Saro-Wiwa (1994b).
77   Saro-Wiwa (1994a).
78   Shiva (1989).
79   Saro-Wiwa (1994b); see also Saro-Wiwa (1994a).
80   Brooks (1994), ppA1, A4.
81   Brooks (1994), ppA1, A4.
82   Brooks (1994), ppA1, A4.
83   Brooks (1994), ppA1, A4.
84   Brooks (1994), ppA1, A4.
85   Brooks (1994), ppA1, A4.
86   Brooks (1994), ppA1, A4.
87   Brooks (1994), ppA1, A4.
88   Saro-Wiwa (1994b).
89   *The Globe and Mail* (1995) pA17.
90   Brooks (1994), ppA1, A4.
91   Brooks (1994), ppA1, A4.
92   *The Globe and Mail*, Canada, 21 Nov. 1995, pA17.
93   Westra and Wenz (1995).
94   Shrader-Frechette (1991), esp chapter 10.
95   Jonas (1984).
96   Sagoff (1988); see also Goodland and Daly (1995.) pp102–124.
97   Westra and Wenz (1995).
98   Wackernagel and Rees (1996).
99   Wackernagel and Rees (1996).
100 Westra and Wenz (1995).
101 Wackernagel and Rees (1996).
102 Kamm and Greenberger (1995), p10.

103   Kamm and Greenberger (1995), p10; see also French (1995) pA1, A13.

104   Epstein (1989).

105   *Rome Statute*, in force, July 12, 2002.

106   Westra (2004a), chapter 7.

107   Heath (2001).

108   Downs (1993), p351.

109   G.A.Res.2200A, U.N. GAOR, 21st Sess., Supp.No.16 at 52, U.N.Doc.A/6316(1966), 999 U.N.T.S. 171, in force March 23, 1976.

110   G.A.Res.2200A, U.N.GAOR, 21st Sess., Supp.No.16 at 49, U.N.Doc.A/6316 (1966), 993 U.N.T.S. 3, in force January 3, 1976.

111   Shue (1996a).

112   Downs (1993).

113   *Alien Torts Claims Act*, 28 U.S.C. 1350 (1789).

114   United States District Court S.D. Florida, *Sinaltra the Estate of Isidro Sequndo Gil, Plaintiffs v. Coca Cola Company et. al.,* 256 F.Supp.2d 1345.

115   Westra (1998), chapter 5

116   Westra (2004a).

117   *Convention on the Prevention and Punishment of the Crime of Genocide* (1951), 78 U.N.T.S. 277.

118   Westra (2004a); see also Brown (2000).

119   Cooney et al (1996), p20.

120   Cooney et al (1996), p20.

121   Cooney et al (1996), p23.

122   *Ocean Dumping Act* (1971), 33 U.S.C. § 1411(a).

123   Cooney et al (1996), p23, n155.

124   Cooney et al (1996), p23.

125   Cooney et al (1996), p18.

126   Cooney et al (1996), p27.

127   Cooney et al (1996), p29.

128   Cooney et al (1996), p30.

129   Cooney et al (1996), p30.

130   *United States v. Britain*, 731 F.2d 1413, 21 E.L.R. 21092 (10th Cir. 1991).

131   Lazarus (1995), p9.

132   Schabas (2000), p206.

133   Schabas (2000), p207.

134   Westra (2004a), pp203ff.

135   Healy (1993), p265.

136   Edgerton (1928), p849.

137   Westra (2004a), chapter 3.

138   Feb. 28, 2002, *Wiwa v. Royal Dutch Petroleum Co.*

139   Bederman (2001), p176.

140   Bederman (2001), p176.

141   Kindred et al (2000), p11.

142   Bederman (2001), p173.

143   Bederman (2001), p179.

144   2002 U.S. Dist.LEXIS 3293, Feb.22, 2002.

145   Reinisch (2001).

146   Postiglione (2001).

147   Westra (1998), chapter 5.

148   Westra (1998), chapter 5.

149   Westra (1998), chapter 5, cp. 'Amended Complaint', www.earthrights.org/shell/complaint.html

150 Westra (1998), chapter 5.

151 *Council Directive* 83/129, 1983 O.J. (L 91)30; Charnovitz (1994).

152 Shue (1996a).

153 Dhoge (2003), pp782–833.

154 Westra (2004); I proposed six categories of ecocrimes: (a) ecocrimes as a form of unprovoked aggression; (b) ecocrimes as attacks on the human person; (c) ecocrimes as a form of genocide; (d) ecocrimes as a breach of global security; (e) ecocrimes as attacks on the human environment; (f) ecocrimes as breaches of global justice.

155 *Filartiga v. Pena-Irala*, 630 F.2d 876 (2d Cir. 1980); *Kadic V. Karadzic*, 70 F.3d 232 (2d Cir.1995); to rape, murder and genocide (*Wiwa v. Royal Dutch Petroleum Co.*, 226 F. 3d 88 (2d Cir., 2000) (Nigeria)); and labour rights and other breaches related to the operation of corporate and industrial enterprises (*Beanal v. Freeport-McMoran, Inc.*, 197 F.3d 161 5th Cir. 1999 (Indonesia)); *United States District Court S. D. Florida, Sinaltral v. Coca Cola Company*, 256 F.Supp. 2d 1345 (S.D.Fla.2003) (Columbia).

156 Dhoge (2003).

157 Dhoge (2003), p51.

158 Dhoge (2003), p51; in June 1999, the US Food and Drug Administration issued a public health advisory on liver toxicity associated with oral and intravenous usage of Trovan.

159 Kingsbury (2005).

160 Kingsbury (2005), p10.

161 Falk (1998).

162 Kinsbury (2005), p10.

163 Westra (2004a), chapter 8.

Ecojustice and Industrial Operations: Irreconcilable Conflict or Possible Coexistence?

INTRODUCTION

The last section of Chapter 7 raised the question of a conflict that cannot be reconciled with today's existing legal instruments and forms of governance. Because 'living with chemistry' and, in general, living in a world dominated by corporate goals is far more hazardous than most believe, far more so even that the possibility of being exposed to an occasional disaster, this is a question that, politically correct or not, needs careful reflection. The present status quo represents a daily proven, well-researched exposure to harm to normal human function and health. This exposure affects different persons in different ways, as it varies according to age, quantity and quality of exposure, individual predisposition and lifestyle.

Yet neither lifestyle nor possible predisposition are sufficient to excuse the industrial exposures that trigger individual pathologies. An analogy in law may be found in the courts' treatment of sexual assaults. Neither a woman's provocative behaviour nor mode of dress may influence the court's assessment of a man's unwanted sexual acts, although often the defence advances such arguments.[1,2] Hence an individual may be more or less susceptible to chemical exposures, because of an immune system affected by obesity, or by a smoking habit (leaving aside for the moment the deliberately addictive aspects of the latter). Neither 'condition', however, should be used in the defence of corporate activities, or to diminish their responsibility for resulting 'harms'. Indeed it is the presence of these inequalities that make the present status quo hard to eliminate: the argument used in defence of corporate industrial activities may be that although some appear to suffer grave harms, not everyone, either in the same area or under the same conditions of exposure, may be equally affected.

This could be one specific instance when the argument for using the 'first generation', understood as children before and after birth, gives the strongest reason for a radical revision of all laws governing chemical and other industrial corporate activities. The grave harms described in Chapter 1, based on the research of the WHO, ensure that a solid basis underlies all arguments for the cessation, or at least the radical modification of present practices of commercial operations. In fact the appeals to the WHO research are particularly important, not only for the thoroughness of their studies or their choice of focus on children of all ages, but also the use of their international, but independent, presence.

In contrast and on the topic of independence, it is important to consider recent critiques of US science research in relation to the policies of the present administration. A recent article describes how 'the Bush government is not simply catering to society's most conservative members, but capitalizing on its wider scientific discomfort'.[3] Abraham relates how the endangered Florida panther has managed to survive in an increasingly shrinking habitat, as 'Shopping malls, roads and golf courses have devoured the roaming grounds of the endangered big cat at the rate of 30,000 acres a year.'[4]

Yet when a biologist with the US Fish and Wildlife Service decided to write yet another (seventh) report on wildlife endangerment, he received 'high level instructions' not to write the reports on the area's 68 endangered species. He continued, however, to report his concerns, and was fired three days after Mr Bush's re-election.[5]

The defence of our own habitat through the presence of large areas of ecological integrity[6,7,8,9] has been the topic of much of my earlier work and of the scientific work of conservation biologists and ecologists. But it is not only wilderness preservation that is at issue. There is also the problem of the consequences, of the very corporate activities that displace or eliminate wildlife habitat: even golf courses and roads bring in overwhelming pesticide use for the former, and air pollution for the latter. Both are ongoing sources of exposure and of indisputable harms, but neither represent accidents, let alone disasters.

For instance, pesticides for individual households were eliminated in Quebec and, in 2004, municipalities in Toronto eliminated routine spraying of common green areas, although individual households still have the option of using chemicals and – of course – golf greens are still not only permitted, but encouraged. Florida biologist Eller, noted:

> *The tension that comes from pro-development interests has always been there, but if there are no reports on threats [to a species], then there is no reason to say no to development.*[10]

And development as such, when unrestrained and not supported by research intent on conservation, needs to be critically examined and – for the most part – either radically modified or eliminated. These are fighting words, no doubt, for most North–West capitalists and industries. But if the alternative is consequences that cause gross and ongoing breaches of human rights through environmental means, or 'ecocrimes' as I have termed these actions,[11] then the present proliferation of human rights should not be limited as it seems to be today, to gender-related issues or politically motivated harms, but should extend to the universal rights to non-interference with normal human function.

There are a great number of activities that are viewed as 'normal' or routine business practices, but that are such that they hide harmful results, under the benign masks of 'progress' or 'advancement' or 'economic opportunities'. It might be interesting to examine some of these routine activities, starting with the most basic one of all, agriculture and the food industry in general. Keeping food healthy and water safe seems to be a basic responsibility of governments in democratic countries. Water and food are basic necessities for all human beings. In Third World countries they may be scarce or even non-existent in some cases. But wealthy, developed countries offer no guarantees in this regard either.

In the next section we will consider the case of Walkerton, Ontario and the terrible results of business as usual, and a government that gave primacy to the protection of business interests over the health and safety of citizens: a common scenario in North America.

RESPONSIBILITY AND ACCOUNTABILITY FOR ECOVIOLENCE: THE EXAMPLE OF WALKERTON

Negligent motoring and negligent manufacturing significantly threaten the public interest; yet Western judges seem more comfortable punishing counterfeiters and prostitutes than imposing sanctions against those who inadvertently take unreasonable risks.[12]

In May 2000, an outbreak of the deadly E. coli virus struck Walkerton, Ontario, a small rural town, killing as many as 18 people at the latest count although, according to later official sources, the total deaths acknowledged by Provincial authorities was only seven. The initial public outrage started with a question: how could this happen in an affluent democracy like Canada's Ontario Province? In early June, the banner headlines multiplied, as the circumstances, background and implications of the case became clear: 'Ontario ignored water alert'[13] is a typical report of the crisis: 'Ontario's Environmental Ministry warned as early as 1997 that shutting down its water testing labs could lead to the kind of water disaster that has hit Walkerton, Ont. and killed at least seven people, internal documents show.' Ontario's Premier, Mike Harris, had pursued a policy of (1) privatizing water testing services without ensuring that medical officers of health were informed if harmful bacteria were detected; (2) revising 'Ontario Drinking Water Objectives', shifting the treatment costs to municipalities, without guaranteeing that smaller municipalities would continue to keep tabs on water quality; (3) disbanding 'teams charged with inspecting municipal water treatment plants';[14] (4) giving priority to 'infrastructure projects to aid economic development'.[15] As a general policy, Mike Harris had clearly stated that provincial debt reduction would be his main objective, not the protection of environmental and public health, repeatedly, as part of his election platform.

Despite the opposition of the Liberal Party and the many environmental and human rights groups who protested, Mike Harris was re-elected for a second term in 1999 precisely on his 'pro business/lower taxes' platform. But the general public would assume that basic safety would be ensured for all citizens, that public health would not be or become an issue. Yet it would be difficult for Harris to claim ignorance of the present trends in Canadian water issues.

This example is of a case unexpected in a country like Canada, especially in one of its richest and most populous provinces. It is important to keep in mind, however, that the Walkerton case study cannot be fully written yet, as its history is still unfolding at this time. Even more important, at this time, (1) Walkerton is only described as an example of an ecodisaster that can happen anywhere, even in a democratic country, and close to home, not only in a developing country under a military regime; and (2) Walkerton is also different in that the ecocrimes committed are systemic, institutional and the result of practices some of which are legal, taken for granted, not the result of specific activity by a specific actor or actors, as is often the case in other case studies, such as those written on Bhopal,[16] or the Saro-Wiwa case in Ogoniland.[17]

Normally case studies include a clear chronology and perhaps details not only about the facts at issue, but also about the individuals or companies involved. Hence, although we will describe, broadly speaking, some of the political and regulative background against which the Walkerton events unfolded, no effort will be made to provide a specific chronology of events, or to indict a specific individual, company or group, as is normally done in case studies. What we hope to do is to show the nature of the sort of 'ecocrimes' that are systemic, diffuse and institutional; Walkerton is a clear example of this sort of disaster.

Hence, I will argue that (1) breaches of environmental regulations are ecocrimes and ought to be treated as such, not only as quasi criminal; and (2) the 'emergent risks'[18] posed by ecocrimes are not easily dealt with either by tradition, regional/national means, let alone by a weakening system supporting deregulations as we will argue below; ecocrimes are not sporadic, occasional offences, they are instead institutional forms of violence often practised through non-point pollution, that is, pollution that does not come from one, identifiable source, in the careless and often negligent pursuit of other goals, mostly economic ones. Then we will turn to the question of moral and legal responsibility, and the way these regulatory breaches are viewed in common law. It is important to understand these breaches as real crimes: unlike other ecodisasters, primarily in developing countries,[19,20,21] or in North American minority neighbourhoods,[22,23,24] Walkerton is an example of the results of legal, institutionalized practices, without illegal acts being committed or the taint or racism.

After considering the governance aspect, and the regulatory framework, the first section of this chapter will turn to the question of corporate responsibility for ecoviolence: this responsibility does not rest equally on corporations and on businesses in general and does not have the good of the people as its primary concern. Whether or not the area megafarms or a single farm operation were the major trigger for the disaster at Walkerton, the relationship between democratic governments, their regulatory systems and public safety must be re-examined, for their failure to meet their protective obligations.[25]

The economic interests of institutions, corporations and individuals, appear to pose the gravest threats to the possibility of achieving environmental security. Some argue that the root of the problem is the form of governance of the country affected by environmental disasters. But, as we shall see, even in a country with no dictator or other repressive form of governance, citizens may be at serious risk.

We will consider the example of Walkerton, together with the ostensible reasons for permitting, in fact encouraging, practices that have documented harmful effects. The desired results intended in this case are the ability of industry to provide abundant meat at low prices, thus enabling everyone to buy and eat as much as they desire. But, although catering to public preferences is often viewed as one of the goals of liberal democratic governance, in this case, the 'preference' is in direct conflict with the public good. In brief, a diet based on animal meat and fat, laced with various chemicals, as required by factory farming conditions, and by the economic interests of industrial producers, is not 'good': it is as harmful to humankind as are illegal drugs. Not only is it harmful to public health, it carries serious implications for public health services, strained to the limit by the recurrence and growth of 'Western man diseases',[26] such as cancers and heart disease.

The true beneficiaries of factory farming are the corporate owners of these operations and, perhaps, the bureaucracies that may get rewarded for their support of these operations. The relation between these operations and farming in general will be discussed with the thrust to deregulation and the support for markets rather than citizen's safety.

After much prevarication and name calling among politicians, the problem came to a head on the front page of Canada's most conservative and pro-business newspaper (a victory in itself). Citing *The Globe and Mail* once again, on 7 June 2000, Andrew Nikiforuk's special report entitled 'National Water Crisis Forecast – Study Blames Declines Supply on Lax Attitudes, Climate Change', placed the finger right on the problem. Canada's foremost water ecologist, David Schindler (University of Alberta) predicts that:

> *the combined effects of climate change, acid rain, human and livestock wastes, increased ultraviolet radiation, airborne toxins and biological invaders will result in the degradation of Canadian freshwater on a scale hitherto unimaginable.*[27]

Once again, as it had happened for many years, the underlying ecoviolence was not isolated as a major issue, and the list of problems Schindler outlines have been, at best, viewed as separate problems, each requiring an individualized response. Schindler, correctly, views all separate effects as arising from a combined, unified cause. I have called the 'cause' disintegrity, or that condition of climate, air and land that engenders and sustains multiple water disasters. The lax attitudes cited by Schindler are also the basis of much of the stress that fosters climate change, so that a lack of moral imperatives, demanding responsibility, not only rights, and supporting appropriate laws and regulations is fundamentally at fault.

We need at least a certain percentage[28,29] of the Earth to be left wild or undeveloped, in order to provide all life with nature's services.[30,31,32] We also need to keep the rest, both land and water, in a state of health.[33,34] Most of all, we need to accept, as Schindler does, the ecosystem approach as a holistic means to understand the problems and to design and implement a solution.

Walkerton is an example of the acceptance of practices and policies chosen under the same problematic conditions as those outlined in our discussion of contingent valuations.[35] We can address the choices that have resulted in the litany of disasters Schindler describes. In most cases, including that of Walkerton, reductionist, rather than holistic, end of pipe solutions were (and are) sought and the institutional response is limited to an effort to isolate the failures of government, bureaucrats, or others to monitor the grave conditions of the natural systems involved, including air, water and land. But no effort or even mention is made of isolating the underlying causes, the practices and choices that North Americans (in this case, Canadians) have made over the years, that have brought these environmental matters to a head. Schindler says: 'People don't appreciate the impact of multiple stressors on our water supply and we have a history of underestimating problems. And when you put all these things together, nasty things tend to happen'.[36] Only the holistic approach truly captures the reality of what is happening. Hence, so long as we continue to view each problem as arising from a separate stressor, we will accept individualized, fragmented responses as adequate. I am arguing that only when we understand the role of multiple stressors on a system, that is on a whole, can we start to move to appropriate public policies.

The Walkerton disaster shows precisely the role of multiple stressors on ecosystems, as well as the multiple instances of violence arising from these stresses. The violent attacks combine to affect human health at most obvious levels. An outbreak of disease (engendered by E. coli) in the water supply and the resulting infection, morbidity and fatality for men, women and children, is undeniably a violent attack, fostered by disintegrity including the lack of appropriately sized natural, wild areas, and environmental degradation.

Diet choices, preferences and megafarms

This section will not address the indefensible violence against non-human animals in factory farms: these have been documented all too well in many books, and evaluated and discussed by many ethicists. Descriptive works like *Slaughterhouse*[37] or *Prisoned Chickens, Poisoned Eggs*,[38] or *Milk, The Deadly Poison*[39] tell a shocking story of violence and inhumanity. Philosophical works like *The Case for Animal Rights*,[40] *Animal Liberation*,[41] discuss and analyse the practices that support our preferred affluent Western diets. Jeremy Rifkin's *Beyond Beef: The Rise and Fall of Cattle Culture* (1992), ties in the unethical diet choices to the global injustices engendered by overuse and overconsumption that are as hazardous to our environment as it is to our health and to the survival of those in impoverished countries in the South–East. Aside from questions relating to the responsibility and accountability of bureaucrats, businesses and institutions of Walkerton, there is a question that was not raised in the newspapers, why that sort of hazardous business was encouraged to locate in the area, without imposing limits or other regulatory restraints to where and how it should operate. The underlying motive can be primarily economic, when we consider the single and the corporate business operations involved. When we consider the motivation of the Ontario government, the economic motive, even if present through business support, is normatively insufficient and legally suspect. Governments should not licence or permit to operate, operations that do not function for the public good, or – at least – that do not impose public harms.

Examples of environmentally hazardous operations may be the opening up of high-ways with multiple lanes, or even the presence of large hospitals, sources of copious toxic wastes. Both examples indicate that the side effects, intrusion into the wild for the former, hazardous waste for the latter, should be mitigated; but in both cases the public good is served by both operations. Clearly, both should take steps to function in a more environmentally safe manner, in order not to give rise to 'double effect' harms to the public. But the basic usefulness of both cannot be denied.

In the same way, we need to consider the question of diet preferences leading the desirability not only of farms producing meat in traditional ways, that is, keeping animals in natural conditions of life, but also factory farms, intended to produce large quantities of meat at prices low enough to enable most citizens of affluent Western democracies to eat abundant meat at all meals. But factory farming raised animals must be fed large amounts of antibiotics and other chemicals to keep them alive in unnatural conditions of confinement, and they are also fed growth hormones and other medicines to bring them as soon as possible to full size and the market. The question then is whether this progress is indeed in the public interest, or whether the harms imposed are significant enough to justify legal countermeasures to control these practices.

In relation to both human rights to be free from harm, and the justice dimensions of environmental effects of the 'cattle culture', Rifkin outlines the effects, such as famine, in developing countries. When cattle are fed grains that would feed hundreds of thousands of people in the South, and instead produce meat for the taste preferences of those who can afford it, this is not only an environmental wrong, but also a breach of justice. Of course, even turning everyone in developed countries to vegetarianism, in the interest of global justice, would not be enough, unless the monumental distribution and political problems were settled first.[42] The science supporting this position is readily available,[43,44,45,46,47] and so are the normative analysis of these practices.

For most of the philosophers, it is the unspeakable violence against the individual animals that is the target of their arguments. I will accept these arguments as given and will not attempt to compare or evaluate them, as there is an abundant literature that has already done much of that work. I will use their joint (though nuanced) agreement that the violence perpetrated upon animals in the quest of consumer preferences is immoral, and use that as a starting point for the arguments of this chapter and this section.

The result of accepting that argument is to accept that what takes place in factory farming is institutionalized, legal violence. What we must add is that the violence eventually returns to us, magnified and unexpected, when we exercise our right to enjoy what we prefer to consume. The ecoviolence that boomerangs back to us follows through these considerations: (1) ecoviolence through animal, agricultural practices; this leads to (2) ecoviolence through ecosystem disruption, representing both violence to the system; and (3) to us through resulting health effects; the consequence is ecoviolence against (4) both individual and public health. The latter in turn includes several interrelated but separate attacks. It is both sad and puzzling that we accept these attacks fostered by a global economic enterprise that supports a hazardous diet for all who want it and can afford it, without regard for the resulting 'Western man's diseases' or for the violence upon which the diet itself is based.

Thus, beyond the violence against so called 'farm' animals, the question about the common good raised in the previous section demands answers: it is not enough to say, look at what happened at Walkerton, and what the government of Ontario or of Canada did or did not do.

Why did we empower politicians, freely and democratically chosen, to support such hazardous choices? These choices are, at the same time, a threat to our health, to other living creatures, and to our joint habitat. Of course, another question comes first: can we truly claim that our preferences are truly ours and freely chosen? Does our knowledge of the consequence of our preferences, spotty and incomplete though it is, render us complicit in the violent results of those preferences? And, most puzzling of all, what leads even the citizens of democratic countries, where at least some information is available to them in principle, to participate in practices that are ultimately going to harm them?

Diet choices are manipulated by those who gain from selling food that is harmful when it is grown, processed and even consumed.[48] This touches each one of us as closely as we can be touched: our immediate survival depends both on our nourishment and on our habitat. Both are under attack, as we are, from current diet choices. We are bombarded with advertisements about fatty, unhealthy food choices we know are harmful to our health and to that of our children. In addition, at least in North–West democracies, we also know that our government's bureaucracies have other priorities than the protection of human health. In the introductory section of this chapter, we saw that Canadian Mike Harris (Ontario's Premier), candidly admitted that his priority was reducing the debt and supporting business. This frank confession was uttered while a television interviewer raised questions about the unprecedented spread of disease, the mounting number of deaths, and while yet another agricultural community, St Thomas, discovered E. coli in the water of a local nursing home.

The connection between diet choices and the E. coli outbreak starts with the existence of megafarms that produce what we believe we need and we are entitled to have, together with the morally culpable negligence of those whose responsibility it is to ensure protection for our life and physical integrity. This example (Walkerton) shows the factual sequence leading to the disaster that occurred.

The first step lies in a political system that only pays lip service to the common interest in ecological/health protection, as legally established by national environmental acts, such as *Canadian Environmental Protection Act* (CEPA) (1999) and by the binational (Canada/US) regulatory mandates of the *Great Lakes Water Quality Agreement* (GLWQA (1978, ratified 1987)), but does not really incorporate the binding requirement 'to protect and restore the integrity' of the Great Lake Waters and of that basin, with all that it would imply for the conduct of business in the area.

The second step may be considered the election of a government that implements disastrous ecological and health deregulation, under the heading of bringing about a 'common sense revolution', that places openly economic interests above environmental protection and the basic rights of Ontario's Canadians. Note that each step can be deemed to be 'normal' 'routine', a legal aspect of institutionalized practices. But the 'megafarms' raise public and individual health problems that do not arise from small family farm operations such as the ones that were present in that Ontario region for years. Consider for instance hog farming. In a feature titled 'Fear of Farming', Alana Mitchell, John Gray and Real Seguin cite some 'Porcine Statistics':

- 12 million: Canada's current (record) hog population
- 36,000: number of hog farms in 1986
- 13,000: number of hog farms today
- 280: pigs per farm in 1986
- 917: pigs per farm today (*The Globe and Mail*, July 3, 2000, A11).

Similar percentages are present in Ontario and in Quebec and bovine statistics report equally large numbers and rapid growth. The phenomenal growth of the megafarms reflects public and individual health problems that do not arise from the operation and the products of the small family farms operations of the past. The epidemic proportions of 'Western man's diseases', all fostered by cheap, available fat and meat products is related to our diet. The World Health Organization (WHO) has publicized the 'Mediterranean diet', in stark contrast with the practices of affluent Western countries (with the exception of Italy, a country that boasts the most longevity in the world today). We are taught, enticed and convinced to prefer unsafe diets, whereas what is healthy and safe is the opposite: meat never, or no more than once a month at best, chicken (normally raised or free range) once a week, at most, for the rest, fruits, vegetables, olive oil, grains and natural starches, and fish.

We reap the result of ignoring the reality of our needs and our best interests at our own cost, and at the cost of those who are disproportionately affected by our practices. These injustices range from the use of grain protein (thus limiting protein intake to those who can afford it in its form as meat). This practice, as many have shown, deprives those who are starving of possible available grains, to satisfy our taste preferences.[49] We also reap the results at many other levels, as agribusiness and factory farms have grown enormously. Farmers themselves suffer, at the very least, noxious odours and other discomforts:

> The Hern family has watched the factory farm evolution up close. For the better part of 140 years, they happily farmed 20 acres near Kirkton, 50 kilometers north of London, Ont. Then some newcomers moved into the neighbourhood. 'I now have 10,000 hogs one mile from my bedroom,' David Hern says. The result is waste equal to that produced by 40,000 people.

But, of course, there is more involved than a bad smell: the threat to the near neighbours and to the rest of us is just as real: hog waste, like cattle manure is not treated. Cattle and hogs can transmit E. coli through their faeces, or from cattle hides after butchering. Some US research shows that cattle raised in overcrowded feedlots in Nebraska and in general fattened at Midwest feedlots are breeding grounds for E. coli, that is actually found in 72 per cent of the lots investigated.[50]

The factory farm is therefore the source of severe individual and public health threats, but it is also at the same time the source of serious environmental damage, and the epitome of gross disregard for the life, health and integrity of individual animals. There is more than a casual connection between these forms of violence, and the harm that eventually rebounds upon us reaches beyond the savage treatment of so called 'farm animals'. It is worth noting that J. Baird Callicott in his classic treatment of the topic, 'Animal Liberation: A triangular affair',[51] although he does not argue on the side of animal ethics, strongly indicts agribusiness practices. He says, of the consumption of meat:

> Meat, however, purchased at the supermarket, externally packaged and internally laced with petrochemicals, fattened in feed lots, slaughtered impersonally and, in general, mechanically processed from artificial insemination to microwave roaster, is an affront not only to physical metabolism and bodily health, but to conscience as well.[52]

We distance ourselves from the violent treatment meted out to animals that we only encounter, eventually, as slabs in a supermarket cooler. Similarly we tend to think of agribusiness as just business, that is, as something unrelated to suffering or violence, just a normal, legal part of everyday life. In fact we admire and even treat as celebrities those whose business thrives and becomes increasingly larger and more profitable year after year. Even environmental damage is often thought to be something else, something other than and unrelated to the concern with violence, or with our health.

When we see (1) animal violence; (2) environmental violence; and (3) violent attacks on our health, for what they really are, the connection becomes clear, as does the cause and effect sequence, and the eventual deadening of our ability to be morally awake and emotionally sensitive to violence in all its forms. Eventually the violence has a boomerang effect as it rebounds on us. Difficult questions remain unanswered: for instance, why do we continue to accept as inevitable this (meat based) diet, these practices with their tripartite violence: to non-human animals, to natural systems to human organisms? Underlying all three, there is also a global injustice in the pursuit of institutional practices that decimate biodiversity, despoil nature, and reduce those in developing countries to famine-stricken masses.[53,54,55]

It might be possible to at least understand, if not condone, such a cluster of immoral choices and preferences, if the results produced unadulterated good for the choosers. However, the opposite is true. Given what goes into the meat and the milk we consume, the hormones, antibiotics, and other chemicals, together with the dirt and contamination to which all these products are exposed through the slaughtering and butchering processes,[56,57,58] it is clear that they present grave threats to health, even beyond diet considerations.

For the latter, Jeremy Rifkin reports on an accidental experiment as it happened to Danish nationals. Due to the naval blockade of 1917,

> *the Danes were cut off from incoming shipments of food. The government was subsequently forced to begin to ration out food, and encourage the country to give up its meat, and eat mainly a potato based diet. In time, some three million people became vegetarians and the death rate from disease fell some 35%.*[59,60]

The reverse is shown by the increase in cancer and heart disease in Japan, as that country moves away from its traditional low meat diet. Of 2.1 million deaths in the US, 1.5 million are due to dietary factors, primarily high consumption of cholesterol and fat in meat. The hormones, synthetics and other substances including bioengineered and transgenic substances that are present in the feed, hence, in the animals we eat, add to the now well-documented health risks. Perhaps the most publicized of these recent times has been the presence of Bovine Growth Hormone (BGH) followed by the infamous outbreak of 'mad cow' disease.[61]

In conclusion, the violence practised on animals to support our choices and preferences for certain foods, is tied to the violence we receive from these choices and preferences in our diet.

The impact of deregulations and other effects of the common sense revolution

> *Each offence must be sentenced in accord with its specific facts but pollution offences must be approached as crimes, not as morally blameless technical breaches of a regulatory standard. (R. v. United Keno Mines, (1980) 10 C. E. L.R. 43 (Terr. Ct.*

of Y.T.). Chief Judge Stewart, at 47; cited in *R. v. Village of 100 Mile House,* (1993) B.C.J. No. 2848 DRS 94 07390, 22 W.C. B (2d), 131)

One of the key elements in the Walkerton tragedy may well be the present legislative and regulatory framework in Ontario. Even before the tragedy happened, Canadian Environmental Law Association's (CELA) *Intervenor* described the situation in Ontario's farming communities in 'Rural Ontario: Industrial hog barns, industrial waste' (Bruckmann, 2000). In the previous section, we described some of the effects of having industrial hazardous facilities in farming areas. We did not enumerate in detail all the human health problems arising from this form of violence against animals. Antibiotics are fed to pigs, as 'thousands of animals are kept together in huge barns, sows producing more piglets, and piglets fattened by the shortest possible time before slaughter.'[62] Animals under these violent, inhumane and unnatural conditions require antibiotics to survive to market. The graphs overleaf shed further light on these issues.

A recent issue of *Nucleus*, the magazine of the Union of Concerned Scientists, makes the same point in 'Hogging It'.[63] Too many antibiotics that can be considered 'key' to human medicine, are 'routinely fed to livestock'; some of these are tetracycline, penicillin and erythromycin, all of which are used for healthy livestock. While the European Union has banned growth hormones, promoting uses of antibiotics that are used for humans, in the US, for instance, their use has increased by 50 per cent.[64]

It is almost obscene to think of using medication in this way, for the profit of some, when children in developing countries are dying from the lack of some of the same medications. Nevertheless these statistics further support the point made in the *Intervenor*. Even more immediately hazardous are the other threats arising from 'intensive livestock facilities':

> *Intensive livestock facilities produce enormous quantities of highly toxic manure. A single hog will produce two tons of manure per year. Ontario's 4 million hogs produce as much raw sewage as the entire human population of the province, without the benefit of a single sewage treatment plant.* (Bruckmann, 2000)

This represents the most hazardous aspect of these industrial farming operations, later confirmed by the general conditions and background to the events in Walkerton. In addition, 'the odour associated with a hog barn is dramatically worse than the odour which comes with a normal farming environment',[65] and this odour of manure itself, can have 'severe health impacts.' Bruckmann adds:

> *Manure contains over 150 gaseous compounds, including hydrogen sulfide, ammonia, carbon dioxide and methane. Residents living near intensive livestock facilities report headaches, nausea, and the exacerbation of asthma and respiratory problems.*[66]

Even before the Walkerton tragedy, it was clear that the existing regulations were totally inadequate: as long as what amounts to a hazardous industrial operation continues to be improperly defined as farming, the nature of the actual operation is not properly understood and cannot be controlled realistically, as I argued in the previous section. In fact, the regulatory infrastructure intended to support 'small scale farms and other

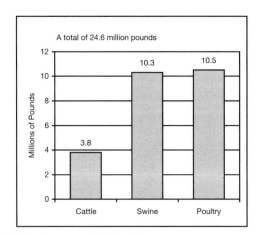

Amount of antibiotics fed to healthy livestock each year during the 1990s

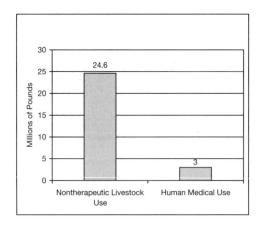

Antibiotics fed to healthy livestock compared with antibiotics used to treat people

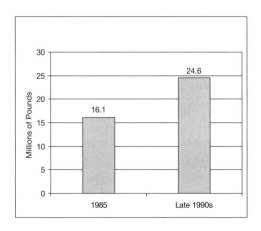

Increase in nontherapeutic antibiotic use in livestock since 1985

rural residents', in effect harms them by supporting and protecting large corporate operations and industrial interests instead. The latter are in conflict with the economic interests of small Ontario farmers, and with the right to life, security and health of all Ontario citizens.

The problem is and has been a two-pronged one: on one hand, the regulatory framework itself is deeply flawed as we will argue below, as it is unclear, imprecise and couched in language that cannot provide clear and tight guidelines. On the other, the deregulations imposed during the last five years by the government of Mike Harris have removed whatever measure of security was provided by monitoring and controls in previously existing laws. Ontario's Environmental Protection Act (OEPA) (1990) lags behind the 1999 CEPA, as we will see in the next section; many of the concepts present in the latter are still absent from the former, for example a reference to the precautionary principle. But deregulation, instead of keeping pace with science's recent discoveries, including scientific recognition of its own inability to be fully predictive,[67] virtually eliminates the monitoring and controls that protected the public before its inception.

The problems generated by specific industrial practices masquerading as 'farming', represent the most evident and obvious cause of the contamination resulting in the Walkerton tragedy. The CELA 'Five Year Report'[68] clearly shows no less than ten areas where the so-called 'Common Sense Revolution' has aggravated, multiplied or fostered environmental problems in the province. The authors list the 'Top 10 Things Wrong with Environmental' protection:

1   Ministries and agencies who protect the environment have too few staff and too few funds to do their job.
2   The government loads environmental responsibilities on small municipalities on one hand and limits their ability to protect the environment (e.g. in 1998 the Provincial Government enacted protection to large scale, industrial livestock facilities with the Farming and Food Production Act but after Walkerton, the province has temporarily relented and permitted municipalities to pass interim control by laws to limit further factory farm development).
3   The Common Sense Revolution thinks environmental protection is red tape: In fact in 2000, the 'Red Tape Commission' became a permanent legislative body.
4   New laws and regulations do not adequately protect the environment (as an example, although under the Living Legacy Strategy (July 1999) almost 400 new 'protected areas' will be created, mining and sport hunting may be permitted there).
5   The government beefs up enforcement, but will not commit to prevention and planning.
6   Under the Common Sense Revolution, protected areas are not protected.
7   The provincial government refuses to act when it should to protect the environment (with reference to Walkerton and the protection of 'large scale industrial facilities', 'the province was reluctant to even consider a regulation to protect the environment and human health from the farm emissions').
8   Industry self regulation and self monitoring increase the risk of environmental damage.
9   Common Sense protects game animals and commercial fisheries, not wildlife ... (The Ministry of Natural Resources (MNR) issued *Beyond 2000*, 'a strategic directions

document' of its management activities. Its tone and emphasis is on 'management and consumption of natural resources, and insufficient emphasis on the protection and conservation of natural systems.')

10   The Revolution fumbles national and international environmental protection initiatives (This point emphasizes non-compliance with GLWQA and the expiration of the Canada Ontario Agreement regarding the Great Lakes Ecosystem (March 2000); as 'the major obstacle on a Federal/Provincial agreement on Climate Change'.[69]

After this initial introductory chapter, the second chapter of the document, on 'water', indicates many of the failures that eventually led to Walkerton. Ostensibly, the 'Ontario Drinking Water's Objectives (1994)' state: 'if the water contains any indicators of unsafe water quality, ... the laboratory will immediately notify the MOE District Officer, who will immediately notify the Medical Officer of Health'.

Unfortunately, however, 'Not following these guidelines is not against the law. The guideline itself is not enforceable'.[70] But Ontario's water problems, although most evident in water quality issues, are equally real in relation to water quantity: 'Throughout the summer of 1999, Great Lakes levels and levels in watersheds throughout the province reached historic lows'.[71]

Yet permits are routinely given to bottling companies to remove water from Ontario's aquifers. When this reduction in availability is coupled with continued and largely uncontrolled pollution, the future for Ontario's water is as grim as that for Canada as a whole.[72]

The desperate need for regulatory action to control 'nutrient runoff from agricultural operations', was noted as early as 1995, when Walkerton was identified by Health Canada as a 'high-risk area for infection from e-coli because of the large local density of cattle operations.[73] But the agency charged with the regulation of farming operations, OMAFRA, has a 'primary client group ... the Ontario farm industry.' The Special Report of the Environmental Commissioner of Ontario (27 July 2000) adds: 'It is open to question whether the ministry can overcome this conflict of interest and effectively regulate this same industry.'[74]

Even aside from bias, lack of resources and of determination to truly eliminate the grave water problems besetting Ontario, any new initiatives are kept reactive, aimed at fixing problems rather than preventing them, thus little hope can be had that Ontario will lose its place as 'North America's third worst polluter'.[75]

Although all ten points noted are highly relevant, some aspects of this list are particularly important, not only for understanding Walkerton, but also for the overall argument of this chapter: they are (3), (5), (8), (9) and (10), above (and the last two are closely related to (6)).

The first, (3), above, deals with 'decision-making' discussed in Chapter 3 of the Five Year Report. In line with the basic understanding of that chapter, most of the problems discussed in this section are indicative of a basic underlying approach: the primacy of economic and business interests not only over environmental protection, but over health and safety of Ontarians and people in general. The *Intervenor* describes the government's approach in the five years of the 'common sense revolution' as 'deregulation, defunding and devolution', and the emphasis on facilitating business enterprise, regardless of its impact on natural systems and, through them, on human life as well. The consistent elimination of red tape, giving rise to an act for its implementation, is a clear commitment to declaring a democratic government that owes its political legitimacy, in principle, to the promotion of the citizens' common good,[76] to business and corporate interests instead.

Efficiency, at the cost of stakeholders' participation[77] and at the cost of expert information, is a serious flaw, not a desirable government goal. Public accountability, according to Carl Dombeck, Chair of Appeal and assessment Boards, means that 'the boards must account to politicians for cost reduction and expediting hearings', for the ultimate aim of 'reducing the cost of doing business in Ontario'.[78] In addition, even the Environmental Commissioner, originally with first incumbent Eva Ligeti, a position intended as a watchdog and control on government's activities, is now filled by a personal friend of the Premier, a man who is involved in that political party.[79] The negative impact of Gordon Miller's personal bias on his role, was obvious after Walkerton, as he repeated and emphasized the human error statement Mike Harris endorsed as 'explanation' and as attempt of exculpation of the government's pivotal role in the tragedy.

Beyond eliminating careful and serious study of all issues, as evidenced by their redefinition of red tape, there are at least two other grave problems in the decision-making structure of Harris' government: the promotion of industry's self-regulation (see also (8) above), and the corresponding quest for a 'balance of industry and non industry representation' on Boards and technical advisory committees (such as the Technical Standards Safety Act (1999)).[80]

There is no possibility of a 'partnership of trust and a balance between voluntary and regulatory actions' (REVA, August 1999) between parties who share little other than unequal power, where one party is most often the attacker (environmentally speaking), and the other, the victim. If we acknowledge the existence of ecoviolence, from local to global threats and health effects on all populations,[81] then it is not possible to pair as partners–actors with such disparate interests, goals and powers. As one would not expect abusers to help to define, enforce, and punish assaults on women and children, so too it is naive to expect such partnerships to yield desirable results in the protection of all life. It may be naive to hope that business would be excluded completely from either the domestic or the international law regime formation. But the international approach to exclude corporate interests at least from NGO status, hence from open participation in treaties and the discussions that give rise to them, at least shows that the influence of these economic interests may be unavoidable in practice, but it is, and should not be openly welcome, in principle.

The present state of the global commons[82,83] attest to the unreality of such a partnership as a goal (see also (8) above). The final remarks of this section will address the problematic relationship between Ontario's revolution and the commitment of Ontario and Canada, to the vital global goals of protection of natural systems. 'Protected areas are not protected', and 'lands for life and Ontario's Living Legacy Strategy' are both misleading and public relation slogans, far from the reality of the situation. The language employed appears to refer to the necessity to protect systemic integrity, in a specific percentage of any region, as science has convincingly proven the importance of preserving unmanipulated and unexploited lands in order to ensure the presence of nature's services as Gretchen Daily explains.[84] Reed Noss has also shown the necessity of keeping large percentages of lands wild, in order to conserve the natural diversity that best supports megafauna and, through it, all life and nature's services on land[85]; James Karr has made the same point with strong scientific evidence in regard to inland waters and rivers[86,87] and Daniel Pauly has done the same for marine reserves.[88]

The necessity for areas of ecological integrity in order to support all life within and without their boundaries, is also present in the regulations, vision and mission statements and constitutions of most nations, including the Liberal Policy Book (where, following Monte Hummel's suggestion, only 12 per cent is listed as the required percentage).[89] After the first appearance of the language of integrity in the Clean Water Act (US, 1972) integrity has appeared in any number of preambles, regulatory documents and legal or programmatic statements, from the Constitution of Brazil (Chapter 6, 'Meio Ambiente') to the statement of the 'Union of Concerned Scientists', to the final draft of the Earth Charter.[90,91]

The 'Global Ecological Integrity Project' has united a number of scientists to study and define the concept, while detailing the consequence that follows upon that understanding. The work of that group and their arguments cannot be repeated at this time and it is available in print.[92] Nevertheless, it is clear that (1) there are compelling scientific reasons for understanding, protecting and restoring, as much as possible, ecological integrity in appropriately sized areas in all regions including Ontario; (2) simply referring to 'healthy' systems is insufficient, because ecosystem health is compatible with careful use and manipulation, whereas integrity supports total lack of human activity in the protected areas, and correspondingly safe practices everywhere else, in order not to have a deleterious impact on protected areas through hazardous activities elsewhere; and therefore (3) integrity (and health) related language should be carefully defined because of the pivotal role they play in various acts, including the GLWQA where integrity is also left undefined.[93] It is not possible to follow a mandate the goal of which is left unclear and undefined. Taking the integrity mandate seriously would entail 'living in integrity',[94] that is, ensuring that (1) appropriately sized wild areas be established or reestablished everywhere; and (2) commercial and urban activities be judged acceptable only if they have no seriously adverse effect on both wild (core) areas, and in the buffer zones established, like half-way houses, around the core, permitting healthy use of natural systems.[95,96]

Although the CELA document does not refer to integrity specifically, it appears to support the measures that are conducive to its implementation: true conservation, respect for protected areas, and concern for national and international obligations, all require ecological integrity as a basic goal. For instance the GLWQA states:

> *The purpose of the parties is to restore and maintain the chemical, physical and bio-logical integrity of the waters of the Great Lakes Basin Ecosystem where the latter is defined as: The interacting components of air, land, water and living organisms including humans within the drainage basin of the St Lawrence River.*[97,98]

However the CELA document refers without comment to the *Beyond 2000* list of 'desired outcomes' that include, 'the long term health of ecosystems'.[99] But health is a component of integrity and necessary though not sufficient to achieve the goals that the CELA document itself argues ought to be achieved. For instance, no recreational activities in protected areas, no hunting or fishing in natural reserves, goes beyond the goal of health: an organic farm is based on a healthy system, so is an area devoted to sustainable and organic forestry practices. But integrity requires no utilization whatever, in order to preserve the natural services referred to earlier.[100,101,102,103]

LESSONS FROM THE WALKERTON CASE

What can be learned from this Canadian case, beyond the obvious importance of a safe, healthy environment as the foundation of human rights in general? Several issues emerge to demonstrate that Seveso, Bhopal or Sandoz, well-known disasters, are not the only way to produce disastrous conditions that impose grave harms on children and future generations. A regular, industrial operation is hazardous to environmental and human health on its own, even before human error may occur to compound the problem. At first sight, Walkerton too is a 'disaster'. But the presence of normal, accepted practices, licensed and promoted by a government that viewed 'cutting red tape' and facilitating business operations as their first priority, rather than the protection of citizens from harm, tells a different story.

That unfortunate prioritization remains the underlying cause of both 'disasters' and regular business operations where neither the health nor the safety of the public are viewed as the main responsibility of democratic institutions that owe their very existence and 'raison d'être' to the public it is elected to protect. The argument that can be used against Walkerton's many factory farm operations is the same as those that can be brought to bear against industrial chemical, pesticide and other harmful activities. Although these may offer increased consumer choices and low price products, essentially they are not in the best interest of most citizens, at least not with the conditions under which they operate.

Earlier I indicated the deleterious effects of the increased availability of an unhealthy diet, based on too much fatty protein, laced with the antibiotics and other chemicals necessitated by the conditions of mass production. Thus this availability is not a benefit but a hazard for most citizens, and the same can be said of many other chemicals designed to make smells or dirt disappear with ease, or weeds to be eliminated from our lawns and golf courses, or even to kill indiscriminately insect predators together with those best adapted to safe crop rotation. Even the greater availability of out of season fruits and vegetables, part of our 'ecological footprint' damage to developing countries, as it goes hand-in-hand with the elimination of local traditional agricultural practices,[104] is not quite the boon to our health it appears to be, as these are most likely laced with chemical residues and far lower in nutritional value than normally grown food has been. Some fungicides and other chemicals are increasingly added to prolong the shelf life of products that are neither grown nor manufactured as required (e.g. bread) in the same area where they are grown.

But the obligations of legislators and monitoring officials are clear in these and all similar cases, to ensure that the public health is protected at the source, by not permitting chemical companies to perform in-house assessment of their products, but rather to demand testing by independent agencies. Academics who would publish their work, or defend a doctoral thesis, are forced to name and accept only the reviews of referees and examiners they have kept 'at arm's length', so that no bias or cronyism may interfere with the quality of their work. How much more important to ensure that the general public should not be harmed by inappropriate relations between the 'testers' of products and processes and the industrial giants that produce and direct them. It is wrong to mislead the public, no doubt, but it is even more wrong to poison or otherwise physically harm an unsuspecting citizen or – even worse – a child.

The responsibilities of these outside 'guardians' should include a thorough examination of all products and processes from cradle to grave, but also it should require that corporate citizens be kept away from these procedures, and not allowed to sit at a 'negotiating' table, as the interests of the general public and that of corporations are not at the same level. Because of their immense economic power, their advertising and marketing campaigns, intended to promote not simply to inform, and the presence of protective trade secrets laws, the public itself is never participating in these discussions of policies as free and informed.

Thus the tragedy at Walkerton is not only a tragedy due to human error: it is instead due to systemic practices, for the most part, and their negligent and violent results. These practices are founded on the total disregard for basic human rights to safety and health as primary obligations of law and governance.

Supporters of the status quo will respond by saying that many of the products that are hazardous both in their manufacture and use are vitally important not only to the economy of nations, but also to the good of humankind, such as plastics, medicines and medical equipment, used in hospitals and elsewhere; additives to make food safer in the long term; cheaper, mass produced cars, information equipment and so on. The question, however, remains: who decides, where and how even ostensibly beneficial products are made, and who controls and enforces their continued safety.

In Walkerton, roughly as many people were killed or severely and irreversibly harmed as in the infamous 9/11 attack in New York. Yet no 'war' on unsafe industry has been instituted and – in fact – the exponential growth of the military establishment in the West is on the rise, to add to the industrial violence to which we are already exposed. It is noteworthy that global change is a further exacerbating factor everywhere, as it was in Walkerton, where the unusually heavy rains led to the spread of contaminants to the affected wells. All industrial enterprises depend on oil as a basic source of energy, and the recent decisions of the Bush administration to open up Alaska for exploration will further destabilize the climate and increase all the present risks especially in developing countries, while postponing sounder decisions that might promote alternative energy sources and even alternative less consumerist lifestyles.

The conflict, as suggested earlier, is between the freedom of certain groups to pursue their interests as they see fit, and the public interest, as discussed in Chapter 5. This conflict is further complicated by the fact that many grey areas are present within it: for instance, many 'consumers' would probably choose their freedom even over the security and safety not only of distant peoples, but even of those in their own community: they may not be prepared to question the ultimate wisdom of the choices they embrace, or the moral implications of such choices.

The lessons that can be learned from Walkerton demonstrate some basic points that are largely forgotten in the current fragmentation of regulatory regimes, most of which appear to have been thought out (or negotiated) in isolation from considerations drawn from the areas governed, by other ministries, other legal instruments and in general, other areas of research. For instance, speaking of the Canadian Charter of

Rights and Freedoms, basic to Canadian law but of limited impact on children, Jenkins and Houbé say:

> *The question arises as to whether it is necessary to have a separate Code of Health Rights, or are common law actions such as negligence and trespass of the person; and existing legislation, Privacy legislation, and legislation governing different medical practitioners, sufficient.*[105]

It is easy to see how insufficient all these instruments are (and have been) when one compares what happened in Walkerton (2000), with this review dated four years later. This 'review' mentions nether public health law nor criminal law, as possible means to protect the child.

Human Rights instruments indeed exist, but they are increasingly viewed as extensions of the right to liberty, without much appreciation of the face that liberty itself, well-protected as it is, may be one of the contributing factors to harm for children, not for their protections.[106] It was unregulated 'freedom' and unrestrained 'rights' that, as we saw, were the main causes of the public health disaster that ensued. In fact it is the 'right' regulation that is often the problem, not the solution: the instruments that support rights are not nuanced enough to help, despite the fact that the ratification of the CRC has engendered an obligation the state should be committed to meet. The EU is at the forefront of ensuring that its legal regimes and regulatory mechanisms comply with the CRC obligations (see for instance the 2001/1701/EC Council Resolution on Pediatric Medical Products).

Returning to the Charter, Section 7, Jenkins and Houbé note that:

> *[it] may apply whenever State requirements or prohibitions affect important and fundamental life choices which include choices involving physical and psychological integrity.*[107]

But despite the requirements of justice and equality present in Section 15(1), the possibility of non-inclusion of potential right-holders is not really envisaged, and that is the main problem that children's rights encounter, where so many other groups take precedence. No arguments are offered on the question of why certain groups and persons are included, and others are not and – as we saw in earlier chapters – the case law refers to the instruments and cites precedent but seldom engages in the discussion of foundational issues. Throughout this discussion and through several chapters, we have been pitting some rights against some other rights, without fully addressing the issue of the concept of rights and why they are fundamental to both morality and the administration of justice, and this topic must be discussed in detail, and we will do so to conclude this chapter.

Before turning to that difficult issue, there is another aspect of the problem that should be discussed. We have considered wider questions of globalization, politics and economics, as well as the legal implications of international instruments. There is one more area that needs to be taken into consideration: public health instruments and regulations. Rather than consider any specific country's positive law in that regard, perhaps we should take an overview of the topic in order to better understand the role it could and perhaps should play in relation to children's health.

PUBLIC HEALTH: ITS MEANING AND ROLE

(Public Health Law) should not be confused with medical jurisprudence, which is concerned only in legal aspects of the application of medical and surgical knowledge to individuals... Public health law is not a branch of medicine, but a science in itself.[108]

Although conceptually international law appears to be connected to public health and it is in fact well able to demonstrate the responsibilities of government institutions to their citizens, in contrast 'health law' and 'public health law' may be less clear in regard to the responsibility to citizens. In fact, while the international responsibility, as noted, is fully accepted both in the soft law instruments I have cited and, as we shall see below in the next section, in binding law as well, the case is quite different for national institutions instead.

Political entities, especially in democratic countries, must accept this responsibility, and that is indeed the commitment of the signatories to the CRC. This commitment is not readily accepted everywhere yet, however, and this is perhaps a form of 'work-in-progress' in developing countries, who have signed on without a clear availability of the necessary funding and infrastructure at the time. The case is quite different for the US, and it will be instructive to consider that case first, in order to better understand what aspects of the commitment to health might be in jeopardy in that case. Lawrence Gostin says:

> *Meaningful protection and assurance of the population's health require communal effort. The community as a whole has a stake in environmental protection, hygiene and sanitation, clean air and surface water, uncontaminated food and drinking water, safe roads, end products and the control of infectious diseases. These collective goods can be secured only through organized action on behalf of the population.*[109]

Speaking of health, we noted earlier the role of health and normal function as absolutely necessary preconditions for the exercise of one's rights, be they civil, political or other. Hence it appeared that the basic rights to 'security and subsistence', including health and normal function, precede, at least conceptually any other rights. As all rights are interdependent and interrelated the right to health may be viewed as already enshrined in international law:

HUMAN RIGHTS
- *Are guaranteed by international standards;*
- *Are legally protected;*
- *Focus on the dignity of human beings;*
- *Protect individuals and groups;*
- *Oblige states and state actors;*
- *Cannot be waived or taken away;*
- *Are interdependent and interrelated;*
- *Are universal. (Administrative Committee on Coordination (ACC); The UN*

System of Human Rights; Guidelines and Information For the resident coordin-
ator System; approved on behalf of the ACC by the Consultative Committee on
Programme and Operational Questions (CCPOQ) at its 16th Session, Geneva,
March 2000).

We will return to a detailed defence of human rights below, as the present focus is on
an introductory discussion of public health and public health law.

As the subtitle of Gostin's influential work indicates, the relation between government institutions and public health, include conflicts of rights, as in the cases where
restraint is indicated, for instance when infectious diseases require quarantine or
isolation, thus interference with individual rights to mobility and self-determination; in
those cases, 'the use of coercion must be part of an informed understanding of public
health law'.[110]

Public health's primary role is 'to restrict human freedoms and rights to achieve
a collective good'.[111] In that case the responsibilities of governments in that regard
would appear to be as clear as their obligations under international law. Nevertheless
not all governments accept their responsibility for the protection of health, and the
Constitution of the US is a clear example of this conflict:

> *(Nothing) in the language of the Due Process Clause itself requires the State to protect*
> *the life, liberty and property of citizens against the invasion by private actors. The*
> *Clause is phrased as a limitation to the State's power to set, not as a guarantee of*
> *certain minimal levels of safety and security.*[112]

The absence of the government's duty to intervene in cases where harm to children is
present, will certainly help to clarify the limited role of the US in enacting protective
policies regarding children's health and environmental damage, such as the ones
recommended by the WHO's research (as we saw in earlier sections of this chapter), and
in the discussion of general policies discussed in Chapters 5 to 8. In regard to children
as well as all vulnerable populations, the problem becomes acute when 'omissions' or
'non-interventions' become the source of grave harms, and even the Supreme Court
of the US remains faithful 'to the negative constitution at all costs'.[113] The Case of
DeShaney v. Winnebago County Department of Social Services (489 U.S. 189), concerned a
one-year-old boy, Joshua, whose father gained custody after a divorce, and retained it
despite reports of physical abuse, duly noted by the social authorities, without however
action being taken:

> *Eventually at 4 years of age Joshua was beaten so badly he suffered permanent brain*
> *damage. He was left profoundly retarded and institutionalized.*[114]

The Court found no obligation on the part of the government to protect children
from harms (unspecified), and – although this is a case of deliberate malfeasance
rather than a general health threat, a fortiori the latter would fare no better in the
protection of the child. The theory upon which this well-accepted principle is based
represents, according to Justice Blackmun, 'a sad commentary upon American life and
constitutional principles'.[115]

In sum then, a State's omission to protect, or non-feasance is constitutionally right in the US, despite the fact that they do use the *parens patriae* doctrine to protect specific 'incompetent individuals', as well as the general community interest in health and welfare, including public health issues in quarantine cases and the like.[116]

Thus we need to understand the obligation to protect not as absolute, but as a variable in certain countries, such as the US. This Constitutional reality may also help to understand that country's unwillingness to sign on to the CRC, thus avoiding not only the original commitment but also the ensuing duty to report on improvements on a regular basis, a fundamental part of the obligation of all signatories.

Thus the children's right to health protection is dependent on several non-technical factors, although technical and economic issues play a significant part in the ability of various countries to improve their present circumstances in that regard.

Each country must have, first of all, a government committed to the protection of human rights through public health, with special emphasis on vulnerable populations, including children. The simple commitment not to cause harm on the part of a government is clearly insufficient and this point will have to be kept in mind as we consider countries' constitutional frameworks and their legal instruments concerning children, as we examine their respective reports on compliance with the requirements of the CRC. Yet this positive law analysis neglects to bring fully into focus the implications of these limits. That will be the topic of the next section.

Public health and children: Some basic issues

> *human health and well-being are the ultimate goals of development; to focus on children's health is thus to contribute directly to socio-economic development, since the health of the child is the key to the health of the adult.*[117]

Public health has as its goal, in general, the protection of the public from disease and, I would add, also abnormal function, by imposing restraints on certain activities, by regulating processes and products that may have adverse impacts on health, as well as by legislating restraints on individuals for the public good.[118] But early childhood and even perinatal disease and injuries cause a great number of health problems that can be prevented only or optimally at that stage. Fuchs and Galba-Araujo state:

> *Nothing has a greater impact on the essential quality of life as an adult than the diseases and injuries in the perinatal period. This period of life is characterized by more perils to human survival and health than any other.*[119]

Indeed, one of the problems that must be overcome is the present view that adult medicine and public health are distinct and separate from child health, rather than viewing them as a continuum. Hence the complementarity of disciplines such as medicine, biology, ecology and human rights, for instance, should be supplemented by a clear understanding of the continuum of health from the perinatal period to the older child and the adult. Any artificial division between various periods of life is entirely specious and counterproductive and should be eliminated.

Thus commitment to a region's health for all their population starts even before conception, with the obligation to ensure proper nutrition for mothers. As an example, in Brazil:

> A survey of the state of Ceara revealed that for every hundred babies conceived in the study area, 17 will die in utero and 13 of those born alive will die within one year. Given similar conditions in all developing areas of the world, perinatal and infant mortality would account for the loss of some 30 million children in those areas every year.[120]

The main reasons for this ongoing slaughter is hunger and malnutrition, and these are conditions prevailing in sub-Saharan Africa, Asia and South America, hence improvements in those conditions should figure most prominently in the reports of the CRC signatories, at least in the sections entitled 'The Way Forward', although at this time for most of those regions economic conditions may not permit the full elimination of malnutrition. The elimination of hunger worldwide is an urgent need as more than 30,000 children die from it every year, according to FAO statistics.

The need for food and safe water are non-controversial issues, but there are also some more difficult issues that must be addressed: the question of individual choices that may have an adverse impact on the foetus, and subsequently on child and adult health. For instance fetal alcohol syndrome may occur even with moderate alcohol consumption,[121] and the effects of tobacco have been well-documented, as well as the effects of drug abuse in pregnancy.[122] These problems are more likely to occur in developed countries, although even there poverty remains a significant indicator in many cases, as does race.

These situations are problematic because the right to autonomy and choice on the part of the woman come into direct conflict with the goals of public health in general and child health in particular (see Chapters 2–4). Even more significant is the question of heart disease, presently the first cause of mortality in developed countries in the American and European regions, the second cause of death in the Eastern regions of the Mediterranean, and the third in the Western Pacific areas of the WHO.[123]

It is worthy of note that rheumatic heart disease can occur in children as early as 4 or 5 years of age in developing countries. It also affects young pregnant women especially around the time of delivery, thus endangering both mother and child.[124]

Essentially, if heart disease is today's greatest killer of adults, and for most countries that entails large expenditures for treatment as well as for related issues such as inability to work or invalidism, then this appeal to the reality of the progression of this disease must be taken in consideration. In addition even hypertension starts in childhood, although it accelerates as adulthood is reached.[125] Thus the promotion of public health practices starting in early childhood and before leads to the prevention of heart disease in adults, a highly desirable outcome from both a human rights and an economic point of view.

There are also many infections that may affect the foetus, hence that are significant contributors to childhood disease and mortality. There are substantial research data that show 'transplacental infections from enteroviruses, the viruses of mumps, measles, varicella, herpes simplex, hepatitis, smallpox and Western equine encephalitis, as well as ... tuberculosis and malaria' and several other diseases.[126]

Hence it appears that public health concerns about children are indeed not only specific and *sui generis*, but they are basic to the health of all populations: therefore the importance of giving primacy to early childhood health cannot be overestimated.

The human right to health is clearly present in many international and regional instruments, starting with Article 25.1 of the *Universal Declaration of Human Rights* (1948):

> *Everyone has the right to a standard of living adequate for the health of himself and of his family, including food, clothing, housing and medical care and necessary social services.*[127,128,129,130,131]

If the right to health is increasingly being accepted as a fundamental one, then it is important to understand fully what that right entails, for instance the fact that it must include the right to essential medicines.[132] Following upon the language of the 1966 ICESCR (6.12.1), which ensures the right of everyone to the enjoyment of the highest attainable standard of physical and mental health, and A.12.2 that lists the steps to be taken by state parties to fulfil their obligation to ensure:

- maternal, child and reproductive health;
- healthy natural and workplace environments;
- prevention treatment and control of disease;
- health facilities, goods and services

are firmly entrenched in international binding law.

By the end of 2002, 142 state parties have signed and ratified the International Covenant, and 109 countries have the right to health incorporated in their constitution, and 83 countries have ratified at least one of the treaties including the right to health.[133]

THE QUESTION OF RIGHTS

> *If, on the other hand, 'natural' means based on what individual humans and human societies are actually like – what persons need and what enables them to thrive as humans – then rights are natural.*[134]

The first thing to note is that universality is the main characteristic of human rights: universality understood as it is in cosmopolitanism, that is, as the foundation of a concept of global justice that transcends national and regional borders.[135] This aspect of human rights is vital for the temporal thrust of future generations' rights, which, as we argued, include the rights of the first generation as well (see Chapter 6).

Both the synchronic and the diachronic aspect of human rights are equally important today, in the context of weak and mercenary national governments, unable and unwilling to restrain the activities of transnational corporate agents. Their institutions support the primacy of economic rights over any other, including public health.[136] The latter, unfortunately tends to be in direct conflict with economic considerations.[137] Jones outlines the 'four central elements of the concept' of rights:

> *First, there is the right-holder, the possessor of the right ...; secondly, there is the addressee of the right, or right regarder;... Thirdly, there is the content of the right, that which the right is a right to;... fourthly, there is a statement of the normative strength of the right-claim, its capacity to override competing considerations.*[138]

Human rights are necessary for the protection of the 'basic interests of persons',[139] but the question remains about which specific rights should take precedence and why. We can start with a *via negativa* of sorts: rights are not supported by a deductively valid argument; hence rights are not necessarily logically compelling; and, technically, there is 'no limit to the possible contents of rights claims, to the things persons can be said to have a right to'.[140]

The last point is the most troubling one. The list of rights that can be said to have priority is widening every year, but it should be limited somehow: if we maintain that there is no limit to the human rights that can be claimed and to the interests to which people can appeal, then it might be extremely difficult to discover the grounds from which to argue that some, but not others, must be seen as basic, or primary.

For a right to be viewed as basic, it must be such that no other right or interest can exist in its absence, and – in order to compel society as a whole on its behalf – the interest supporting that right must be not only 'vital, but vulnerable', that is, it must be such that the interest it supports is such that no one can protect herself alone from attacks to it.[141] In addition to 'basic rights' supported by interests like physical necessities for survival, neither the exercise of human rationality, surely a most 'basic' defining right of all human beings, nor any other right referring to normal human function, can exist without the protections of its preconditions, that is, without those conditions that ensure the development of both.[142]

Hence the conditions that ensure not only immediate survival, but also subsistence and security, ensure that human beings will not be totally vulnerable and helpless when confronting the multiple threats to which we are exposed. Even the exercise of civil and political rights is totally dependent upon subsistence and security, and the preservation of the preconditions of developing normally and rationally, in the context of health and normal function (see the discussion in Chapter 1).

The right to life is considered to be absolutely basic, and it is entrenched in all international human rights instruments and in national constitutions, and the implications of this universal right are clear:

> *the right to life has much to do with providing the wherewithal to keep people alive, as with protecting them against violent death ... the right to life, if it exists at all, is a right to subsistence as well as to security.*[143]

I have proposed that the right to health must also be included for all citizens, not as a guarantee to freedom from disease for life, a patently impossible goal to impose as an obligation on society but – as a minimum – as the right to biological integrity and normal (initial) function, rather than ongoing assurance that, plainly, cannot be given. To ensure such rights to children, as noted in above also helps to maintain their health through life, although the latter is a condition for which adults must take some responsibility as well.

But the conditions of total vulnerability in the case of the infant, the preborn and further future generations, serve to make these cases the clearest examples of non-derogable duties not to harm, on the part of national governments and international institutions, but most of all, for the industries whose activities present the gravest dangers. The duty is to 'Do No Harm', so it represents a positive obligation to ensure that activities that are not proscribed, do not infringe the rights all humans possess to be, minimally, what they can be.

This argument is clearly Aristotelian and teleological: if Aristotle had considered the protection of trees, for instance, he would have pointed out that interference with an acorn, depriving it of water and other conditions favourable to its growth and development are also examples of harms to the oak tree that the acorn will eventually become. The two sorts of harms are neither separate nor sequential: they are one and the same.

Jones argues that the 'negative/positive rights distinction' needs to be re-examined because both subsistence and security require more than omissions of certain harm-imposing actions. But transferring the full responsibility to ensure subsistence rights to all, makes it difficult to clarify with any precision who holds the duty to comply, and how the obligation is to be met: 'the distinction between negative and positive rights is simply not an accurate rendering of the duties corresponding to any given rights'.[144] Jones explains that there is 'no one-to-one relation between rights and duties', but that each right generates 'waves of duties'.[145] Shue characterizes the required duties as follows:

i.   duties to avoid depriving right-holding individuals of the content of the right,
ii.   duties to protect right-holders from being deprived of the right content, and
iii. duties to aid deprived right-holders when avoidance and protection have
     failed.[146]

These characteristics help to isolate the most 'basic' or fundamental rights such as the ones we have argued are owed to children, the preborn and the future generations. What separates those rights from the ones giving rise to the duties listed by Shue, is that giving aid may be an acceptable move if, say, people are starving today, because both our schemes for 'avoidance' and for 'protection' have failed. At least, it may be more acceptable if malnutrition had not become too advanced, or all our aid may be insufficient to reverse the death they are facing.

But in many of the cases we have discussed in this book, not only starvation, lack of water and shelter, but also the chemical/industrial assaults we have described, are such that once we have failed to 'avoid' and to 'protect', it is too late to reverse the harm, hence the glaring breach of human rights. One terrible example will suffice.

The Environmental Working Group (Washington, DC) tested newborn babies and found an average of over 200 industrial, chemicals, pollutants and pesticides in each baby. As we saw in the research of the WHO (Chapter 1), the young are far more vulnerable than adults to these harms. The environmental group admitted that they might have found more 'but testing for chemicals is difficult':

● Chemical companies are not required to tell the public or government how to detect their chemicals in humans.

- For most chemicals on the markets, there are no methods yet for testing human tissues.
- Only a few laboratories have the equipment and expertise to run the test.
- The few tests laboratories run are often expensive. The tests for cord-blood analysis for this report cost $10,000.00 per sample.[147]

These findings contrast with US Federal policies, such as the Toxic Substances Control Act (1976), which 'exempts 63,000 existing chemicals from safety analysis by declaring them safe as used'.[148]

The point of this example is that once these exposures have occurred, 'aid' is of little use, except to mitigate the financial conditions that may accompany the irreversible conditions engendered by these exposures, which include harms to both the structure and the function of the exposed human (see for instance the discussion of thalidomide exposure in Chapter 2, as well as carcinogenic exposures in Chapter 1).

Perhaps the rights of which we should be speaking first are even more than basic: they are fundamental. The right to free speech, for instance, means little if one cannot reason or speak, or if one's life will be severely shortened by one or several of these exposures. But to speak of fundamental rights is to be forced to accept some form of essentialism, in order to understand the meaning of rights that are fundamental to a human being: harm or reduction of function can only be seen clearly if we start with an understanding of what a human being is and what she can be and do in her development. Essentialism is no longer judged to be philosophically acceptable by many, because it has been viewed as providing a static understanding of human beings, hence as prescribing definitions or concepts that are dated and unable to incorporate the reality of change. In case law, for instance, in cases regarding women's issues, one often finds references to a 'Victorian approach', to indicate a way of thinking that severely limits women's potential and the egalitarian treatment to which they are entitled.

However, this negative assessment of essentialism is often taken for granted without any attempt to fully understand the true import of the notion. If it means a static description of an unchanging state of affairs, say the expression of a notion like 'the earth is flat', then clearly that notion must be eliminated before another, more appropriate one can replace it.

But an essential understanding, even in Aristotle, simply points to the permanence that underlies change, that is, the temporal continuity that makes me, essentially, the same person my mother nursed, sent to school, and that my husband married 50 years ago. Nor is this only a philosophical notion: that is the role DNA plays today in a number of situation including criminal cases. My temporal continuity with a long line of developmental states is only guaranteed by relating the same essential, though changing times/levels to one self.[149]

Hence, essentialism is not in conflict with change: it provides the basis for temporal continuity of a changing entity or concept. Thus without a full understanding of the meaning and role of essentialism, it is easy to dismiss it. Yet, without some fundamental/ essential understanding of humanity, it is not possible to judge when one's rights to human development have been breached.

The essence of what it is to be human, cannot be fully discussed in the present context. But it is undeniable that a clear understanding of what we can be, and how we can expect to function normally when not prevented, is foundational to understanding the meaning of fundamental rights and interests, hence to support the primacy of these rights before all others. But is the claim that we must give primacy to these fundamental rights enough to demonstrate why we should do so? Perhaps a review of the main characteristics of the rights to survival/health/normal functions for which we have argued in this book, may help to indicate the need to give these rights special status, starting with the inherent dignity of each human being that is understood as a premise to any argument about rights. Additionally, the economic and social costs of ignoring fundamental rights to health and to normal function for each human being, also support the importance of the rights I have proposed in a practical way.

These rights are universal; they are primary, as they precede earned rights (such as the right to practise a profession or trade), or other rights dependent on a specific nationality or pertaining to a position or office.

The rights for which I have argued are basic, preceding as we have indicated all other rights; they are also foundational, as they are closest to what it means to be a human being; they are among the most vulnerable rights imaginable, especially at the stages at which we envision them to be primary; finally, most often, breaches of these rights give rise to irreversible harms. Singly and collectively, therefore, these characteristics tend to make these rights unique, and political leaders and especially lawmakers should revise their instruments and institutions to ensure that this primacy is recognized and implemented.

NOTES

1   Westra (2004a), chapter 5.
2   Canadian case *Pappajohn v. the Queen* (1980), 2 S.C.R. 120.
3   Abraham (2005).
4   Abraham (2005).
5   Abraham (2005).
6   Westra (1994).
7   Westra (1998).
8   Noss (1992).
9   Noss and Cooperrider (1994).
10 Cited in Abraham (2005).
11 Westra (2004a), chapters 2 and 7.
12 Fletcher (1971), p401.
13 Bourette (2000).
14 Ibbitson (2000), pA7.
15 Machine (2000), pA7.
16 Baxi (1999).
17 Westra (1998).
18 Hiskes (1998).
19 Gbadegesin (2001).
20 Westra (1998).
21 Baxi (1999).
22 Gaylord and Bell (1995).
23 Westra and Lawson (2001).
24 Bullard (1994).

25 Westra (1998), chapter 3; Pogge (2001b).
26 Burkitt (1991).
27 Schindler (2000), pA5.
28 Westra (1998).
29 Pimentel et al (2000).
30 Daily (1997).
31 Westra (1998).
32 Noss (1992).
33 Rapport (1995).
34 Callicott (1999).
35 Westra (2000b).
36 Schindler (2000).
37 Eisnitz (1997).
38 Davis (1996).
39 Cohen (1998).
40 Regan (1983).
41 Singer (1975).
42 Pogge (2001b).
43 Pimentel and Goodland (2000).
44 Pimentel et al (1998).
45 Daly (1996).
46 Brown (1995).
47 Kendall and Pimentel (1994).
48 Epstein (1989).
49 Rifkin (1992); Singer (1995).
50 *The Globe and Mail,* July 3, 2000, pA11.
51 Callicott (2000).
52 Callicott (2000), p60.
53 Rifkin (1992).
54 Singer (1995).
55 Rachels (1997).
56 Eisnitz (1997).
57 Cohen (1998).
58 Davis (1996).
59 Parsons (2000).
60 Rifkin (1992).
61 McCalman et al (1998).
62 McCalman et al (1998).
63 Mellon and Fondriest (2001).
64 Mellon and Fondriest (2001), p2.
65 Mellon and Fondriest (2001).
66 Bruckmann (2000), p5.
67 Kay and Schneider (1994).
68 Clark and Yacoumidis (2001).
69 Adapted from Clark and Yacoumidis (2001), pp7–14.
70 Clark and Yacoumidis (2001), p17.
71 Clark and Yacoumidis (2001), p20.
72 Barlow (1999).
73 Clark and Yacoumidis (2001), p24.
74 Clark and Yacoumidis (2001), p24, n.61, 101.
75 Clark and Yacoumidis (2001), p26.

76   Gilbert (1994).
77   Gilbert (1994), p34.
78   Gilbert (1994), p2.
79   Gilbert (1994), p36.
80   Gilbert (1994), p40.
81   Westra (2000a).
82   Brown (2000).
83   Pimentel et al (2000).
84   Daily (1997).
85   Noss (1992).
86   Karr and Chu (1995, 1999).
87   Karr (2000).
88   Pauly (2000).
89   Hummel (1989).
90   Westra (1994).
91   Westra (1998).
92   Pimentel et al (2000).
93   Westra (1994).
94   Westra (1998).
95   Noss (1992).
96   Noss and Cooperrider (1994).
97   GLWQA (1978), ratified 1987.
98   Westra (1994), p21.
99   Westra (1994), p79.
100 Noss (1992).
101 Noss and Cooperrider (1994).
102 Ulanowicz (1995).
103 Karr and Chu (1999).
104 Shiva (1989).
105 Jenkins and Houbé (2004).
106 Westra (2004a), chapter 5.
107 Jenkins and Houbé, (2004), p40.
108 Tobey (1926), pp6–7.
109 Gostin (2000), pp7, 8.
110 Gostin (2000), p18.
111 Gostin (2000), p20.
112 Rehnquist (1989).
113 Gostin (2000), p32.
114 Gostin (2000), p33.
115 *Webster v. Reproductive Health Services*, 492 U.S. 490 (1989), a case dealing with discrimination against African Americans in the provision of health services.
116 Seidman and Tushnet (1996), p54; but see also discussion of *parens patriae* in common law in Chapter 5, this book.
117 Petros-Barzavian (1980), pvii.
118 Gostin (2000), pp16–21.
119 Fuchs and Galba-Araujo (1980), p9.
120 Fuchs and Galba Araujo (1980), p16.
121 Hanson et al (1978), p457.
122 Nichterm (1973), p24; Wilson et al (1973), p457.
123 World Health Organization (1980).

124 Strasser (1978), pp18–25; see also 'The prevention of coronary heart disease starts in childhood', 1978, *Postgraduate Medical Journal* 54: 135–230.

125 Brook (1978), pp1–174; Epstein (1979), pp7–12.

126 Remington and Klein (1976), pp1–32.

127 See also *International Convention on the Elimination of all Forms of Racial Discrimination*, A.5 (e)(iv)(1965).

128 *Convention on the Elimination of All Forms of Discrimination Against Women*, A,11.1(f) and 12 (1979).

129 *Convention on the Rights of the Child*, A. 24 (1989).

130 *European Social Charter*, A.11 (revised) (1965).

131 *African Charter on Human and Peoples Rights*, A.16 (1981).

132 Hogerzeil (2003), p25.

133 Hogerzeil (2003) p26.

134 Shue (1996a).

135 Beetham (1995), p47; see also Plant (1991), p290.

136 Jones (2000), p51.

137 Shue (1996a).

138 Jones (2000), pp52–53.

139 Jones (2000), p55.

140 Jones (2000), p56.

141 Shue (1996b), pp114–115.

142 Gewirth (1982); see also Westra (2004a), pp107–120.

143 Vincent (1996), p90.

144 Jones (2000), p62; see also Shue (1979), pp65–84.

145 Jones (2000), p64.

146 Shue (1996a), pp51–64.

147 Houlihan et al (2005).

148 Houlihan et al (2005).

149 Schmitz (2005), pp275–281.

CHAPTER 9

Developmental and Health Rights of Children in Developing Countries: Towards a Model Legislation for the Rights of the Child to Health

United Nations Food and Agriculture Organization (FAO) Statistics:

According to the United Nations Food and Agriculture Organization Statistics (FAO), about 35,615 children died from conditions of starvation on September 11, 2001

RELEVANT STATISTICS

- Victims: 35,615 children (source: FAO)
- Where: Undeveloped (poor) countries
- Specialty programmes: none
- Newspaper articles: none
- Messages from the president: none
- Solidarity actions: none
- Minutes of silence: none
- Rock concerts: none
- Organized forums: none
- Pope messages: none
- Alert level: zero
- Military mobilization: none

Imagine a 'United we stand' effort to eradicate hunger.

INTRODUCTION

In the last chapter we discussed the health impact of diet choice in the Walkerton case in Canada, but the paragraph at the head of this chapter paints a picture that is in many ways diametrically opposed to the one I have been describing as general to North–West countries. Choices and preferences, whether individual or collective, play little or no role in the health of children in the South–East. A month as a volunteer/researcher at the WHO/International in Geneva (30 May–28 June 2005), working on an assigned group of developing countries (see Appendix 2), demonstrated the grave dissonance between the arguments, laws and policies needed to address the right of children to health in the North, and those needed by their counterparts in the South.[1]

For the latter, the main issue, the gravest problem, is survival, not choices. We are routinely bombarded with terrible pictures of starving and sick children in sub-Saharan Africa, from Niger to Darfur and we are made aware of our apparent inability to provide the desperately needed aid in a timely and efficient manner.[2] For children in the South, the first emphasis must be placed on our responsibility, before we can begin to address their rights. Nevertheless the presence of these rights, some of which are outlined in the *Convention on the Rights of the Child* (CRC), imposes certain clear requirements on society:

> *within the health sector, this would include explicit attention to ensure that health data is disaggregated in order to identify and better target discrimination as it would be manifested in laws, policies and practices ... [and] by recognizing children as rights holders, and not relegating them to the status of objects of charity or protection, and with due recognition of their evolving capacities.*[3]

The emphasis of much of the law and policy regarding children in the North, is disproportionately concerned with children's 'participation' in civil society, education and their need to have their opinions respected, as is the case in the CRC itself (see Appendix 1). This is nothing but a version of 'Civil and Political Rights of the Child', leaving aside, for the most part, the legal and policy requirements to ensure the health and normal function that will permit the child to exercise these rights, or even to comprehend them.

This has been the argument of this work in general, and the WHO is valiantly moving towards a 'human rights approach to public health':

> *The Department of Child and Adolescent Health and Development (CAH), located in the WHO Cluster for Family and Community Health, has been at the forefront of those efforts. The work of CAH is based on the firm conviction that all children and adolescents should have the means and opportunity to develop to their full potential. In addition to basic needs, survival, and maximum development, access to health and health services are fundamental human rights.*[4]

In developing countries it is the right to development that is vital to children, as it is to peoples, whereas for developed countries it is the right to protection from violent interference with their health that is primary, as it is a routine threat from industrial activities, and is not based on social or family violence, but additional to it.[5] The latter has been discussed at some length in the previous chapters. The concept of a right to normal development (in both physical structure and function) is a common denominator, something that all children share although attacks on that right assume different aspects for children in the North and those in the South.

It bears repeating: the right to normal health and development and the right to be well-born and to develop normally is shared by all children; for the children in the North, the protection that is required is against attacks based on choices and preferences, and that is extremely hard as these attacks are viewed for the most part simply as the result of routine activities, that do not require special scrutiny or analysis. For the child in the South, it is a question of omission rather than commission, but it is no less a culpable form of violence, perpetrated and perpetuated by carelessness, indifference and neglect.

It is not what society's many activities do to those children, it is what is not done for them that kills them so routinely that these occurrences are not even viewed as newsworthy, most of the time. In some sense, however, the violence is still an indirect effect of Northern, technologically advanced societies. It is the 'trickle down' effect of climate change, creeping desertification and weather extremes,[6,7,8] it is the disposal of hazardous wastes,[9,10] it is the ongoing extraction of oil and the presence of mining activities without the necessary framework of environmentally protective legislation or social and medical assistance to eliminate or at least mitigate the resulting health harms.[11,12] Thus children in the South bear a double burden: still exposed to indirect harms from the North, but without the availability of the North's supportive/protective infrastructure. Hence children from the South may not carry the 'Body Burden' placed on their siblings in the North,[13] but they have no safety net for the 'burdens' that do reach them.

The differences and the overlaps between the two sorts of exposure will need careful analysis and discussion, and this topic will be addressed in the following sections.

NORTH V. SOUTH FOR CHILDREN'S RIGHTS: EXPOSURES, REMEDIES AND OBSTACLES

With a few exceptions, the health equity literature is surprisingly silent on rights...
there is little talk of entitlement or claims – and even less of violations.[14]

A lot can be learned from the simple comparison between the WHO's research on each set of issues for children's health.. In Chapter 1, the threats to children's health were outlined in some detail, based on WHO's 2002 research (Tamburlini et al 2002). Their follow-up document in 2005, *Children's Health and Environment*,[15] reviews the 'environmental risk factors and their effects on children's health', under the following categories:

- Poor indoor air quality;
- Outdoor air pollution;
- Poor water supply and inadequate sanitation;
- Inadequate nutrition;
- Microbiological food contamination;
- Inadequate building standards and unsafe play material;
- Hazardous chemicals;
- Mobility and transport patterns;
- Ionizing and non-ionizing radiation;

- Noise;
- Natural disasters and climate change;
- Occupational risk factors;
- Critically adverse social environments;
- Consequences of armed conflict.[16]

It is obvious how many of these categories do not apply to the child in the South, from 'indoor air quality', to 'inadequate building standards' and 'unsafe play material', from 'noise' to 'occupational risk factors'.[17] But some of the categories need serious considerations everywhere: 'Poor water supply and inadequate sanitations', 'natural disasters and climate change', and the 'consequences of armed conflict', and all clearly present in developing countries, although their presence may manifest itself in somewhat different circumstances.

Finally, 'inadequate nutrition', or 'malnutrition' is indeed *the* major problem of children in the South, as we shall see, but the expression itself has several different meanings when applied to different situations. The language under that category is instructive:

> *Inappropriate diets and eating patterns that include frequent consumption of highly sugared soft drinks and energy dense snacks particularly when combined with insufficient physical activity, contribute to the increased prevalence of overweight and obesity.*[18]

In contrast we can compare at least two applicable Millennium Development Goals:

Goal 1 – Target 1. Halve between 1990 and 2015,the proportion of people whose income is less than $1 a day.
Target 2. Halve between 1990 and 2015 the proportion of people who suffer from hunger.
Goal 4 – Target 5. Reduce by $\frac{2}{3}$ between 1990 and 2015 the under-five mortality rate.

In addition to these obvious applicable goals, Goal 6, 'Combat HIV/AIDS Malaria and Other Diseases', is equally connected to Goals 1 and 4: malnutrition is implicated as it aggravates all other diseases, but 'inadequate nutrition' of children and pregnant women is *not* about poor diet choices in developing countries.

It is about survival for the desperately poor, not obesity, and not only does it contribute significantly to all other major childhood diseases (pneumonia, malaria, measles, diarrhoea), malnutrition is listed as a cause of mortality for children 0–5 on its own.[19] Hence in this category, to seek policies to alleviate 'inadequate nutrition' means to pursue completely different goals for North and South children. For the latter, undernutrition is both a cause of death and a contributing factor for all the other main diseases that lead to mortality:

> *although not listed specifically as a cause of death, undernutrition (low-weight-for-age) contributes greatly to child mortality. Mildly underweight children under age 5 are five times as likely as their nourished peers to die, and severely undernourished children are eight times as likely to do so.*[20] *Overall, 52.5 percent of all post neonatal*

childhood deaths are associated with undernutrition: 60.7 percent of diarrhea deaths, 57.3 percent of malaria deaths, 52.3 percent of pneumonia deaths, and 44.8 percent of measles. Ensuring the adequate nutrition of children under five could prevent more than 2.5 million deaths from these diseases.[21]

Excluding neonatal deaths, the five major conditions that cause deaths to children under five – diarrhoea, pneumonia, malaria, measles and AIDS – are exacerbated by malnutrition before and after birth, so its impact can hardly be overestimated. With the exception of HIV/AIDS, these conditions can easily be prevented: vaccinations, treated mosquito nets and other simple measures are all highly cost-effective, as is hunger and malnutrition alleviation.[22] See the tables below for statistics relating to deaths of children under the age of five.

The six countries with highest number of annual deaths of children under the age of five

Country	Deaths per year (thousands)
India	2402
Nigeria	834
China	784
Pakistan	565
Democratic Republic of Congo	484
Ethiopia	472
Total of six countries above	5541
Global annual deaths	10,800

Source: Black, Morris and Bryce (2003)

Causes of death of children under age five

Disease or condition	Share of under-five deaths
Neonatal	33
Diarrhea	22
Pneumonia	21
Malaria	9
Measles	1
AIDS	3
Other	9

Note: Figures are based on data from the 42 countries that account for 90 per cent of all deaths.
Source: Adapted from Black, Morris and Bryce (2003)

Similar omissions of easily affordable care are present in the category of 'safe water and sanitation': for the North the water may be hazardous to life and health because of nearby industrial activities, or agricultural pesticide contamination. For the South, most often, water is extremely scarce, and contamination arises from 'natural' sources, like inappropriate sanitation practices. The latter can also be mitigated without great expenditures, although hazardous mining and oil extraction practices may add an ulterior 'Northern' component to the plight of children in the South.[23]

Finally, the right to shelter appears explicitly in African regional instruments, whereas in the North, most often, it is not the lack of shelter, but the construction of it that presents the risks to children's health.

Previous chapters have addressed the prevalence of obstacles to children's health and normal function in the North. The obstacles prevailing in the South will be quite different, because of different prevailing circumstances. In the next section some of these obstacles are reviewed, with particular reference to the five sample countries I have researched, in order to best address from the standpoint of practical issues, the universal norms required to ensure that the *Convention on the Rights of the Child* also includes model legislation for the protection of the child's right to health.

'WORLD FIT FOR CHILDREN'? FIRST OBSTACLE: *ENVIRONMENTAL CONDITIONS*

Several of the Millennium Development Goals (MDGs) were discussed in the previous section. Each is listed separately from the others, and not necessarily connected with the rest. In addition, it is clear that each 'Goal' is impeded and constrained in its implementation by a host of obstacles. But before turning to the individual analysis of specific problems, it is important to acknowledge a major obstacle that affects the implementation of all goals as it aggravates or causes each one of the problems we have outlined: the environment.

As an obstacle to the child's right to health, the environment affects a child's circumstances in a number of different ways. It plays a major role from an ecological, biological and political point of view, and it affects children in the North differently from those in the South, as was noted above. For the environment itself, our first concern must be the impact of climate change, as it is felt in different ways in various regions of the world. Yet recent events, however, tend to disprove the separation we have been using between issues affecting children in the North and those affecting children in the South.

Ecology, climate change and global warming

> *what has impressed me most is the distinctive physical ecology, and how it has helped to shape Africa's recent economic history.*[24]

Thus the first thing to note about the extreme burden of disease to which regions like sub-Saharan Africa are exposed, start with their own ecology. The region is exposed to repeated droughts; then, it is, for the most part, a tropical country, a circumstance that is rendered problematic by the presence of global warming. Africa's life and death crises, all of them involving children, are rendered more severe by the presence of climate change. In fact the region's burden of disease is the gravest in the world, and it affects children aged 0–5 and other young children, as well as the life expectancy of all its people:

> *By the turn of the new millennium sub-Saharan Africa's life expectancy stood at forty-seven years, more than two decades lower than in East Asia (sixty-nine years), and thirty-one years lower than the average age in developed countries (seventy-eight years).*[25]

Its climate conditions, harsh and unstable from the outset, render the region particularly vulnerable to global warming, despite the presence of several landlocked countries, and the lack of low-lying coastlines such as other regions, for example the Maldives, the Marshall Islands, and several Caribbean Islands. These regions will disappear altogether unless some measures are taken immediately both locally and globally.[26]

Many other countries are also threatened, including Bangladesh and, as recent events have clearly shown, Florida, Louisiana and Mississippi, in the US. Despite the efforts of the present Bush administration to belittle and ignore its findings, incontrovertible science shows that the increase of global temperatures have already increased global rainfall, steadily increasing loss of sea-ice and high altitude snow and ice cover, and that we can anticipate a rise of sea levels 'by 20cm by 2030, and 65cm by the end of the 21st century'.[27] In fact the US has supported the work of a few dissident scientists such as Richard Lindzen of MIT or the discredited work of Danish Bjorn Lomberg,[28] as it continues to avoid taking any measures to retard global warming or to cut back emissions, although clearly it is itself under threat:

> *Rising sea levels could obliterate the East Coast, as well as the Gulf Coast States of Florida, Alabama, Mississippi, Louisiana, and Texas. The Environmental Protection Agency (EPA) has estimated that a two-foot rise in sea level caused by increased ocean temperatures and melting ice caps would wipe out 17 to 43 per cent of American Wetlands.*[29]

Ironically, it is Katrina, a hurricane repeatedly described by George W. Bush and those in his organization as a 'natural disaster', which confirmed in the most brutal manner, the predictions of the EPA, as well as those of the International Panel on Climate Change (IPCC) and most of the world's scientists. As one of the world's great cities, New Orleans has all but disappeared and the citizens of several states are reduced to refugee status, the role of the warmed sea in whipping a commonplace tropical storm into the greatest disaster in the US cannot be denied.

Perhaps now some of the desperately needed steps will be taken, yet no mention has been made so far in the mainstream media of the vital climate component, while everyone decries the lack of preparedness and timely action b y the US government. As is customary for the news reports from Iraq, the bodies are not shown by US media, and only Euronews so far (6 September) has shown the dead bodies, all but forgotten in the same Superdome in New Orleans, side by side almost with the live refugees.

It is almost incomprehensible how the importance of the climate to a nation, wherever it is located, has not been appreciated or weighed against the immediate economic interests of the prevailing ruling groups, who continue to insist that the environment is 'out there', an issue of interest for some, perhaps one of aesthetics, rather than the most important issue for human rights to life, security and subsistence, and health. Don Brown puts this well:

a nation's climate is an extraordinarily important ingredient in determining a nation's quality of life and its economic possibilities. Because no theory in international relations justifies the right of any nation to act in such a way that it greatly harms another nation's quality of life, those nations that cause global warming violate the most basic international norms. Wars have been fought for much less, and have been viewed as just.[30]

When a country starts, like Africa, with an already underdeveloped economy, minimal to non-existent social infrastructure, and conditions of extreme poverty for most of the population, it is easy to see that it, and other developing countries in similar conditions, cannot even hope to do what the richest country in the world was and is – apparently – unable to do: protect its most vulnerable citizens, including its children. Ross Gelbspan addresses these questions in an article entitled 'Katrina's Real Name':

The Hurricane that struck Louisiana yesterday was nicknamed Katrina by the National Weather Service. Its real name is global warming. When the year began with a two-foot snowfall in Los Angeles, the cause was global warming. When 124-mile-an-hour winds shut down nuclear plants in Scandinavia and cut power to hundreds of thousands of people in Ireland and the United Kingdom, the driver was global warming. When a severe drought in the Midwest dropped water levels in the Missouri River to their lowest on record earlier this summer, the reason was global warming. In July, when the worst drought on record triggered wildfires in Spain and Portugal and left water levels in France at their lowest in 30 years, the explanation was global warming. When a lethal heat wave in Arizona kept temperatures above 110 degrees and killed more than 20 people in one week, the culprit was global warming. And when the Indian city of Bombay (Muambai) received 37 inches of rain in one day – killing 1,000 people and disrupting the lives of 20 million others – the villain was global warming. As the atmosphere warms, it generates longer droughts, more-intense downpours, more-frequent heat waves, and more-severe storms. Although Katrina began as a relatively small hurricane that glanced off south Florida, it was supercharged with extraordinary intensity by the relatively blistering sea surface temperatures in the Gulf of Mexico. The consequences are as heartbreaking as they are terrifying. Unfortunately, very few people in America know the real name of Hurricane Katrina because the coal and oil industries have spent millions of dollars to keep the public in doubt about the issue. The reason is simple: To allow the climate to stabilize requires humanity to cut its use of coal and oil by 70 percent. That, of course, threatens the survival of one of the largest commercial enterprises in history. In 1995, public utility hearings in Minnesota found that the coal industry had paid more than $1 million to four scientists who were public dissenters on global warming. And ExxonMobil has spent more than $13 million since 1998 on an anti-global warming public relations and lobbying campaign. In 2000, big oil and big coal scored their biggest electoral victory yet when President George W. Bush was elected president – and subsequently took suggestions from the industry for his climate and energy policies. As the pace of climate change accelerates, many researchers fear we have already entered a period of irreversible runaway climate change. Against this background, the ignorance of the American public about global warming stands out as an indictment of the US media. When the US press has bothered to cover the subject of global warming, it has *focused almost exclusively on its political and diplomatic aspects and not on what the warming is doing to our agriculture, water supplies, plant and animal life, public health, and weather. For years, the fossil fuel industry has lobbied the media to accord the same weight to a handful of global warming skeptics that it accords the findings of the Intergovernmental Panel on Climate Change – more than 2,000 scientists from 100 countries reporting to the United Nations. Today, with the science having become even more robust – and the impacts as visible as the megastorm that covered much of the Gulf of Mexico – the press bears a share of the guilt for our self-induced destruction with the oil and coal industries.*[31]

Beyond the economic, scientific and political aspects Gelbspan addresses, there is an even darker side to the continued refusal of the US Administration to face the responsibility for the effects of climate change: the faces of the sick, starving, dying and the children in Africa's many drought-induced famines, and those of the crying and desperate people in New Orleans are all black, poor and highly vulnerable. Environmental racism is, as I have argued, as strong in North America as it is in Africa.[32]

Of course global warming severely aggravates a serious situation based on the natural ecology of developing regions such as most of sub-Saharan Africa, or other regions in South America and Asia. The most vulnerable are, as usual, the children, and their plight is totally ignored by the US and a conservative administration intent on overturning *Roe v. Wade*, if at all possible, and on reducing the availability of abortion. However, it appears that what happens to the infants in the womb or after they emerge from it is no longer a serious concern, as business-as-usual assaults and harms the preborn with near impunity and current policies offer no special protection and no health guarantees even after birth, as the situation in both examples under discussion, Africa and the US South, indicates.

Ecology, poverty and children's health

The requirement of the *Convention on the Rights of the Child* (Article 44) is that all countries who have ratified the convention report periodically what they have done to implement that instrument. The understanding is that, in order to harmonize with the Articles of the CRC, all countries are now compelled to put in place legislation to protect the rights of the child as well as maternal/child health protection and a host of other regulations intended to address the specific problems children will encounter in each country. The five countries listed in Appendix 2 (Bolivia, Cambodia, Ghana, Nigeria and South Africa) illustrate well the variety of problems each governing body is expected to address, and the difference between their obligations (and aspirations) and the result on the ground.

The problems to be addressed range from child abductions and sales to the need to respect various traditions that may be deleterious to children's health, from unsterilized birth attendants and equipment to female genital mutilation, to the persistence of practices such as Tro-Kosi in Ghana. The main issue, of course, remains survival and related issues of access to the necessities to support life (water, nutrition, shelter), as well as the necessities to promote and maintain health: that is, vaccinations, medicines, treated bed-nets and the like.

The emphasis of the WHO's research related to maternal and child health,[33] and my own desk analysis of the developing countries listed above, shows the recurrence of several themes, both in the new legislation introduced by the respective governments, and the categories of obstacles encountered in their implementation efforts. For instance, the presence of geographical obstacles is an ongoing thread: neither public transport nor road infrastructures exist to facilitate the attendance of parents and children at newly established clinics. In addition the geography of Bolivia, the harsh weather conditions in Africa, all support the spread of disease, but so does the difficulty of travelling to locations where inoculations, medicines or other public health support may be available.

Speaking of malaria, one of the most widespread diseases in developing countries, Jeffrey Sachs says:

> *Malaria is utterly treatable, yet, incredibly, it still claims up to three million lives per year, mostly young children, about 90 percent of whom live in Africa. Low cost treatments exist, but they do not reach the poor.*[34]

The ecological link here lies in the temperature and in general the climate conditions, as Africa is a tropical continent and malaria, of course, is a tropical disease.[35] In addition, the distance between the availability of treatment in principle and the geographical, logistical and climate obstacles in practice, is a fact of life in all five developing countries I have researched, as is the chronic and persistent underfunding of all governmental institutions charged with enforcing and monitoring all legal instruments and initiatives for children's health.

The main, basic reason for this distance is poverty as even organizations charged with providing funds for assistance often neglect many of the interrelated issues that exacerbate the problems they are attempting to mitigate:

> *The IMF has overlooked urgent problems involving poverty traps, agronomy, climate, disease, transport, gender and a host of other pathologies that undermine economic development.*[36]

Another problem is the lack of education that renders many mothers suspicious of 'modern' medicine and the prevalence of traditional practices, as well as the lack of technical abilities, and properly trained personnel. These obstacles militate against the implementation of maternal/infant and early childhood health regulations.

The desk research I conducted for WHO in Geneva was based on the information provided by the five developing countries listed above, and research on legal databases, under ten separate headings:

1   International Legal Instruments;
2   Regional Instruments;
3   National Legal Instruments;
4   The Definition of the Child and Birth Registration;
5   Child and Maternal Health;
6   Public Health Law;
7   Social Security Issues;

8   Anti-Discrimination Law;
9   Customary Traditional Law;
10 Other Relevant Legislation.

The all-important fourth category in the above list is discussed in the following section, with reference to the five countries examined in Appendix 2.

THE DEFINITION OF THE CHILD AND BIRTH REGISTRATION: IMPACTS ON HEALTH

One of the most important basic issues related to child health is that of birth registration. A country cannot begin to assess its child health needs if it does not have records of how many children are born and where they are. A census is not possible without this information, and neither is the issue of free primary care cards or the organization of vaccination clinics, or the monitoring of perinatal conditions, unless women attend mother and infant clinics, and children are registered at birth. There is no need at this time to revisit the question of the definition of the child, as was done in earlier chapters, in relation to pre-birth exposures and maternal and corporate choices.

The length of 'childhood' instead presents some interesting anomalies to which I shall return below, but the main problem is birth registration. In South Africa, as well as the other countries researched, mobile clinics and hospitals are necessary to improve birth registration percentages, as too many are never registered. In Ghana, birth registration is not legally enforced, and the same is true in Cambodia. In Bolivia, however, the *Code for Children and Adolescents* (1999), Article 97, states that all children must receive a free birth registration 'immediately' after birth although, according to UNICEF, at least 778,000 children are not registered (0–14 years of age) and 42 per cent of these are under one year of age. Obstacles to birth registration include the fact that, traditionally, children are only registered if they survive to age 2 or 3, hence cultural reasons as well as ignorance about the importance of that document pose obstacles to the registration of births.

The definition of the child is also problematic as the average age of majority is 18, but that legal limit is often undermined by conflicting regulations concerning marriage, sexual consent or work. In South Africa, according to their constitution (Article 28(3)), child means a person under the age of 19, but the age of sexual consent is 12 for girls and 14 for boys. In Nigeria, there is no uniform definition of the child: compulsory education ends at age 15, early employment or 'apprenticeship' is allowed; for the *Immigration Act*, everyone under the age of 15 is a minor; the age of sexual consent varies from 13 (in two states) to 18, or 16 in other states; in the North-East, the Islamic religion does not allow sexual consent.

In Ghana, although childhood has a single definition (age 18), children between 14 and 18 have no legal status or social protection; many children between 14 and 18 work in the domestic or agricultural sectors; and there are no statistics on the number of street/working children, in the cities. In Cambodia, the present age of majority is 16, but there are plans to reduce it to 14 so that children can help their families; although the age of marriage is 18 for girls (20 for boys), if the girl becomes pregnant, parents or guardians may consent to an earlier marriage. For Bolivia, children are subject to protection 'from conception to the end of their 12th year and adolescents from 12 to 18 years';[37] the marriage age is 14 for girls and 16 for boys.

It is easy to see the impact on child health of all these obstacles and additional problems will emerge as we turn to maternal and child health.

Child and maternal health and public health: Issues and obstacles

The work of the WHO on the Millennium Development Goals emphasizes the importance of the 'health system as a core social institution',[38] in contrast with 'market-based' health systems. The latter are systematically depriving the poor of their rights to equal access. In addition, according to the WHO's research, the current situation is also deleterious to the legitimacy of the state and its ability to perform its regulatory and governance functions.

This position, however, is in direct conflict with what has emerged from our research in the earlier chapters, where the situation of child health and protection in the North–West developed countries was discussed. In some sense the aetiology of the loss of relevance and legitimacy of the state are similar it both regions: in both cases the multiple corporate pressures affect the health of the poor through promises to increase the efficiency of health services delivery through markets. In contrast, corporate activities have generated or exacerbated many of the health problems discussed in the earlier chapters, through multiple hazardous exposures on one hand, and through costly and often untried pharmaceuticals, on the other.[39,40]

In developed countries the presence of corporate interests and their impact on public health, whether direct, that is through the result of their harmful activities, or indirect, through their well-orchestrated campaigns to discredit scientific evidence contrary to their economic interests,[41] are too powerful in most states to allow complete reliance on domestic regulatory regimens (see Chapters 5 and 7). Hence we argued for appeals to international and supranational law, both of which at least had the potential to by pass or to defeat the oppressive market influence on national laws.

Hence to ensure the presence of an argument that is truly universal, as it applies to both North and South in some way, it might be best to be cautious about 'strengthening the state', unless there are corresponding assurances about internal equity and respect for human rights. An example of this difficulty can be noted in the Nigeria section of Appendix 2, where some states in the Nigerian Federation do not recognize the right to consent to sexual activity, or permit Sharia laws in certain states to set aside judgements of the regular courts in defence of women's rights. The other four templates also include similar issues and difficulties.

Another significant problem involving the role of the state is the question of the allocation of funds to support and implement the legal infrastructure imposed by the ratification of the CRC. Again in Nigeria, at the time of their report (2003) only 17 per cent of Nigerians had access to health facilities, despite the language of the *Bamako Initiative* (1999), guaranteeing access to health care for children from disadvantaged families. Even when international organizations provide funds earmarked for pubic health expenditures, or specifically for child/maternal health, it is not always possible to ensure that social spending is given primacy over other government expenditures and programmes.

In Bolivia, municipalities are allocated funding for basic health insurance, but often these funds are diverted to other expenditures. But the problems are not only due to wrong choices by local functionaries, they are endemic to countries where the economy is failing because of other intrinsic problems, such as 'its geography, the great social and economic inequalities that divide the country; and regional political relations fraught with difficulty, particularly with Chile, Brazil and Argentina'.[42] And most other developing countries in this group present similar problems.

Maternal/child health issues include the transmission of HIV/AIDS which is perhaps the most costly health problem, as malaria, tuberculosis, pneumonia and diarrhoea are far less costly to treat, hence this section focused on the economic aspects of the situation.

Returning to Bolivia's situation, it is a landlocked country, hence it is extremely difficult for Bolivia to establish the trade relations that might help to reduce poverty and help to establish the basic public health organization that is desperately needed. Without debt elimination or reduction and substantial help from abroad, even the best intentions and the introduction of protective regulatory regimes will not succeed to protect maternal and child health.

Thus there can be no complacency in simply observing the improvements introduced and the changes instituted by government instruments when the situation on the ground does not and will not reflect major changes. These changes will not happen unless the economies of each country cannot support the measures that have been legislated, and the wealthy countries refuse to shoulder their obligations.[43]

Social security issues, other types of legislation

Perhaps the discussion in the last few paragraphs belongs in this section rather than in the previous one. But it is extremely useful to see the impact of social and economic issues on our main topic: child survival and health. On the topic of the difference between ratification of the CRC and the commitment to implement, and real actual implementation, we can also compare some of the language of the major international covenants, ratified by these five countries, and the reality of the situation as reported by the committee on implementation to the UN

For instance, Nigeria has ratified CEDAW (4 January 1969), but only a few of its states prohibit female genital mutilation; only two states prohibit street hawking or begging by school-age girls, and one state only prohibits it during school hours; in some states the Sharia courts overturn court decisions concerning women and children reached by other courts. Ghana was the first country to ratify the CRC, but it has no laws forbidding cruel, inhuman and degrading treatment against children, and the number of 'street children' in the cities attest to the fact that very little has been done to mitigate the conditions that force children to the streets, so that 'the best interest of the child principle' does not appear to be well-established.

In Cambodia, the demilitarization of child-soldiers is progressing 'at the rate of 10,000 per year', indicating that it remains a serious problem, despite the fact that the country signed the Optional Protocol to the *Convention of the Rights of the Child*, on the involvement of Children in Armed Conflicts. In Bolivia women can still earn a living either as domestic servants, or by procuring young girls for middlemen from the cities, as the sale, trafficking and kidnapping of children is not a criminal offence yet. But when 5 million out of an 8.3 million population are living below the poverty line, it easy to see where the major problems lie, that is in the economic situation, as indicated in the previous sections.

Hence, the very implementation of basic human rights must be seen in the light of North/South interaction in general, and the developing countries' slow and limited compliance in actual terms, that is, beyond the presence of paper commitments, must be understood in the light of the refusal, or negligence of the most powerful Western nations, to meet their obligations. Nor should such obligation be viewed as optional, or charity. It is essentially reparation and restitution, either for the legacy of a colonial past, or for the ongoing exploitation through our ecological footprint, or both.

TOWARDS MODEL LEGISLATION ON THE RIGHTS OF THE CHILD TO HEALTH

The first four chapters of this book emphasized the vital importance of the definition of the child to a fuller understanding of the rights of the first generation. After reviewing the existing definitions in Internal, Civil and Common law and the related case law, in Chapter 5, the 'social construct' approach to the definition of the child was considered, and the possibility of a serious re-examination of accepted definitions was proposed.

Given the special vulnerability of the child in infancy and in the perinatal period in general, two grave problems have emerged in our review of the legal situation of the child.

The first is that the 'inherent right to life', that is Article 6.1, regards that right as common to all human beings, but it does not clearly and unequivocally apply to the child, especially during the most vulnerable period when, according to many, her humanity is in question. The obvious conflict with the women's rights to choice in reproductive matters, prevents the use of strong and unequivocal language of the child, where pre-birth protection is only mentioned in the preambular portion of the instrument.

Hence the right of the child to a safe environment, most conducive to her health and development, is not a binding requirement of any law, international, supernational or domestic. The closest approach to the meaning if not the letter of such a requirement may be found in the disposition of the cases adjudicated by the European Court of Human Rights discussed above, where children's 'biological integrity' is treated as paramount, thus superseding the right of legal persons (corporations and other institutions) to pursue profitable economic activities.

We also noted that the *American Convention on Human Rights* is the only document specific in its language, extending the right to life to conception. But even here, the environment is not a part of any document on the right of the child to health, although several African legal instruments, for instance, make that connection explicit, and the European case law makes it implicitly.

This is a moral, social and legal impasse that will be extremely hard to resolve. I have proposed that the most accepted liberal social definition of the child is viewed as a 'social construct'. In that case, the present flawed and incomplete understanding of the child can and should be 're-constructed' in ways that permit factoring in the latest scientific findings. Then perhaps the rigid limits of 'childhood' could be opened to reasoned argument, rather than remain closed through the unshakeable *fiat* of political correctness.

But there is another problem that needs to be faced before we can hope to design any model legislation: both main terms must be clarified. Not only the definition of the child, but the very definition of health is in need of re-examination. In the case of perinatal issues, both instruments and case law, lacking clarity and precision in the definition of the child, and in that of health itself, resorted to such euphemisms as, for instance, 'the right of the child to be well born'. Health is equivocal in this respect, as what is at issue is the child's biological integrity, in both aspects of structural and functional wholeness, and I defended this position and understanding for individuals in general as 'microintegrity'.[44]

Microintegrity and potency as health components

Second-Order Principles 7: The Interface of Microintegrity and Macrointegrity, and Their Interface, and Second Order Principle 8: Accepting the Potency Thesis
SOP 7 We must respect the individual integrity of single organisms (Micro-Integrity), in order to be consistent in our respect for integrity and also to respect and protect individual functions and their contribution to the systemic whole.
SOP 8 Given the uncertainties embedded in SOPs 1, 2, and 3, the 'Risk Thesis'[45] must be accepted, for uncertainties referring to the near future. We must also accept the 'Potency Thesis' for the protection of individuals and wholes in the long-term.

The emphasis on the whole rather than on individual components, it has been argued, is needed in order to combat the extreme individualism prevalent in our Western democratic societies. It is also necessary because the habitat is primary: no embryo can live except in the uterus; no life can arise and persist in an unsuitable environment.

But the presence of a holistic emphasis should not blind one to the intimate interconnection between individual and whole. To be sure, individual non-human components are necessary to the functioning of the whole structure in various degrees, whereas the humans' role is not as vital, as I argued earlier.

Aside from this acknowledged difference in the relation between human individuals and their habitat, and non-human components of the same natural habitat, the similarity is important, and the emphasis on microintegrity is a vital but neglected area of environmental ethics. In humans, as in animals and natural systems, we now often see something quite different from clear, deliberate and visible harms being perpetrated. Even without the use of guns to kill wild birds or advanced technologies to destroy fish species, the physical integrity of all life may be at stake through subtle attacks. In each case, not only the environment, or the habitat, is imperiled but the innermost being of each individual and species. The structural integrity of an individual human being is affected when her capacities, her potential, and her present and future development are under attack. To be sure, the same can be said about each single plant, insect, or other animal when anthropogenic stress is introduced into its habitat. But these harms are not all of the sort that can be seen as either present or imminent. The consequences may well happen sometime in the future. They may also curtail future capacities that are now only *potentially* present in the affected individual.

An example of this 'harm' perpetrated on a potentiality might be the effect of certain toxic substances on the mental abilities, temperament and attention span a boy would *normally* acquire as he grows. Another example may be found in the *naturally* evolving reproductive capabilities of a female infant. Both of these children have certain abilities *potentially*, as they are clearly present in their respective DNA.[46]

This argument accords with our intuitions that the loss of life is a grave injury, and that the younger the person to whom such loss applies, the worse the injury. In cases of disasters, 'women and children first' is in line with our intuitive belief that it is far more cruel to snuff out a life that is just beginning, or to envisage the termination of a 'future' that has just begun, than to stop a life that is almost played out. In rescuing people from fires or sinking ships, 'children first', not 'grandfathers first', represents the normal practice, and it appears to be morally right.

A similar argument is used by Thomas Murray in defence of foetal rights in the case of maternal/foetal conflicts.[47] Murray argues convincingly that 'the timing of a harm is irrelevant', and that even 'viability is irrelevant for nonfatal harms'. Murray's argument does not address the abortion question at all, as he divides the unborn into two categories: foetuses 'destined to be born' and those 'who will not know extrauterine life.'[48] I find the grounds for this division incoherent and thus insufficient to support the clear distinction Murray needs. Nevertheless, the rest of his argument is far more defensible. He offers an interesting example:

> *Imagine two different cases. In the first, a man assaults a woman with the intention of inflicting grave harm on her fetus. He succeeds, causing permanent, irreparable – but not fatal – damage to the fetus's spinal cord, resulting in paralysis. In the second case, all the circumstances are identical, except that the man attacks an infant rather than a fetus, with the same result – permanent, irreparable paralysis; was the first act any less wrong than the second?*
>
> *In both cases, lifelong harm was done to humans who, whatever your beliefs about when personhood begins, would eventually cross that line and attain full moral status.*[49]

This example leads Murray to conclude that 'the timing of a harm is not morally relevant', and that a harm to a 'not-yet-born-person … is as great a harm as if it were done later.'[50] He maintains the same position in the case of viability, despite the fact that viability serves as a threshold in *Roe v. Wade*, when the 'potentiality of human life', according to the Court, becomes closer to actuality.[51]

In addition, the existence of foetal therapies, foetal surgeries and foetal rights points to the fact that there are good arguments for the protection of the *potential capacities* of individuals and therefore, I have argued, for the criminalization of future harms. These harms will only manifest themselves in the future, through the permanent curtailment of capacities that were only *possible*, or budding, at the time when the attack or injury occurred. In the example Murray presents, a blow affecting the spinal cord will not prevent the foetus from developing and being born, but it will prevent its capacity for self-originating movement in the future, when that capacity should have come to fruition.

The integrity argument and the value of ecological integrity are based on point C, the point of optimum capacities.[52] This is a 'potency' or 'future' argument, at least in part. The other components of C are present, such as the system's ability to withstand stress now and to continue in its own evolutionary path. But the range of evolutionary paths available to the system, and its future capacity to resist anthropogenic stress, can only support 'future' or 'potency' arguments as much as the arguments cited in abortion or foetal rights issues did. A female infant cannot reproduce when she is in the womb or for a long time afterwards. But regardless of whether she will ever choose to do so in the future, if her original capacity for reproduction is eliminated through some chemical exposure, she has suffered a grave harm, and the perpetrators of that harm should be subject to criminal prosecution. Further, the timing of that harm, before or after her birth, ought to be viewed as irrelevant in assessing culpability.[53]

Through these two applications of a 'potentiality' or 'future' argument against certain harms and attacks on individual integrity, I have argued that the defence of individual integrity (structural and functional, C, as I have termed it) exists already in philosophical debates, although these debates have not yet been extended to environmental issues, to my knowledge. In a move that could be based on a similar argument, the Ontario government has moved to criminalize truck safety violations, in the wake of a number of cases in which repeated infractions were dealt with as civil cases through fines and reprimands, without halting the carnage of innocent parties on the highways. The latest accident killed two women in January 1997, as their car was hit by two runaway tires from a large rig with a history of fines and problems. With the support of public opinion, the Ontario Provincial Police now has the power to treat safety failures at the inspection site as criminal acts (similar to driving under the influence of alcohol) and take away an individual's licence and right to operate the vehicle, *even if* no one has been harmed.[54] This is a clear instantiation of the 'Risk Thesis'.

This practical application shows that future-oriented arguments can also be used for environmental issues, in two ways. First, a harm to individual integrity (and capacity) remains such even if it is not immediately visible or provable and even if it will affect the individual or her offspring only in the future. Second, from the standpoint of the perpetrators, the timing of the harm is irrelevant, and therefore it neither diminishes nor eliminates culpability (even if *mens rea*, or the deliberate intent to harm a particular individual, is absent). It could be argued in Murray's case that the attacker had no interest in harming a *specific* individual. Therefore, even a future harm perpetrated on a *present* individual's potential capacity is as much a culpable act as if it had occurred when the full extent of the harm would be disclosed and evident. Hence, I have argued that the 'Risk Thesis' ought to be accepted, and I have proposed an additional thesis, the 'Potency Thesis', to account for environmentally imposed harms with future effects.

It is easier to appreciate the import of the 'Potency Thesis' when human individuals are concerned, but the thesis is equally valid when we apply it to individuals from other species whose (micro-)integrity is under attack. Not only should their individual capacities – hence their own unfolding future – be respected, but we also need to acknowledge the role their individual function performs within the whole of which they are a part. In other words, their individual integrity, or microintegrity (as optimum individual capacity *c*) is valuable in and of itself; but it is also valuable for the contribution of each undiminished individual to the macrointegrity, or optimum capacity of the whole (*C*), within which it dwells.

At that time, my work centred on the ecological integrity, that is on macro-integrity, or the structural and functional integrity of ecosystems, the latter defined in details in the joint work of the Global Ecological Integrity Group.[55] Its central meaning was the optimum capacity of specific systems to continue their evolutionary paths, according to their time and location, and the emphasis is on the whole, rather than on individuals. The latter is the main focus now, in fact a specific group or population of individuals: the children.

Health as the structural and functional basis for optimum capacity

If a developmental process in the brain is halted of inhibited, there is little chance for repair, and a small change may have substantial consequences for lifetime brain functions. Evidence is accumulating that pre- and early post-natal exposure to industrial chemicals can contribute to neurodevelopmental impairment.[56]

Presented at a meeting of the Collegium Ramazzini, appropriately titled 'Living in a Chemical World', Philippe Grandjeans's presentation adds a chilling rejoinder to a long list of perinatal and childhood harms perpetuated through various substances, untested, or not fully tested globally (other presenters at the same congress, and on related topics were: Giorgio Tamburlini 'New developments in children's environmental health in Europe'; Mathuros Ruchirawat, 'Environmental impacts on children's health in Southeast Asia'; Raul Harari, 'Children's health and the environment in Latin America'; Ralph Trapp, 'Worldwide governmental efforts to locate and destroy chemical weapons and weapon materials: Minimizing risk in transport and destruction').

When we add the impressive scientific evidence presented at that meeting to (a) the pharmaceutical hazards discussed in Chapter 2, with its focus on thalidomide: and (b) the harms imposed by 'choices', such as tobacco, alcohol or glue sniffing (see Chapter 5), and the vast literature on occupational exposures, the mass of scientific evidence is so overwhelming that to simply propose the use of the precautionary principle in policy making, seems like proposing the use of a pea-shooter to halt or divert a charging wild elephant.

The science is here, solidly present in the well-researched work of major doctors and epidemiologists in the world today. It is not recent or unsupported hypotheses: it is science with a long history, and a comparison with the effects of the products of the tobacco industry come to mind. No one today proposes 'more studies' or just the use of the precautionary principle to combat tobacco's well-proven harms. Tobacco corporate bodies are to be found, increasingly, in the courts, where the harms imposed by their 'enhanced', addictive products are treated as they should be, as crimes.

Yet those harms are, at least minimally and initially the product of choices. The 'choice' involved is indeed limited, given the lack of information and the costly, manipulative marketing campaign mounted to convince vulnerable populations of the desirability of cigarette smoking, despite the assurance of morbidity and early premature mortality these products engender.

Thus the comparison with the products of chemical industries reveals two major disanalogies, both of which render the case for certainty (as compatible with science in general) rather than just precaution, and for criminalization even more urgent and appropriate for the latter than for the former. Those who still today 'choose' tobacco (even acknowledging fully the limits of such 'choice'), are not totally vulnerable and helpless as the first generation at the perinatal, infant and early childhood stages.

So, the first disanalogy is the target of the attacks. While some may argue that the tobacco industry provides a product that society's young people and adults desire, the same cannot be said for any chemical product: pesticides and other toxics are no one's drug of choice, although they may be used in otherwise useful products. Hence this may be termed a double disanalogy: the target's inability to choose, and the utter undesirability of the product per se, regarding the very possibility of such choice.

The second disanalogy lies in the impossibility of reversing the effects of many if not most chemical exposures. Smoking, while hard to quit, inflicts harms that may be mitigated if the addict manages to remain smoke-free for a number of years. But, as the initial quote indicates as well as the discussion of thalidomide's effects in Chapter 2, there is a window of 'opportunity', so to speak, when the preborn may be harmed. When that happens, for instance, when there is the loss of a limb through a specific event when an endocrine disruptor prevents the normal development of the foetus, that limb can never be regrown as is possible for fruit flies.[57]

The same is true of the loss of brain function, as Grandjean indicated (Grandjean, 2005). Hence the biological integrity of the child, a concept that the European Court of Human Rights for instance, extends analogically from the right to life,[58] should be explicitly extended to include both the normal structure and function of each child. To deprive an individual of a limb through a violent attack, is an act that is viewed as criminal, for the most part, although in some cases, such as the conduct of a just war, the event may simply give rise to civil responsibility. One fails to see what is different when the attack is on the same individual, but at a much earlier time, such as pre-birth as well as pre-viability, when those exposures are proven to produce the most extensive harms.[59]

Therefore, without some added specificity, 'health' even with the addition of well-being, is insufficient to ensure that legal instrument and judges understand the true import of health enough to protect the child, mainly through prevention of irreversible harms, and the criminalization of harmful practices.

REQUIRED ELEMENTS FOR A PROPOSED MODEL LEGISLATION ON THE RIGHTS OF THE CHILD TO HEALTH

First step: What is health?

Health is a state of complete, physical, mental and social well-being and not merely the absence of disease or infirmity.[60]

This definition has been criticized by many, but it has not been changed since 1948, at the time when most of the new chemicals started being unleashed upon the world, with the health effects we have noted. Hence, just as the rule of *infans conceptus* was initially necessary to prove that – in fact – there was a child developing in the mother's womb (see Chapter 2), a requirement since supplanted by routine prenatal tests everywhere in the world, that definition is now inappropriate and anachronistic.

Not only is it inappropriate because it does not take into consideration the effect of all the recent chemical 'discoveries', for the last 50 years, but also its focus on 'well-being', a subjective condition that may owe a lot to social circumstances, is misleading today. For instance, a well-adjusted Down's Syndrome child or young adult may well experience 'physical, mental and social well-being', as would a child unaware of the import of limbs lost through his mother's thalidomide exposure. In fact, one can adapt and be content experiencing general well-being in a number of cases where one's biological integrity has been breached.

Another example may be the inability to conceive or to father a child, or even being born with a less than expected intelligence, all because of various chemical exposures. Well-being is compatible with adjustment, and the acceptance of a diminished physical or mental capacity. But the negligence or wilful blindness that engendered that condition ought not to be tolerated because it may be possible for those affected to be unaware of the aetiology of their altered abilities, or to have the temperament to adapt to them.

A better unofficial definition may be the one found in the *Journal of Community Health* (1982):

> *A state characterized by anatomic, physiological and psychological integrity, ability to perform personally valued family, work and community roles; ability to deal with physiological, biologic, psychologic and social stress; a feeling of well-being, and freedom from the risk of disease and untimely death.*[61]

This definition clearly includes integrity and makes it primary, whereas another definition states:

> *A state of equilibrium between humans and the physical biologic and social environment, compatible with fully functional activity.*[62]

And the *Dictionary of Epidemiology*[63] provides an 'ecological definition':

> *A sustainable state in which humans and other living creatures with which they interact can coexist indefinitely in equilibrium. The word health is derived from Old English hal, meaning whole, sound in mind and limb.*

The last two definitions are far superior even to the 1984 WHO 'discussion document' defintion, listed in the *Dictionary of Epidemiology*, and 'abbreviated to':

> *The extent to which an individual or group is able to realize aspirations and satisfy needs and to change or cope with the environment. Health is a resource for everyday*

life, not the objective of living; it is a positive concept, emphasizing social and personal resources as well as physical capabilities.[64]

The social component of this 'discussion document' definition renders it incompatible with a definition that is factual as well as just: the ability of a mentally handicapped person to access community services to 'satisfy needs' and 'social resources', has little or nothing to do with identifying and eliminating the activities and the products that cause her retardation in the first place. Similarly, the mandated presence of ramps and other special facilities is not satisfactory as the *only* response to the lack of physical and biological integrity of someone who lacks one or more limbs because of unrestrained chemical hazards, to which she was exposed pre-birth. Essentially, all socially oriented definitions tend to group together all pathologies regardless of origin and of the possibility of eliminating their causes.

The other definitions I have listed refer to one's 'biologic' or 'physiologic' integrity, thus placing the emphasis on normal structure and function as needed. If we consider the results of the products of the tobacco industry, we can argue in a similar vein, that the availability of oxygen and other conditions supported by social security to enable someone with tobacco induced emphysema to function, is not enough to call the person 'healthy' in any sense of the term. While social services are necessary for those who are already affected, to place the emphasis exclusively on services required after the fact is to by pass the most important thing: human beings should not be exposed to harm-causing agents as a routine part of modern life, and those who cause the exposures should be treated as criminals, because they are in breach of basic human rights.

Second step: Why is another definition of health necessary?

In this section we shall simply review the reasons why a child should be entitled to the right to health that have emerged from our discussion so far, and why that entitlement needs to include a better understanding of health. The argument I propose is not that it would be nice, or good or even right for the child to have such a right: the argument is that it should be illegal for a child not to have such a right, given the presence of related, implicit and explicit legislative instruments.

In Chapter 1 we noted that presence of international instruments that mandate that laws and policies be instituted according to the principle of 'the best interest of the child',[65] whereas Article 6.1, 'State Parties recognize that every child has the inherent right to life'; and Article 8.1 assures the child of her right to identity and a nationality. Unfortunately, the more controversial statement regarding the child's need for protection can only be found in the Preamble of this document:

> *Bearing in mind that, as indicated in the 'Declaration of the Rights of the Child,' the child, by reason of his physical and mental immaturity, needs special safeguards and care including appropriate legal protection, before as well as after birth.*

Although it is acknowledged that preambular statements do not carry the same weight as other articles within an instrument, in practice, neither articles nor Preambles are enforceable, so that the distinction between the two areas reflects a metaphoric rather than an actual difference in status.

However, the requirement for the child's identity and nationality carries its own weight (Chapter 1). Nationality implies the duty to extend physical protection on the part of the state, and this duty cannot be set aside except for extreme cases, such as treason, a category obviously inapplicable to the child. Children as a group represent an extremely vulnerable population, one whose rights are clearly not well-established. That said, the 'duty to intervene' was proposed to replace the sovereignty of individual state parties, when the latter are not proven to be effective defenders of children's rights (Chapter 1).

When we turn from international to domestic law, the situation is even more controversial, as neither civil nor common law is explicit and decisive on the question of the child's 'inherent right to life', let alone the possibility to consider such a right as well as the right to health in general, for the whole prenatal period. The specific case of thalidomide, a clear case of unacceptable harm imposed before birth gave rise to appropriate legislation for the protection of the child; but it remained limited to the specifics of the case rather than extend generally, as it should, to all chemical and pharmaceutical products that permanently harm the preborn and the very young child.

Laws regarding the protection of children's life and health are far from clear and well-designed. Some cases and instruments are indeed protective, but that is only true for the most part, of case of third-party harms, not maternal/foetal conflicts (Chapter 3). In contrast, the civil law traditional child's right as *infans conceptus* to retain any right that might accrue to her after birth, is not as clear-cut on the question of the right to life (Chapter 2). One could almost say that, in contrast with the pronouncements of international law, domestic laws are either incoherent or deliberately self-contradictory on the topic of children's rights.

Nevertheless, despite the presence of grave disagreements, confusion and self-contradiction, it can be argued that there is a strong enough legal voice to permit one to conclude that these confusions and self-contradictions should be openly confronted and resolved. In no other area of law, to my knowledge, is such vagueness and uncertainty permitted, so that explicit review of present instruments appears to be indicated.

Third step: Present circumstances that demand urgently the re-examination of present legal infrastructure (North–West Countries)

In the earlier sections of this chapter a great deal was said about the problems faced by the child in developing countries. In this section we will sum up and reconsider the child's hazards in developed countries. There seem to be three major categories of actual problems that demand the urgent re-examination of present legal instruments regarding children's rights:

(1)   the accumulated research of the WHO regarding the presence of 'windows of vulnerability', or times when the child is most susceptible to exposure to materials that will produce irreversible harms (see Chapter 1);

(2) the proliferation of hazardous industrial practices and product, from thalidomide to VOCs, to pesticides and phthalates, as we are presently living in a chemical world; and

(3) the oppressing presence of another anachronism: the 'legal personhood' of the corporation, still unexamined since 1886,[66] with the corollary of its largely unrestrained 'personal freedom' rights.

In Chapter 1, the confirmation of years of medical and epidemiological research was summarized by the WHO[67] document on that topic. Their findings are clear; the child is not a small adult, the physiology, metabolism and general development of the child are different in kind not in degree, from that of adults. Hence the urgent need to design model legislation that protects the life and health of the child, rather than simply relying on existing human rights instruments, which are neither explicit nor clear in themselves. The latter cannot simply be adapted and applied to the child, without interjecting major changes and emendations. This was also noted in this chapter in the discussion of the vast differences between the explicit health needs of children in North–West countries and those in the South–East.

These differences emerge principally when we consider category (2) in the list above, as the WHO has done in 2002 (Tamburlini et al, 2002) and again in 2005,[68] as was discussed in detail in the present work. There is a strong thrust today to ensure that legislative bodies produce instruments and adjudicate cases in ways that keep pace with social developments and beliefs. It is no less important to ensure that instruments and judgements should equally keep pace with developments and discoveries of the physical and natural sciences.

The dissonance between the rush to render adequate justice in the light of social developments in Canada, for instance in the areas of family and gender law, has been emphasized in the work of the Hon. Justice L'Heureux-Dubé.[69] I characterized the impact of her work under four specific headings, as I extended her approach analogically to environmental issues.

The essence of L'Heureux-Dubé's work can be understood and characterized under four main headings:

1 the quest for substantive justice;
2 the elimination of discrimination;
3 the focus on the 'rule of reason' over precedent in judgement (a conceptual approach);
4 the importance of going beyond case law in the judgments, by considering more than just the actions involved, that is, taking 'judicial notice' of social facts and common knowledge, and looking to:
   (a) the context of the actions,
   (b) the effect of the actions,
   (c) the harms arising from the actions.

All of these categories, both conceptual and factual, can be used analogously beyond the human rights and family law setting that represents the main focus of L'Heureux-Dubé's work.[70]

Thus a legally accepted designation of health cannot represent the reality of today's world without incorporating the recognition of new and proliferating hazards, just like a current judgement in family law must represent current women's rights legal developments. The chemical hazards are caused by substances that, for the most part, did not exist in 1948, and the damages to health and normal function that they produce could not have been acknowledged at that time. That excuse, however, is no longer valid, as the products and processes now exist almost everywhere in developed countries and their effects have been fully documented by scientists everywhere including the WHO.

Finally, the anachronistic and dangerous untouchability of the theory of the 'legal personhood' of the corporation. Once again, something that originally might have served a useful purpose, now also supports numerous public harms, including and especially, irreversible harms to health. As we noted in Chapter 4, the protection of a legal person's freedom is often in direct conflict with the principle of 'the best interest of the child'. In Chapter 5, we also argued against the role of consumerism promoted by corporate interests, and supported by marketing and media campaigns, as the latter can be viewed as attacks on the health and normal function of the child.

We can conclude that for these clusters of reasons, factual or conceptual, the definition of health is as much in need of redefinition as the definition of the child. Recognizing the presence of these altered circumstances must precede any effort to re-open the question of what health is. Until that has been done, it will be very difficult to truly and effectively protect the child from harm.

A QUESTION OF ECOJUSTICE: REVIEWING THE BURDEN OF EXPOSURE (NORTH) AND THE BURDEN OF DISEASE (SOUTH)

Article 24
1. State Parties recognize the right of the child to the enjoyment of the highest attainable standard of health and to facilities for the treatment of illness and rehabilitation of health. State Parties shall strive to ensure that no child is deprived of his or her right to access to such health care services.

This is the article that addresses specifically the child's right to health, and the language of the first few lines, if truly applied and practised, might be sufficient to limit and perhaps even eliminate the burden of exposure we have discussed, especially when combined with Article 24.2:

(d) to ensure appropriate pre-natal and post-natal care for mothers. . .
(f) to develop preventive health care, guidance and family planning education and services.

Nevertheless the rights here indicated are not entirely rights of children, despite the fact they are placed in a convention dedicated to their rights. The language is such that the mandates of this article may benefit children, but they are not exclusively or even primarily in their interest. The main beneficiaries are women instead. Even Article 24.2(f) is not intended to reduce or eliminate harmful pre-birth exposures, but to consider whether children should be born at all. Article 27 includes some helpful statements:

> *Article 27.1 State Parties recognize the right of every child to a standard of living adequate for the child's physical, mental, spiritual and moral development.*

But, as for Article 24.2 (f), we would need to stretch the language of the article almost beyond recognition to understand it to include safer environmental conditions and protection from industrial harms. Therefore the child in the North, the child living 'in a chemical world' not of his own making or choice, is not fully protected by these statements: the instrument lacks any language that would alleviate what the child born in affluent countries is expected to bear.

Nor is there any other language more specifically intended to address the situation. Routine industrial practices and products continue to attack the child's biological integrity, his emotional equilibrium, his mental activity, with almost complete impunity. As we noted, existing legal standards are – for the most part – unsafe for the young child, especially in the perinatal period. Generally speaking, these standards are negotiated, rather than based on independent scientific research, and the fact that each product is not used in isolation, but it is one of many whose interaction is not researched at all, any more than its cumulative effects are, is not taken into consideration within the standards themselves.[71]

A legal instrument specifically designed for the protection of the child, such as the CRC, ought not to focus so much as this one does on the civil and political rights of the child, that is it should not devote its attention for the most part to the older child, with hardly any consideration for either the vulnerable preborn and infant's health and biological integrity, or for that of the adult to come who, as we saw, will also bear the brunt of the effects of early exposures.

Before the child can exercise her right to 'freedom of thought, conscience and religion', or the right to 'freedom of association and freedom of peaceful assembly' (Article 14.1 and Article 15.1), and before she can exercise the 'right to receive and impart information and ideas of all kinds' (Article 13.1), the child has to be in a mental and physical condition such that it will enable her to understand, think and express herself. Once again the child is viewed primarily as a 'little adult', with the same interests and needs as a fully developed adult, but without any consideration of the special needs basic to her age.

The utmost vulnerability and the immaturity of the child, and the delicacy of the conditions of the developing child, are totally disregarded, after the brief reference in the Preamble that we noted. Articles 19.1 and 2 address the question of protection 'from all forms of physical or mental violence, injury or abuse, neglect or negligent treatment, maltreatment or exploitation' (Article 19.1), and propose 'protective measures,' including 'as appropriate, ... effective procedures for the establishment of social programmes', after the fact, and for 'other forms of prevention and for identification, reporting, referral, investigation, treatment and follow-up of instances of child maltreatment...' (Article 19.2).

These articles envision single attacks, not institutionalized 'ecoviolence' as I have termed present harmful environmental conditions.[72] Hence any understanding of the wholesale, indiscriminate harm produced by the regular operations of industries, and the 'externalities' they anticipate and condone (aside from occasional disasters), is not even on the horizon of the drafters of the Convention.

In the previous section point (2) advocated the mandatory training of legislators and judges, so that, besides being appraised of general social advances, they could be made fully aware of the advances of science and technology. No legislation could be formulated today by jurists who lacked the basic understanding of women's rights or gay rights, and who simply resorted to legal formulas dated 45–50 years earlier in their work. Equally, the understanding of scientific and technological innovations and their impact on the child should not be ignored by regulatory instruments and judgements that do not recognize the import of changes that occurred in the last 50 years.

The child born in the South fares marginally better in the convention as the basic conditions needed for survival (in existence from the origin of manmade laws for the most part) are stated more clearly and explicitly at several points in the CRC. Returning once again to Article 24, for instance:

> 2. *State Parties shall pursue full implementation of this right and in particular, shall take appropriate measures:*
>   (a) *to diminish infant and child mortality;*
>   (b) *to ensure the provision of necessary medical assistance and health care to all children with emphasis on the development of primary health care;*
>   (c) *to combat disease and malnutrition, including within the framework of primary health care, through inter alia, the application of readily available technology and through the provision of adequate nutritious food and clean drinking water, taking into consideration the dangers and risks of environmental pollution;*

As we saw earlier, malnutrition and the disease corrected by primary health care as well as the provision of clean drinking water (protected from environmental pollution), are the major problems besetting the child in developing countries. In additionl, Article 24.3 requires State Parties 'to take all effective and appropriate measures, with a view to abolishing traditional practices prejudicial to the health of children'.

The awareness of these issues affecting the life and health of children in the South, however, is not paralleled by an equal awareness of the gravest obstacles to children's life and health and normal function, as they are in peril from routine 'traditional' practices in the North.

Hence, regard and care for the future must start with respect for all children, in the first generation. The latter in turn, must start with an urgent and thoughtful, in depth revision of what is truly necessary to protect that generation and the future. Ecojustice demands that intragenerational and intergenerational rights starting from and interwoven with the rights of the child, MUST start with the review of laws and policies especially those in the three major areas listed above: (1) the definition of health; (2) the awareness of recent science and technology 'advancement' ensuring that these are reflected fully in all human rights instruments, especially in the *Convention of the Rights of the Child*; (3) the removal of the problematic ascription of all the rights and freedoms of natural persons, to legal persons as well. In addition, a full revision of the definition of the child in international and domestic instruments would be useful as well.

Either a new version of the CRC or, better yet, a new convention including Model Legislation on the Right of the Child to Health, is desperately needed to protect today's and tomorrow's children; hence, our future.

NOTES

1   I am extremely grateful to Dr Marcus Stahlhofer for his help and guidance during my month at the WHO. He selected the five countries I researched – South Africa, Nigeria, Ghana, Cambodia and Bolivia – and proposed the categories for the relative Templates.
2   Sachs (2005).
3   Gruskin (2001), pp1–7.
4   Turman et al (2001), pp147–154
5   Westra (2004a), chapter 2.
6   Pimentel et al (1998), pp817–816.
7   McMichael (1995a).
8   McMichael (1995b),
9   Lagrega et al (1994).
10 Soskolne (2001), pp3–9.
11 Westra (1998) pp111–122.
12 Seck (1999), pp139–221
13 Houlihan et al (2005).
14 Freedman et al (2005), p31.
15 Licari et al (2005).
16 Licari et al (2005), pp13–22.
17 Licari et al (2005), pp13–22.
18 Licari et al (2005), p15.
19 Freedman et al (2005), p132; Caulfield et al (2004), pp193–198.
20 Pelletier et al (1993), pp1130–1133.
21 Freedman et al (2005), p55; Caulfield et al (2004), pp193–198.
22 Pogge (2001a), p6.23; Sachs (2005), p188–209.
23 Westra (1998), chapter 5; Seck (1999).
24 Sachs (2005), p192.
25 Sachs (2005), p194.
26 Sands (2005), p77.
27 Sands (2005), pp77–78; *IPCCb Synthesis of Technical and Scientific Information* (available at www.ipcc.ch/pub/sarsyn.htm).
28 Sands (2005), p91.
29 Shiva (2002), p43.
30 Brown (2000), p86.
31 Gelbspan (2005).
32 Westra and Lawson (2001).
33 Freedman et al (2005).
34 Sachs (2005), p196.
35 Sachs (2005), p198.
36 Sachs (2005), p79.
37 *Code for Children and Adolescents (1999), Article 2.*

38 Freedman et al (2005), p13.
39 Thompson et al (2001).
40 Harjuila (2005).
41 Michales (2005), pp96–101.
42 Sachs (2005), p106.
43 Sachs (2005), pp357–358.
44 Westra (1998), pp236–240.
45 Thomson (1990).
46 Grandjean (2005).
47 Murray (1996), pp464–472.
48 Murray (1996), p465.
49 Murray (1996), p466.
50 Murray (1996), p466.
51 Murray (1996), p467.
52 Westra (1994), chapter 2.
53 Murray (1996).
54 *The Globe and Mail* (Toronto) (January 3, 1997), pA3.
55 Pimentel et al (2000), chapter 2.
56 Grandjean (2005).
57 Colborn et al (1996).
58 Article 2, European Charter of Human Rights; see for instance *Guerra v. Italy*, 116/1996/735/ 932, 19 February 1998.
59 Tamburlini et al (2002).
60 Preamble to the constitution of the World Health Organization, as adopted by the International Health conference, New York, 19 June–20 July, 1946; signed on 22 July 1946 by the representatives of 51 states; Official Records of the World Health Organization, no. 2, p100 and entered into force on 7 April 1948. The definition has not been amended since 1948.
61 Stokes et al (1997).
62 Last (1997).
63 Last (2001).
64 Lopen (1987), pp5–28.
65 CRC, Article 3.
66 *Santa Clara v. Southern Pacific R.R. Corp.*, 1886.
67 Tamburlini et al (2002).
68 Licari et al (2005); see also, Gordon et al (2004).
69 Westra (2004b), pp81–84.
70 *Egan v. Canada*, (1993), 2 S.C.R. 513; *Moge v. Moge*, (1992) 3 R.F.L. 3d 345; *Trinity Western*, (1996) 27 O.R. 3d, 132 D.L.R. 4th; *A.G. Canada v. Mossop*, (1993) 1 S.C.R. 554; *Vriend v. Alberta Alta*, (1994) 6 1 S.C.R. 493.
71 Westra (2004a), chapter 4.
72 Westra (2004a).

Convention on the Rights of the Child

Adopted and opened for signature, ratification and accession by General Assembly resolution 44/25 of 20 November 1989
Entry into force 2 September 1990, in accordance with article 49

Preamble

The States Parties to the present Convention,

Considering that, in accordance with the principles proclaimed in the Charter of the United Nations, recognition of the inherent dignity and of the equal and inalienable rights of all members of the human family is the foundation of freedom, justice and peace in the world,

Bearing in mind that the peoples of the United Nations have, in the Charter, reaffirmed their faith in fundamental human rights and in the dignity and worth of the human person, and have determined to promote social progress and better standards of life in larger freedom,

Recognizing that the United Nations has, in the Universal Declaration of Human Rights and in the International Covenants on Human Rights, proclaimed and agreed that everyone is entitled to all the rights and freedoms set forth therein, without distinction of any kind, such as race, colour, sex, language, religion, political or other opinion, national or social origin, property, birth or other status,

Recalling that, in the Universal Declaration of Human Rights, the United Nations has proclaimed that childhood is entitled to special care and assistance,

Convinced that the family, as the fundamental group of society and the natural environment for the growth and well-being of all its members and particularly children, should be afforded the necessary protection and assistance so that it can fully assume its responsibilities within the community,

Recognizing that the child, for the full and harmonious development of his or her personality, should grow up in a family environment, in an atmosphere of happiness, love and understanding,

Considering that the child should be fully prepared to live an individual life in society, and brought up in the spirit of the ideals proclaimed in the Charter of the United Nations, and in particular in the spirit of peace, dignity, tolerance, freedom, equality and solidarity,

Bearing in mind that the need to extend particular care to the child has been stated in the Geneva Declaration of the Rights of the Child of 1924 and in the Declaration of the Rights of the Child adopted by the General Assembly on 20 November 1959 and recognized in the Universal Declaration of Human Rights, in the International Covenant on Civil and Political Rights (in particular in articles 23 and 24), in the International Covenant on Economic, Social and Cultural Rights (in particular in article 10) and in the statutes and relevant instruments of specialized agencies and international organizations concerned with the welfare of children, '

Bearing in mind that, as indicated in the Declaration of the Rights of the Child, 'the child, by reason of his physical and mental immaturity, needs special safeguards and care, including appropriate legal protection, before as well as after birth',

Recalling the provisions of the Declaration on Social and Legal Principles relating to the Protection and Welfare of Children, with Special Reference to Foster Placement and Adoption Nationally and Internationally; the United Nations Standard Minimum Rules for the Administration of Juvenile Justice (The Beijing Rules) ; and the Declaration on the Protection of Women and Children in Emergency and Armed Conflict,

Recognizing that, in all countries in the world, there are children living in exceptionally difficult conditions, and that such children need special consideration,

Taking due account of the importance of the traditions and cultural values of each people for the protection and harmonious development of the child,

Recognizing the importance of international co-operation for improving the living conditions of children in every country, in particular in the developing countries,

Have agreed as follows:

PART I

Article 1

For the purposes of the present Convention, a child means every human being below the age of eighteen years unless under the law applicable to the child, majority is attained earlier.

Article 2

1. States Parties shall respect and ensure the rights set forth in the present Convention to each child within their jurisdiction without discrimination of any kind, irrespective of the child's or his or her parent's or legal guardian's race, colour, sex, language, religion, political or other opinion, national, ethnic or social origin, property, disability, birth or other status.

2. States Parties shall take all appropriate measures to ensure that the child is protected against all forms of discrimination or punishment on the basis of the status, activities, expressed opinions, or beliefs of the child's parents, legal guardians, or family members.

Article 3

1. In all actions concerning children, whether undertaken by public or private social welfare institutions, courts of law, administrative authorities or legislative bodies, the best interests of the child shall be a primary consideration.

2. States Parties undertake to ensure the child such protection and care as is necessary for his or her well-being, taking into account the rights and

duties of his or her parents, legal guardians, or other individuals legally responsible for him or her, and, to this end, shall take all appropriate legislative and administrative measures.

3. States Parties shall ensure that the institutions, services and facilities responsible for the care or protection of children shall conform with the standards established by competent authorities, particularly in the areas of safety, health, in the number and suitability of their staff, as well as competent supervision.

Article 4

States Parties shall undertake all appropriate legislative, administrative, and other measures for the implementation of the rights recognized in the present Convention. With regard to economic, social and cultural rights, States Parties shall undertake such measures to the maximum extent of their available resources and, where needed, within the framework of international co-operation.

Article 5

States Parties shall respect the responsibilities, rights and duties of parents or, where applicable, the members of the extended family or community as provided for by local custom, legal guardians or other persons legally responsible for the child, to provide, in a manner consistent with the evolving capacities of the child, appropriate direction and guidance in the exercise by the child of the rights recognized in the present Convention.

Article 6

1. States Parties recognize that every child has the inherent right to life.

2. States Parties shall ensure to the maximum extent possible the survival and development of the child.

Article 7

1. The child shall be registered immediately after birth and shall have the right from birth to a name, the right to acquire a nationality and. as far as possible, the right to know and be cared for by his or her parents.

2. States Parties shall ensure the implementation of these rights in accordance with their national law and

their obligations under the relevant international instruments in this field, in particular where the child would otherwise be stateless.

Article 8

1. States Parties undertake to respect the right of the child to preserve his or her identity, including nationality, name and family relations as recognized by law without unlawful interference.

2. Where a child is illegally deprived of some or all of the elements of his or her identity, States Parties shall provide appropriate assistance and protection, with a view to re-establishing speedily his or her identity.

Article 9

1. States Parties shall ensure that a child shall not be separated from his or her parents against their will, except when competent authorities subject to judicial review determine, in accordance with applicable law and procedures, that such separation is necessary for the best interests of the child. Such determination may be necessary in a particular case such as one involving abuse or neglect of the child by the parents, or one where the parents are living separately and a decision must be made as to the child's place of residence.

2. In any proceedings pursuant to paragraph 1 of the present article, all interested parties shall be given an opportunity to participate in the proceedings and make their views known.

3. States Parties shall respect the right of the child who is separated from one or both parents to maintain personal relations and direct contact with both parents on a regular basis, except if it is contrary to the child's best interests.

4. Where such separation results from any action initiated by a State Party, such as the detention, imprisonment, exile, deportation or death (including death arising from any cause while the person is in the custody of the State) of one or both parents or of the child, that State Party shall, upon request, provide the parents, the child or, if appropriate, another member of the family with the essential information concerning the whereabouts of the absent member(s) of the family unless the provision of the information would be detrimental to the well-being of the child. States Parties shall further ensure that the submission of such a request shall of itself entail no adverse consequences for the person(s) concerned.

Article 10

1. In accordance with the obligation of States Parties under article 9, paragraph 1, applications by a child or his or her parents to enter or leave a State Party for the purpose of family reunification shall be dealt with by States Parties in a positive, humane and expeditious manner. States Parties shall further ensure that the submission of such a request shall entail no adverse consequences for the applicants and for the members of their family.

2. A child whose parents reside in different States shall have the right to maintain on a regular basis, save in exceptional circumstances personal relations and direct contacts with both parents. Towards that end and in accordance with the obligation of States Parties under article 9, paragraph 1, States Parties shall respect the right of the child and his or her parents to leave any country, including their own, and to enter their own country. The right to leave any country shall be subject only to such restrictions as are prescribed by law and which are necessary to protect the national security, public order (ordre public), public health or morals or the rights and freedoms of others and are consistent with the other rights recognized in the present Convention.

Article 11

1. States Parties shall take measures to combat the illicit transfer and non-return of children abroad.

2. To this end, States Parties shall promote the conclusion of bilateral or multilateral agreements or accession to existing agreements.

Article 12

1. States Parties shall assure to the child who is capable of forming his or her own views the right to express those views freely in all matters affecting the child, the views of the child being given due weight in accordance with the age and maturity of the child.

2. For this purpose, the child shall in particular be provided the opportunity to be heard in any judicial and administrative proceedings affecting the child, either directly, or through a representative or an appropriate body, in a manner consistent with the procedural rules of national law.

Article 13

1. The child shall have the right to freedom of expression; this right shall include freedom to seek, receive and impart information and ideas of all kinds, regardless of frontiers, either orally, in writing or in print, in the form of art, or through any other media of the child's choice.

2. The exercise of this right may be subject to certain restrictions, but these shall only be such as are provided by law and are necessary:
(a) For respect of the rights or reputations of others; or
(b) For the protection of national security or of public order (ordre public), or of public health or morals.

Article 14

1. States Parties shall respect the right of the child to freedom of thought, conscience and religion.

2. States Parties shall respect the rights and duties of the parents and, when applicable, legal guardians, to provide direction to the child in the exercise of his or her right in a manner consistent with the evolving capacities of the child.

3. Freedom to manifest one's religion or beliefs may be subject only to such limitations as are prescribed by law and are necessary to protect public safety, order, health or morals, or the fundamental rights and freedoms of others.

Article 15

1. States Parties recognize the rights of the child to freedom of association and to freedom of peaceful assembly.

2. No restrictions may be placed on the exercise of these rights other than those imposed in conformity with the law and which are necessary in a democratic society in the interests of national security or public safety, public order (ordre public), the protection of public health or morals or the protection of the rights and freedoms of others.

Article 16

1. No child shall be subjected to arbitrary or unlawful interference with his or her privacy, family, home or correspondence, nor to unlawful attacks on his or her honour and reputation.

2. The child has the right to the protection of the law against such interference or attacks.

Article 17

States Parties recognize the important function performed by the mass media and shall ensure that the child has access to information and material from a diversity of national and international sources, especially those aimed at the promotion of his or her social, spiritual and moral well-being and physical and mental health. To this end, States Parties shall:

(a) Encourage the mass media to disseminate information and material of social and cultural benefit to the child and in accordance with the spirit of article 29;

(b) Encourage international co-operation in the production, exchange and dissemination of such information and material from a diversity of cultural, national and international sources;

(c) Encourage the production and dissemination of children's books;

(d) Encourage the mass media to have particular regard to the linguistic needs of the child who belongs to a minority group or who is indigenous;

(e) Encourage the development of appropriate guidelines for the protection of the child from information and material injurious to his or her well-being, bearing in mind the provisions of articles 13 and 18.

Article 18

1. States Parties shall use their best efforts to ensure recognition of the principle that both parents have common responsibilities for the upbringing and development of the child. Parents or, as the case may be, legal guardians, have the primary responsibility for the upbringing and development of the child. The best interests of the child will be their basic concern.

2. For the purpose of guaranteeing and promoting the rights set forth in the present Convention, States Parties shall render appropriate assistance to parents and legal guardians in the performance of their child-rearing responsibilities and shall ensure the development of institutions, facilities and services for the care of children.

3. States Parties shall take all appropriate measures to ensure that children of working parents have the right to benefit from child-care services and facilities for which they are eligible.

Article 19

1. States Parties shall take all appropriate legislative, administrative, social and educational measures to protect the child from all forms of physical or mental violence, injury or abuse, neglect or negligent treatment, maltreatment or exploitation, including sexual abuse, while in the care of parent(s), legal guardian(s) or any other person who has the care of the child.

2. Such protective measures should, as appropriate, include effective procedures for the establishment of social programmes to provide necessary support for the child and for those who have the care of the child, as well as for other forms of prevention and for identification, reporting, referral, investigation, treatment and follow-up of instances of child maltreatment described heretofore, and, as appropriate, for judicial involvement.

Article 20

1. A child temporarily or permanently deprived of his or her family environment, or in whose own best interests cannot be allowed to remain in that environment, shall be entitled to special protection and assistance provided by the State.

2. States Parties shall in accordance with their national laws ensure alternative care for such a child.

3. Such care could include, inter alia, foster placement, kafalah of Islamic law, adoption or if necessary placement in suitable institutions for the care of children. When considering solutions, due regard shall be paid to the desirability of continuity in a child's upbringing and to the child's ethnic, religious, cultural and linguistic background.

Article 21

States Parties that recognize and/or permit the system of adoption shall ensure that the best interests of the child shall be the paramount consideration and they shall:

(a) Ensure that the adoption of a child is authorized only by competent authorities who determine, in accordance with applicable law and procedures and on the basis of all pertinent and reliable information, that the adoption is permissible in view of the child's status concerning parents, relatives and legal guardians and that, if required, the persons concerned have given their informed consent to the adoption on the basis of such counselling as may be necessary;

(b) Recognize that inter-country adoption may be considered as an alternative means of child's care, if the child cannot be placed in a foster or an adoptive family or cannot in any suitable manner be cared for in the child's country of origin;

(c) Ensure that the child concerned by inter-country adoption enjoys safeguards and standards equivalent to those existing in the case of national adoption;

(d) Take all appropriate measures to ensure that, in inter-country adoption, the placement does not result in improper financial gain for those involved in it;

(e) Promote, where appropriate, the objectives of the present article by concluding bilateral or multilateral arrangements or agreements, and endeavour, within this framework, to ensure that the placement of the child in another country is carried out by competent authorities or organs.

Article 22

1. States Parties shall take appropriate measures to ensure that a child who is seeking refugee status or who is considered a refugee in accordance with applicable international or domestic law and procedures shall, whether unaccompanied or accompanied by his or her parents or by any other person, receive appropriate protection and humanitarian assistance in the enjoyment of applicable rights set forth in the present Convention and in other international human rights or humanitarian instruments to which the said States are Parties.

2. For this purpose, States Parties shall provide, as they consider appropriate, co-operation in any efforts by the United Nations and other competent intergovernmental organizations or non-governmental organizations co-operating with the United Nations to protect and assist such a child and to trace the parents or other members of the family of any refugee child in order to obtain information necessary for reunification with his or her family. In cases where no parents or other members of the family can be found, the child shall be accorded the same protection as any other child

permanently or temporarily deprived of his or her family environment for any reason, as set forth in the present Convention.

Article 23

1. States Parties recognize that a mentally or physically disabled child should enjoy a full and decent life, in conditions which ensure dignity, promote self-reliance and facilitate the child's active participation in the community.

2. States Parties recognize the right of the disabled child to special care and shall encourage and ensure the extension, subject to available resources, to the eligible child and those responsible for his or her care, of assistance for which application is made and which is appropriate to the child's condition and to the circumstances of the parents or others caring for the child.

3. Recognizing the special needs of a disabled child, assistance extended in accordance with paragraph 2 of the present article shall be provided free of charge, whenever possible, taking into account the financial resources of the parents or others caring for the child, and shall be designed to ensure that the disabled child has effective access to and receives education, training, health care services, rehabilitation services, preparation for employment and recreation opportunities in a manner conducive to the child's achieving the fullest possible social integration and individual development, including his or her cultural and spiritual development

4. States Parties shall promote, in the spirit of international cooperation, the exchange of appropriate information in the field of preventive health care and of medical, psychological and functional treatment of disabled children, including dissemination of and access to information concerning methods of rehabilitation, education and vocational services, with the aim of enabling States Parties to improve their capabilities and skills and to widen their experience in these areas. In this regard, particular account shall be taken of the needs of developing countries.

Article 24

1. States Parties recognize the right of the child to the enjoyment of the highest attainable standard of health and to facilities for the treatment of illness and rehabilitation of health. States Parties shall strive to ensure that no child is deprived of his or her right of access to such health care services.

2. States Parties shall pursue full implementation of this right and, in particular, shall take appropriate measures:

(a) To diminish infant and child mortality;

(b) To ensure the provision of necessary medical assistance and health care to all children with emphasis on the development of primary health care;

(c) To combat disease and malnutrition, including within the framework of primary health care, through, inter alia, the application of readily available technology and through the provision of adequate nutritious foods and clean drinking-water, taking into consideration the dangers and risks of environmental pollution;

(d) To ensure appropriate pre-natal and post-natal health care for mothers;

(e) To ensure that all segments of society, in particular parents and children, are informed, have access to education and are supported in the use of basic knowledge of child health and nutrition, the advantages of breastfeeding, hygiene and environmental sanitation and the prevention of accidents;

(f) To develop preventive health care, guidance for parents and family planning education and services.

3. States Parties shall take all effective and appropriate measures with a view to abolishing traditional practices prejudicial to the health of children.

4. States Parties undertake to promote and encourage international co-operation with a view to achieving progressively the full realization of the right recognized in the present article. In this regard, particular account shall be taken of the needs of developing countries.

Article 25

States Parties recognize the right of a child who has been placed by the competent authorities for the purposes of care, protection or treatment of his or her physical or mental health, to a periodic review of the treatment provided to the child and all other circumstances relevant to his or her placement.

Article 26

1. States Parties shall recognize for every child the right to benefit from social security, including social insurance, and shall take the necessary measures to

achieve the full realization of this right in accordance with their national law.

2. The benefits should, where appropriate, be granted, taking into account the resources and the circumstances of the child and persons having responsibility for the maintenance of the child, as well as any other consideration relevant to an application for benefits made by or on behalf of the child.

Article 27

1. States Parties recognize the right of every child to a standard of living adequate for the child's physical, mental, spiritual, moral and social development.

2. The parent(s) or others responsible for the child have the primary responsibility to secure, within their abilities and financial capacities, the conditions of living necessary for the child's development.

3. States Parties, in accordance with national conditions and within their means, shall take appropriate measures to assist parents and others responsible for the child to implement this right and shall in case of need provide material assistance and support programmes, particularly with regard to nutrition, clothing and housing.

4. States Parties shall take all appropriate measures to secure the recovery of maintenance for the child from the parents or other persons having financial responsibility for the child, both within the State Party and from abroad. In particular, where the person having financial responsibility for the child lives in a State different from that of the child, States Parties shall promote the accession to international agreements or the conclusion of such agreements, as well as the making of other appropriate arrangements.

Article 28

1. States Parties recognize the right of the child to education, and with a view to achieving this right progressively and on the basis of equal opportunity, they shall, in particular:

(a) Make primary education compulsory and available free to all;

(b) Encourage the development of different forms of secondary education, including general and vocational education, make them available and accessible to every child, and take appropriate measures such as the introduction of free education and offering financial assistance in case of need;

(c) Make higher education accessible to all on the basis of capacity by every appropriate means;

(d) Make educational and vocational information and guidance available and accessible to all children;

(e) Take measures to encourage regular attendance at schools and the reduction of drop-out rates.

2. States Parties shall take all appropriate measures to ensure that school discipline is administered in a manner consistent with the child's human dignity and in conformity with the present Convention.

3. States Parties shall promote and encourage international cooperation in matters relating to education, in particular with a view to contributing to the elimination of ignorance and illiteracy throughout the world and facilitating access to scientific and technical knowledge and modern teaching methods. In this regard, particular account shall be taken of the needs of developing countries.

Article 29   *General comment on its implementation*

1. States Parties agree that the education of the child shall be directed to:
(a) The development of the child's personality, talents and mental and physical abilities to their fullest potential;

(b) The development of respect for human rights and fundamental freedoms, and for the principles enshrined in the Charter of the United Nations;

(c) The development of respect for the child's parents, his or her own cultural identity, language and values, for the national values of the country in which the child is living, the country from which he or she may originate, and for civilizations different from his or her own;

(d) The preparation of the child for responsible life in a free society, in the spirit of understanding, peace, tolerance, equality of sexes, and friendship among all peoples, ethnic, national and religious groups and persons of indigenous origin;

(e) The development of respect for the natural environment.

2. No part of the present article or article 28 shall be construed so as to interfere with the liberty of individuals and bodies to establish and direct educational institutions, subject always to the observance of the principle set forth in paragraph 1 of the present article and to the requirements that the education given in such institutions shall conform

to such minimum standards as may be laid down by the State.

Article 30

In those States in which ethnic, religious or linguistic minorities or persons of indigenous origin exist, a child belonging to such a minority or who is indigenous shall not be denied the right, in community with other members of his or her group, to enjoy his or her own culture, to profess and practise his or her own religion, or to use his or her own language.

Article 31

1. States Parties recognize the right of the child to rest and leisure, to engage in play and recreational activities appropriate to the age of the child and to participate freely in cultural life and the arts.

2. States Parties shall respect and promote the right of the child to participate fully in cultural and artistic life and shall encourage the provision of appropriate and equal opportunities for cultural, artistic, recreational and leisure activity.

Article 32

1. States Parties recognize the right of the child to be protected from economic exploitation and from performing any work that is likely to be hazardous or to interfere with the child's education, or to be harmful to the child's health or physical, mental, spiritual, moral or social development.

2. States Parties shall take legislative, administrative, social and educational measures to ensure the implementation of the present article. To this end, and having regard to the relevant provisions of other international instruments, States Parties shall in particular:

(a) Provide for a minimum age or minimum ages for admission to employment;

(b) Provide for appropriate regulation of the hours and conditions of employment;

(c) Provide for appropriate penalties or other sanctions to ensure the effective enforcement of the present article.

Article 33

States Parties shall take all appropriate measures, including legislative, administrative, social and educational measures, to protect children from the illicit use of narcotic drugs and psychotropic substances as defined in the relevant international treaties, and to prevent the use of children in the illicit production and trafficking of such substances.

Article 34

States Parties undertake to protect the child from all forms of sexual exploitation and sexual abuse. For these purposes, States Parties shall in particular take all appropriate national, bilateral and multilateral measures to prevent:

(a) The inducement or coercion of a child to engage in any unlawful sexual activity;

(b) The exploitative use of children in prostitution or other unlawful sexual practices;

(c) The exploitative use of children in pornographic performances and materials.

Article 35

States Parties shall take all appropriate national, bilateral and multilateral measures to prevent the abduction of, the sale of or traffic in children for any purpose or in any form.

Article 36

States Parties shall protect the child against all other forms of exploitation prejudicial to any aspects of the child's welfare.

Article 37

States Parties shall ensure that:

(a) No child shall be subjected to torture or other cruel, inhuman or degrading treatment or punishment. Neither capital punishment nor life imprisonment without possibility of release shall be imposed for offences committed by persons below eighteen years of age;

(b) No child shall be deprived of his or her liberty unlawfully or arbitrarily. The arrest, detention or imprisonment of a child shall be in conformity with the law and shall be used only as a measure of last resort and for the shortest appropriate period of time;

(c) Every child deprived of liberty shall be treated with humanity and respect for the inherent dignity of the human person, and in a manner which takes into account the needs of persons of his or her age. In particular, every child deprived of liberty shall be separated from adults unless it is considered in the child's best interest not to do so and shall have the right to maintain contact with his or her family through correspondence and visits, save in exceptional circumstances;

(d) Every child deprived of his or her liberty shall have the right to prompt access to legal and other appropriate assistance, as well as the right to challenge the legality of the deprivation of his or her liberty before a court or other competent, independent and impartial authority, and to a prompt decision on any such action.

Article 38

1. States Parties undertake to respect and to ensure respect for rules of international humanitarian law applicable to them in armed conflicts which are relevant to the child.

2. States Parties shall take all feasible measures to ensure that persons who have not attained the age of fifteen years do not take a direct part in hostilities.

3. States Parties shall refrain from recruiting any person who has not attained the age of fifteen years into their armed forces. In recruiting among those persons who have attained the age of fifteen years but who have not attained the age of eighteen years, States Parties shall endeavour to give priority to those who are oldest.

4. In accordance with their obligations under international humanitarian law to protect the civilian population in armed conflicts, States Parties shall take all feasible measures to ensure protection and care of children who are affected by an armed conflict.

Article 39

States Parties shall take all appropriate measures to promote physical and psychological recovery and social reintegration of a child victim of: any form of neglect, exploitation, or abuse; torture or any other form of cruel, inhuman or degrading treatment or punishment; or armed conflicts. Such recovery and reintegration shall take place in an environment which fosters the health, self-respect and dignity of the child.

Article 40

1. States Parties recognize the right of every child alleged as, accused of, or recognized as having infringed the penal law to be treated in a manner consistent with the promotion of the child's sense of dignity and worth, which reinforces the child's respect for the human rights and fundamental freedoms of others and which takes into account the child's age and the desirability of promoting the child's reintegration and the child's assuming a constructive role in society.

2. To this end, and having regard to the relevant provisions of international instruments, States Parties shall, in particular, ensure that:

(a) No child shall be alleged as, be accused of, or recognized as having infringed the penal law by reason of acts or omissions that were not prohibited by national or international law at the time they were committed;

(b) Every child alleged as or accused of having infringed the penal law has at least the following guarantees:

(i) To be presumed innocent until proven guilty according to law;

(ii) To be informed promptly and directly of the charges against him or her, and, if appropriate, through his or her parents or legal guardians, and to have legal or other appropriate assistance in the preparation and presentation of his or her defence;

(iii) To have the matter determined without delay by a competent, independent and impartial authority or judicial body in a fair hearing according to law, in the presence of legal or other appropriate assistance and, unless it is considered not to be in the best interest of the child, in particular, taking into account his or her age or situation, his or her parents or legal guardians;

(iv) Not to be compelled to give testimony or to confess guilt; to examine or have examined adverse witnesses and to obtain the participation and examination of witnesses on his or her behalf under conditions of equality;

(v) If considered to have infringed the penal law, to have this decision and any measures imposed in consequence thereof reviewed by a higher competent, independent and impartial authority or judicial body according to law;

(vi) To have the free assistance of an interpreter if the child cannot understand or speak the language used;

(vii) To have his or her privacy fully respected at all stages of the proceedings.

3. States Parties shall seek to promote the establishment of laws, procedures, authorities and institutions specifically applicable to children alleged as, accused of, or recognized as having infringed the penal law, and, in particular:

(a) The establishment of a minimum age below which children shall be presumed not to have the capacity to infringe the penal law;

(b) Whenever appropriate and desirable, measures for dealing with such children without resorting to judicial proceedings, providing that human rights and legal safeguards are fully respected.

4. A variety of dispositions, such as care, guidance and supervision orders; counselling; probation; foster care; education and vocational training programmes and other alternatives to institutional care shall be available to ensure that children are dealt with in a manner appropriate to their well-being and proportionate both to their circumstances and the offence.

Article 41

Nothing in the present Convention shall affect any provisions which are more conducive to the realization of the rights of the child and which may be contained in:

(a) The law of a State party; or

(b) International law in force for that State.

PART II

Article 42

States Parties undertake to make the principles and provisions of the Convention widely known, by appropriate and active means, to adults and children alike.

Article 43

1. For the purpose of examining the progress made by States Parties in achieving the realization of the obligations undertaken in the present Convention, there shall be established a Committee on the Rights of the Child, which shall carry out the functions hereinafter provided.

2. The Committee shall consist of ten experts of high moral standing and recognized competence in the field covered by this Convention. The members of the Committee shall be elected by States Parties from among their nationals and shall serve in their personal capacity, consideration being given to equitable geographical distribution, as well as to the principal legal systems. (amendment)

3. The members of the Committee shall be elected by secret ballot from a list of persons nominated by States Parties. Each State Party may nominate one person from among its own nationals.

4. The initial election to the Committee shall be held no later than six months after the date of the entry into force of the present Convention and thereafter every second year. At least four months before the date of each election, the Secretary-General of the United Nations shall address a letter to States Parties inviting them to submit their nominations within two months. The Secretary-General shall subsequently prepare a list in alphabetical order of all persons thus nominated, indicating States Parties which have nominated them, and shall submit it to the States Parties to the present Convention.

5. The elections shall be held at meetings of States Parties convened by the Secretary-General at United Nations Headquarters. At those meetings, for which two thirds of States Parties shall constitute a quorum, the persons elected to the Committee shall be those who obtain the largest number of votes and an absolute majority of the votes of the representatives of States Parties present and voting.

6. The members of the Committee shall be elected for a term of four years. They shall be eligible for re-election if renominated. The term of five of the members elected at the first election shall expire at the end of two years; immediately after the first election, the names of these five members shall be chosen by lot by the Chairman of the meeting.

7. If a member of the Committee dies or resigns or declares that for any other cause he or she can no longer perform the duties of the Committee, the State Party which nominated the member shall appoint another expert from among its nationals to serve for the remainder of the term, subject to the approval of the Committee.

8. The Committee shall establish its own rules of procedure.

9. The Committee shall elect its officers for a period of two years.

10. The meetings of the Committee shall normally be held at United Nations Headquarters or at any other convenient place as determined by the Committee. The Committee shall normally meet annually. The duration of the meetings of the Committee shall be determined, and reviewed, if necessary, by a meeting of the States Parties to the present Convention, subject to the approval of the General Assembly.

11. The Secretary-General of the United Nations shall provide the necessary staff and facilities for the effective performance of the functions of the Committee under the present Convention.

12. With the approval of the General Assembly, the members of the Committee established under the present Convention shall receive emoluments from United Nations resources on such terms and conditions as the Assembly may decide.

Article 44

1. States Parties undertake to submit to the Committee, through the Secretary-General of the United Nations, reports on the measures they have adopted which give effect to the rights recognized herein and on the progress made on the enjoyment of those rights:

(a) Within two years of the entry into force of the Convention for the State Party concerned;

(b) Thereafter every five years.

2. Reports made under the present article shall indicate factors and difficulties, if any, affecting the degree of fulfilment of the obligations under the present Convention. Reports shall also contain sufficient information to provide the Committee with a comprehensive understanding of the implementation of the Convention in the country concerned.

3. A State Party which has submitted a comprehensive initial report to the Committee need not, in its subsequent reports submitted in accordance with paragraph 1 (b) of the present article, repeat basic information previously provided.

4. The Committee may request from States Parties further information relevant to the implementation of the Convention.

5. The Committee shall submit to the General Assembly, through the Economic and Social Council, every two years, reports on its activities.

6. States Parties shall make their reports widely available to the public in their own countries.

Article 45

In order to foster the effective implementation of the Convention and to encourage international co-operation in the field covered by the Convention:

(a) The specialized agencies, the United Nations Children's Fund, and other United Nations organs shall be entitled to be represented at the consideration of the implementation of such provisions of the present Convention as fall within the scope of their mandate. The Committee may invite the specialized agencies, the United Nations Children's Fund and other competent bodies as it may consider appropriate to provide expert advice on the implementation of the Convention in areas falling within the scope of their respective mandates. The Committee may invite the specialized agencies, the United Nations Children's Fund, and other United Nations organs to submit reports on the implementation of the Convention in areas falling within the scope of their activities;

(b) The Committee shall transmit, as it may consider appropriate, to the specialized agencies, the United Nations Children's Fund and other competent bodies, any reports from States Parties that contain a request, or indicate a need, for technical advice or assistance, along with the Committee's observations and suggestions, if any, on these requests or indications;

(c) The Committee may recommend to the General Assembly to request the Secretary-General to undertake on its behalf studies on specific issues relating to the rights of the child;

(d) The Committee may make suggestions and general recommendations based on information received pursuant to articles 44 and 45 of the present Convention. Such suggestions and general recommendations shall be transmitted to any State Party concerned and reported to the General Assembly, together with comments, if any, from States Parties.

PART III

Article 46

The present Convention shall be open for signature by all States.

Article 47

The present Convention is subject to ratification. Instruments of ratification shall be deposited with the Secretary-General of the United Nations.

Article 48

The present Convention shall remain open for accession by any State. The instruments of accession shall be deposited with the Secretary-General of the United Nations.

Article 49

1. The present Convention shall enter into force on the thirtieth day following the date of deposit with the Secretary-General of the United Nations of the twentieth instrument of ratification or accession.

2. For each State ratifying or acceding to the Convention after the deposit of the twentieth instrument of ratification or accession, the Convention shall enter into force on the thirtieth day after the deposit by such State of its instrument of ratification or accession.

Article 50

1. Any State Party may propose an amendment and file it with the Secretary-General of the United Nations. The Secretary-General shall thereupon communicate the proposed amendment to States Parties, with a request that they indicate whether they favour a conference of States Parties for the purpose of considering and voting upon the proposals. In the event that, within four months from the date of such communication, at least one third of the States Parties favour such a conference, the Secretary-General shall convene the conference under the auspices of the United Nations. Any amendment adopted by a majority of States Parties present and voting at the conference shall be submitted to the General Assembly for approval.

2. An amendment adopted in accordance with paragraph 1 of the present article shall enter into force when it has been approved by the General Assembly of the United Nations and accepted by a two-thirds majority of States Parties.

3. When an amendment enters into force, it shall be binding on those States Parties which have accepted it, other States Parties still being bound by the provisions of the present Convention and any earlier amendments which they have accepted.

Article 51

1. The Secretary-General of the United Nations shall receive and circulate to all States the text of reservations made by States at the time of ratification or accession.

2. A reservation incompatible with the object and purpose of the present Convention shall not be permitted.

3. Reservations may be withdrawn at any time by notification to that effect addressed to the Secretary-General of the United Nations, who shall then inform all States. Such notification shall take effect on the date on which it is received by the Secretary-General

Article 52

A State Party may denounce the present Convention by written notification to the Secretary-General of the United Nations. Denunciation becomes effective one year after the date of receipt of the notification by the Secretary-General.

Article 53

The Secretary-General of the United Nations is designated as the depositary of the present Convention.

Article 54

The original of the present Convention, of which the Arabic, Chinese, English, French, Russian and Spanish texts are equally authentic, shall be deposited with the Secretary-General of the United Nations.

IN WITNESS THEREOF the undersigned plenipotentiaries, being duly authorized thereto by their respective governments, have signed the present Convention.

Implementation of the *Convention on the Rights of the Child* in Selected Countries

This Appendix examines five developing countries in respect of their implementation of the *Convention on the Rights of the Child* (CRC), using their own information about that implementation (which they are required to report under Article 44 of CRC). Additional information from legal databases has also been incorporated. For each of the five countries, the ten specific areas are addressed in turn:

1   International Legal Instruments
2   Regional Instruments
3   National Legal Instruments
4   The Definition of the Child and Birth Registration
5   Child and Maternal Health
6   Public Health Law
7   Social Security Issues
8   Anti-Discrimination Law
9   Customary and Traditional Law
10 Other Relevant Legislation

BOLIVIA

GENERAL REMARKS

- From the legal viewpoint, the main achievement of the period 1997–2002 of the Bolivian Government was the promulgation of the Code for Children and Adolescents (1999) as an instrument for the implementation of children's rights. It seeks to protect children under eighteen and all vulnerable children: the challenge is the implementation (A.4);
- However, the Code should promote all three national languages, as well as Spanish (Aymara, Quechua and Guarani) (A.14);
- Regional differences remain as well as vast differences between urban and rural areas (A.25);
- The principles of 'the best interest of the child' and that of 'respect for the views of the child' are hard to implement as they run counter to the traditional ways of dealing with children in Bolivia;
- There are only 111 institutions for homeless children, and the conditions there are not always conducive to the health and development of children (A.29, 31);
- Although there is no war in Bolivia at present, the programmes to eradicate cultivation of coca have caused insecurity and human rights violations, although there are plans to protect the rights of children affected by the conflict (A.41);
- Landmines exist between Bolivia and Chile and talks are taking place to deal with that problem (A.42);
- The Code does not address the problem of sale, trafficking and kidnapping of children, sometimes disguised as 'adoption', although there are plans to make these activities criminal (A.45);
- Child abductions are reported routinely, especially in the cities (A.3);
- The country is very diverse geographically, and the indigenous populations live mostly in the Altiplano region, the population in the low-lying areas (a very hot region) are mostly Spanish speaking (A.50);
- The last census (2001) shows that 19.3% of the population is under age 6 (A.53);
- The Andean region's lack of infrastructure, roads and irrigation have impeded the efforts to improve living conditions, and have led to migration to cities: 62% of Bolivians now live in the cities (A.56–57);
- The poverty rate was 59% in 2002, a four point decrease since 1997: five million people are poor out of a total population of 8.3 million, of those, 2.5 million are under 18, and 500,000 under 5 (A.76);
- Rural areas show most extreme poverty (59%) as opposed to urban areas (22%) (A.2);
- Children are placed in jails with their parents unless there is family available to take care of them: in 1999 there were 1,000 children living in prison with their parents; these children have low development rates and little access to health as well as exposure to violence and abuse from other inmates (A.245).

(1) International Legal Instruments

International Covenant on Economic, Social and Cultural Rights   Ratified October 29, 1993
(ICESCR (1966) U.N.T.S.3)

A.10.2. Special protection should be accorded to mothers during a reasonable period before and after childbirth. During such period working mothers should be accorded paid leave or leave with adequate social security benefits.

A.12.2 The steps to be taken by the State Parties to the present Covenant to achieve the full realization of this right shall include those necessary for:

(a) The provisions for the reduction of the stillbirth rate and of infant mortality and for the healthy development of the child;

(b) The improvement of all aspects of environmental and industrial hygiene;

(c) The prevention, treatment and control of epidemic, endemic, occupational and other diseases;

(d) The creation of conditions which would assure to all medical service and medical attention in the event of sickness.

The International Covenant on Civil and Political Rights   Ratified October 29, 1993
(ICCPR (1966) 999 U.N.T.S.171)

A.6.1. Every human being has the inherent right to life. This right shall be protected by law. No one shall be arbitrarily deprived of his life.

A.6.4. Sentence of death shall not be imposed for crimes committed by persons below 18 years of age and shall not be carried out on pregnant women.

The International Convention on the Elimination of all Forms of Racial Ratified January 4, 1969
Discrimination (CERD) (U.N.Doc.A/6014 (1966), 660 U.N.T.S. 195)

The Convention on the Elimination of All Forms of Discrimination Against Women Ratified January 14, 1996
(CEDAW) (U.N.Doc.A/48/49(1993)

A.5.(b) To ensure that family education includes a proper understanding of maternity as a social function and the recognition of the common responsibility of men and women in the upbringing and development of their children, it being understood that the interest of the children is the primordial consideration in all cases.

A.12.1. State Parties shall take all appropriate measures to eliminate discrimination against women in the field of health care in order to ensure, on a basis of equality of men and women, access to health care services, including those related to family planning.

A.12.2. Notwithstanding the provisions of paragraph 1 of this Article, State Parties shall ensure to women appropriate services in connection with pregnancy, confinement and the post-natal period, granting free services where necessary, as well as adequate nutrition during pregnancy lactation.

The Optional Protocol to the *Convention on the Elimination of All Forms* Ratified February 22, 2004
of Discrimination Against Women (CEDAW-OP)

Convention Against Torture and Other Cruel, Inhuman or Degrading Ratified July 28, 2001
Treatment or Punishment (U.N.Doc.A/39/51(1984))

Convention on the Rights of the Child (CRC) Ratified April 18, 2001
(U.N.Doc.A/RES/44/25/25, 20 November, 1989), 16 July 1995

A.3.1. In all actions concerning children, whether undertaken by public or private social welfare institutions, courts of law, administrative authorities or legislative bodies, the best interests of the child should be the primary consideration.

A.6.1. State Parties recognize that every child has the inherent right to life.

A.6.2. State Parties shall ensure to the maximum extent possible the survival and development of the child.

A.24.1. State Parties recognize the right of the child to the enjoyment of the highest attainable standard of health and to facilities for the treatment of illness and rehabilitation of health. State Parties shall strive to ensure that no child is deprived of his or her right to access to health care services.

A.24.3. State Parties shall take all effective and appropriate measures with a view to abolishing traditional practices prejudicial to the health of children.

Optional Protocol to the *Convention on the Rights of the Child* on the Signed September 8, 2000
involvement of children in armed conflicts (CRCOPAC)
(U.N.Doc.A/54/49/Vol.III (2000))

Optional Protocol to the *Convention on the Rights of the Child* on the Signed September 8, 2000
sale of children, child prostitution and child pornography
(CRCOPSC) (U.N.Doc.A/54/49, Vol. III (2000))

(2) Regional Instruments

Organization of American States (OAS) Into force November 29, 1999, Ratified January 7, 2000

A.5. Survival and Development

1. Every child has an inherent right to life. This right should be protected by law.

2. State Parties to the present Charter shall ensure that, to the maximum extent possible, the survival, protection and development of the child.

A.13. Handicapped Children

1. Every child who is mentally or physically disabled shall have the right to special measures of protection in keeping with his physical and moral needs and under conditions which ensure his dignity, promote his self-reliance and active participation in the community.

A.14. Health and Health Services

1. Every child shall have the right to enjoy the best attainable state of physical, mental and spiritual health.

2. State parties to the present charter shall undertake to pursue the full implementation of this right and in particular shall take measures:

   (a) to reduce infant and child mortality rate;

(b) to ensure the provision of necessary medical assistance and health care to all children with emphasis on the development of primary health care;

(c) to ensure the provision of adequate nutrition and safe drinking water;

(d) to combat disease and malnutrition within the framework of primary health care through the application of appropriate technology;

(e) to ensure appropriate health care for expectant and nursing mothers;

(f) to develop preventive health care and family life education and provision of service;

(g) to integrate basic health service programmes in national development plans;

(h) to ensure that all sectors of the society, in particular, parents, children, community leaders and community workers are informed and supported in the use of basic knowledge of child health and nutrition, the advantages of breastfeeding, hygiene and environmental sanitation and the prevention of domestic and other accidents;

(i) to ensure the meaningful participation of non-governmental organizations, local communities and the beneficiary population in the planning and management of a basic service programme for children;

(j) to support through technical and financial means, the mobilization of local community resources in the development of primary health care for children.

(3) National Legal Instruments

The Constitution of Bolivia

(with Amended Text of 1995 and Reforms of 2002 and 2004).

Article 6 – Personhood and judicial powers.

1. All human beings have personhood and judicial power, according to the laws. They enjoy the rights, freedoms and guarantees recognized by this constitution, without any distinction of race, sex, language, religion, political opinion, or other, origin, economic and social condition or any other.

2. The dignity and the liberty of persons are inviolable. To respect and protect them is the first duty of the State.

Article 7 – Fundamental Rights.

● All persons have the following fundamental rights, in conformity with the laws that regulate their exercise.

(a) to life, health and security.

Chapter II – The Public Defender

Article 127 – The Defender of the People

● … At the same time, he guards the defence, promotion and publicizing of human rights.

Article 158 – Social Security.

1. The State has the obligation human capital by defending the health of the population; to ensure the means of subsistence and rehabilitation of invalids; it will also tend to improve the living conditions of family groups.

2. The regulations of social security will be inspired by the principles of universality, solidarity, unity of management, economy, opportunity and efficiency, thus dealing with the contingencies of infimity, maternity, professional risks, invalidity, death and others…

Article 199 – Protection by the State of the physical, moral and mental health of childhood.

1. The State will protect the physical, mental and moral health of childhood, and will protect the rights of the child to education.

2. A special code will regulate the protection of minors in harmony with general legislation.

(4) The Definition of the Child and Birth Registration

The Code for Children and Adolescents (1999)

Fundamental Principles

Article 1 – The Object of the Code

● The present Code establishes and regulates a regime of prevention, protection and attention that the State and Society must guarantee to all children and adolescents, in order to ensure them a physical, mental, moral, spiritual and emotional and social development, under conditions of liberty, respect, dignity, equity and justice.

Article 2 – Subjects of Protection
- We consider children all human beings from conception to the end of their 12th year, and adolescents from 12 to 18 years.
- In cases especially singled out by the Law, the following dispositions will apply to persons from 18 to 21 years of age.

Article 5 – Guarantees
- Children and adolescents, as subjects of rights, will enjoy all the fundamental rights and constitutional guarantees applicable to all persons, without prejudice regarding the integral protection instituted by this Code.

Article 8 – Primacy of Attention
- All children and adolescents have the right to be assisted first by judicial and administrative authorities.

Article 13 - Guarantee of State Protection
- All children and adolescents have the right to life and health. The State has the obligation to guarantee and protect these rights, by implementing social policies that will establish conditions of dignity for gestation, birth and full development.

Article 14 – Universal Access to Health
- The State, through the appropriate organizations, must ensure to all children and adolescents, universal and equal access to all services to promote, protect and regain health, even to free access, if they do not have sufficient means, of medicines, and all other forms or medical treatment, to habilitate or rehabilitate, as necessary.

Article 105 – Respect
- Consists in the inviolability of the physical, psychic and moral integrity of the child, or adolescent…
- No Child or adolescent may suffer discrimination, on ethnic, gender, or social grounds, or for reason of religious beliefs. The State has the obligation to guarantee a treatment based on respect and equality to all children and adolescents who live in the national territories.

Article 106 – Dignity
- It is everyone's duty to watch for the dignity of children and adolescent and to keep them safe from any inhuman, violent or dehumanizing treatment, and to denounce to the appropriate authorities all cases of suspected or confirmed maltreatment.

Article 108 – Maltreatment
- All acts of violence by fathers constitute maltreatment. Other responsible adults and/or institutions, through abuse, actions or omissions, whether habitual or occasional, which go against the rights recognized to children and adolescents by this Code and other laws; also violence that causes them damage or that is prejudicial to their health, physical, mental or emotional.
- The cases of maltreatment which represent a crime, will be passed on to general justice provisions according to the law.

Article 109 – Circumstances
- A child or adolescent is considered to be victim of maltreatment when:
  1. Physical, mental or moral damage has been caused, even if it is inflicted a disciplinary or educational measure.
  2. The discipline does not respect their dignity nor their integrity.
  3. Food, clothing, living necessities, education, or care of their health is not provided adequately according to their available economic means
  4. If they are employed in work that is prohibited or contrary to their dignity, or puts their life or health in danger.

Article 97 – Registration
- All children must be registered in the civil register, and must receive a certificate so stating, gratis, immediately after their birth…
- Family Code (below) stipulates that boys can marry at age 16, and girls at age 14 (A.24);
- As far as registration is concerned 'immediate' birth registration is often not feasible, and alternative language is under review (A.32);
- A large proportion of the population still have no birth certificate; according to UNICE 20% of such cases (778,000), are between 0-14 years old, and 42% are under one year of age (A.228);
- Often the absence of a birth certificate is due to cultural reasons: many people are ignorant of the importance of that document, and the traditional practice is to register children only if they have survived to age 2 or 3 (A.29).

(5) Child and Maternal Health

The Code of Social Security (14 December 1956) has specific provision regarding maternal health:

Section 'B' – Maternity

Article 23

The ensured or the wife or common law partner of the ensured has the right, during the pregnancy, birth and post-partum periods to the necessary medical assistance, including surgery, hospital and medications as required by the patient.

Article 24 Sanitary assistance starts when the association (CAJA) recognizes the pregnancy, until a maximum of 6 weeks after delivery.

Article 25

In case of an abortion procured without medical prescription there is only the right to indispensable medical assistance.

The Code of the Family

Article 4

(Public and Private Protection of the Family).

The family, marriage and maternity enjoy the protection of the State. This protection is effective with the present Code, through special dispositions to provide security and assistance for the family and its members in specific areas.

Article 14

(Extension of Assistance). Assistance to families includes all that is necessary for the support of the family, shelter, clothing, and medical attention.

- The Promulgation of the Offences Against Sexual Freedom Act (Protection of Victims) (No. 2033 of 1999) has been amended to include the rape of children and adolescents (A.66);
- A national child and mother benefit scheme (now Basic Health Insurance) was introduced to promote the health of mothers and children (A.89), and its main object is to reduce maternal and infant mortality (A.91);

The Code for Children and Adolescents (1999)

Article 15   Protection of Maternity

It is the duty of the State to protect maternity by means of health organizations and to guarantee:

1. Free attention to the mother in all steps from pre-natal, birth, and after birth, with medical treatment and specialized provision of medicines complementary examinations and nutritional support;
2. For pregnant women in prison, all the services listed in no. 1. The judge in her case, and those in charge of penitentiary institutions are responsible for this and all other related dispositions;
3. The health organizations, medical personnel, and paramedics must provide to children and adolescents who are pregnant, priority medical attention for free, as well as medical psychological and social requirements during the pregnancy, birth and post-partum.

- The percentage of women who had antenatal checkups went from 29 to 33 percent in 2000; and the proportion of hospital deliveries from 39% in 1997 to 54% in 2001 (A.130);
- Although the target was a reduction of maternal mortality of 50% from 1994, it only decreased from 416 to 390 per 100,000 live births (A.133);
- Many women find it difficult to make decisions for themselves, as they are used to having others make decisions for them; there is also the perception that many interventions are not appropriate, as they do not take in consideration cultural factors (A.135);

Article 17   Maternal Breastfeeding

- It is the duty of the State and of public and private institutions and of employers in general, to provide conditions adequate for breastfeeding including such cases as those where the mother has been deprived of her liberty.
- In 1998 a Demographic and Health survey (ENDSA) found that 69% of children under 2 months were breastfed, although there is a 23% risk of mortality for babies who are not breastfed under two months, and no data are available after 1998 (A.139);
- AIDS is considered an incipient epidemic, although it is still consider to be fairly low; the presence of STDs is high especially for poor populations in rural areas and a National Programme for STDs and HIV/AIDS operates prevention programmes (A.149–151);
- Under Article XI of the Penal Code, rapists went unpunished when they married their victims, often children of 14 (D.40).

(6) Public Health Law

Code of Social Security (14 December1956)

Article 14

In case of infirmity, recognized by medical services, the ensured and other beneficiaries will have the right to services necessary for the cure of the illness and other medical assistance including medicines...

The beneficiaries of the worker age:

- His wife or common law woman registered...
- His legitimate children, natural children recognized and those who have been adopted up to 16 years, or 19 years if studying at a State institution...
- A Strategy for Comprehensive Health Care for Childhood Illnesses (AIEPI) was incorporated into basic health. Insurance is applied in 60% of primary health care, although the target was 80% by 2000: the strategy covers diarrhea, pneumonia, malaria, measles and malnutrition (A.101);
- These policies results are dependent on the automatic allocation of 6.8% of municipal budgets to basic health insurance (A.102); but there are grave economic difficulties: for the epidemiological shield, only chagas disease had available funds for the second half of 2000;
- The malaria programme only has funding for the two areas with the highest prevalence of the disease, and the tuberculosis programmes were not implemented for a long time as the disease was not considered to have a high priority (A.104);
- Despite major efforts to promote health services for under-fives, demand is still because a) population is not aware of the services, and b) in rural areas, cultural factors are an impediment;
- An 'indigenous insurance scheme' is being put in place working with indigenous doctors (kallawayas) combining traditional and western medicine (A.99);
- First and repeat consultations for children under 5 have improved slightly from 1997 to 2000 (from 1.1 to 1.6);
- Differences remain between vaccination coverages for urban and rural settings, and the mother's educational status plays a large role;
- The Programme for Care for under 6s has played a significant role: 66% of children have completed the vaccination cycle, and 60% have been treated when an illness has been discovered (A.115);
- The Goals for Children include a 50% reduction of general malnutrition over 10 years: by 1998 Bolivia has achieved 30% of target;
- The availability of housing with drinking water has increased from 71% in 1997 to 85% in 2000, but although it is 93% in urban areas in 2000, in rural areas it is still only 69% (A.128);
- The Rural Basic Sanitation Programme (PROSABA) has provided 100,000 with drinking water, 8000 with sanitation and 5,000 with latrines, and there are a total of US$87.5 million earmarked for this project and others of this kind (A.129);
- A major problem is the rate of neonatal mortality, as nationally 40% of deaths under 5 occur within the first month of life, the result of preventable complications, and 57% of total deaths occur with the first week of life (A.137);
- A programme has been introduced giving special vouchers to recent medical graduates who want to work in the countryside, in order to improve the care for children under 5 especially;
- Rates of infant mortality account for 50% of all deaths for the whole population, and Bolivia's mortality is 79 for 1,000, as opposed to the regional average which is 39 per thousand (C.14);
- In January 2005 the 'Government planned to amend legislation to extend health-care insurance to 5 and 6 year olds' (D.53).

(7) Social Security Issues

- See particulars listed under Public Health (Social Security Code).
- The Code does not specify any legal measure against the sale, trafficking and kidnapping of children, and it makes no provisions for the international return of children: a bill has been envisaged to make these practices criminal offences (A.45);
- 6.8% of municipal budgets have been allocated to basic health insurance but many municipalities fail to make the appropriate disbursements (A.102): in general these efforts are not effective enough because of a chronic shortage of equipment and of poorly trained staff (A.103);
- The population of Bolivia does not have social security coverage (The Social Security Code only refers to employed persons), because most of them work in the informal sector, but there are plans to integrate the social into the basic Health Insurance (A.154);

- The code stipulates (Article 115.4) that the state must maintain and staff pre-school centres for children between 4-6 (A.191), and the programme dramatically improves children's language, creativity and psychosocial achievements (A.194), and basic nutrition is also stressed in these programs (A.195);
- Child trafficking is often prompted by parents who seek to ease their poverty, and they allow their children to be taken to the cities, such as La Paz and Santa Cruz; in rural areas, children 'are recruited by travelling middlemen, while others are abducted from their homes, from school or while herding livestock' (A.325);
- Some aspects of social spending are below the Latin American average; such spending increased slightly in 2002, but it declined in 2003 (C.27);
- Street children benefit from a nutritional support programme conducted by private centres with the support from the World Food Programme and the Government of Italy: the National Programme for Assistance to Children (PAN) may not be able to respond to the real needs (D.27).

(8) Anti-Discrimination Laws

- Poverty affects mostly rural populations and those living in the poorest sections of towns: most of these people are of indigenous origin (A.27);
- There is a strong correlation between membership in indigenous groups and social exclusion and poverty (A.82);
- Many women take jobs as domestic workers and some are involved in the trafficking of virgin girls and their exploitation; in addition, some organ trafficking takes place, disguised as illegal adoptions (A.324);
- Serious problems are present in the 300 experimental establishments for the disabled; according to UNESCO only 1% of disabled children receive assistance in Bolivia (D.36).

(9) Customary and Traditional Law

No special mention is made of any traditional laws.

(10) Other Relevant Legislation

- After the Ratification of the Optional Protocol on the sale of children prostitution and child pornography in 2001, a bill was prepared to make these activities criminal offences (A.321).

References

A =   Committee on the Rights of the Child, Consideration of Reports submitted by state parties Under article 44 of the Convention (Third Periodic Report) CRCC/C125/Add.2 13 November 2002 (16 July 2002)

C =   Written Replies by the Government of Bolivia Concerning the List of Issues (CRC/C/Q/BOL/3) received by the Committee on the Rights of the child relating to the third periodic report of Bolivia (CRCC/C/125/Add.2)

D =   Summary Record of the 1020th Meeting: Bolivia 02-02/2005.CRC/C/SR.1020. 25, January 2005.

E =   List of Issues: Bolivia.23/12/92. CRC/C/3WP.1 Pre-Sessional Working Groups 14-18 December 1992.

Note: Translations from the Codegos, Laura Westra with the assistance of Claudia Gomez

CAMBODIA

GENERAL REMARKS
● The Cambodia National Council for Children (CNCC should coordinate better with provincial ministers, as that is a vital link for the implementation of the CRC (A, 14);
● The demilitarization of child-soldiers is progressing at the rate of 10,000 per year;
● The Royal Government needs to take stronger action to protect children from abduction and exploitation (B, 29)

(1) International Legal Instruments
International Covenant on Economic, Social and Cultural Rights   Ratified October 29, 1993
(ICESCR (1966) U.N.T.S.3)

A.10.2. Special protection should be accorded to mothers during a reasonable period before and after childbirth. During such period working mothers should be accorded paid leave or leave with adequate social security benefits.

A.12.2 The steps to be taken by the State Parties to the present Covenant to achieve the full realization of this right shall include those necessary for:

(a)   The provisions for the reduction of the stillbirth rate and of infant mortality and for the healthy development of the child;
(b)   The improvement of all aspects of environmental and industrial hygiene;
(c)   The prevention, treatment and control of epidemic, endemic, occupational and other diseases;
(d)   The creation of conditions which would assure to all medical service and medical attention in the event of sickness.

The International Covenant on Civil and Political Rights (ICCPR (1966)   Ratified October 29, 1993
999U.N.T.S.171)

A.6.1. Every human being has the inherent right to life. This right shall be protected by law. No one shall be arbitrarily deprived of his life.

A.6.4. Sentence of death shall not be imposed for crimes committed by persons below 18 years of age and shall not be carried out on pregnant women.

The International Convention on the Elimination of all Forms of Racial   Ratified January 4, 1969
Discrimination (CERD) (U.N.Doc.A/6014 (1966), 660 U.N.T.S. 195)

The Convention of all Forms of Discrimination Against Women (CEDAW)   Ratified January 14, 1996
(U.N.Doc.A/48/49(1993); 14 January 1996

A.5.(b) To ensure that family education includes a proper understanding of maternity as a social function and the recognition of the common responsibility of men and women in the upbringing and development of their children, it being understood that the interest of the children is the primordial consideration in all cases.

A.12.1. State Parties shall take all appropriate measures to eliminate discrimination against women in the field of health care in order to ensure, on a basis of equality of men and women, access to health care services, including those related to family planning.

A.12.2. Notwithstanding the provisions of paragraph 1 of this Article, State Parties shall ensure to women appropriate services in connection with pregnancy, confinement and the post-natal period, granting free services where necessary, as well as adequate nutrition during pregnancy lactation.

The Optional Protocol to the Convention on the Elimination of All   Ratified February 22, 2004
Forms of Discrimination Against Women (CEDAW-OP)

Convention Against Torture and Other Cruel, Inhuman or Degrading   Ratified July 28, 2001
Treatment or Punishment (U.N.Doc.A/39/51(1984))

Convention on the Rights of the Child (CRC) (U.N.Doc.A/RES/44/25/25,   Ratified April 18, 2001
20 November, 1989), 16 July 1995

A.3.1. In all actions concerning children, whether undertaken by public or private social welfare institutions, courts of law, administrative authorities or legislative bodies, the best interests of the child should be the primary consideration.

A.6.1. State Parties recognize that every child has the inherent right to life.

A.6.2. State Parties shall ensure to the maximum extent possible the survival and development of the child.

A.24.1. State Parties recognize the right of the child to the enjoyment of the highest attainable standard of health and to facilities for the treatment of illness and rehabilitation of health. State Parties shall strive to ensure that no child is deprived of his or her right to access to health care services.

A.24.3. State Parties shall take all effective and appropriate measures with a view to abolishing traditional practices prejudicial to the health of children.

Optional Protocol to the *Convention on the Rights of the Child on the Involvement of Children in Armed Conflicts* (CRCOPAC) (U.N.Doc.A/54/49/Vol.III (2000))	Signed September 8, 2000
Optional Protocol to the *Convention on the Rights of the Child on the Sale of Children, Child Prostitution and Child Pornography* (CRCOPSC) (U.N.Doc.A/54/49, Vol. III (2000))	Signed September 8, 2000

(2) Regional Instruments
No specific information.

(3) National Legal Instruments
The Constitution of Cambodia (with Amendments passed 4 March, 1999)
Article 31   The Kingdom of Cambodia shall recognize and respect human rights as stipulated in the United Nations Charter, the Universal Declaration of Human Rights, the covenants and conventions related to human rights, women's and children's rights.
Article 32
Every Khmer citizen shall have the right to life, personal freedom and security.
Article 34
New (As Amended March 1999): Khmer citizens of either sex at least eighteen year old have the right to vote.
Article 38
The law guarantees there shall be no physical abuse against any individual.
Article 46
The commerce of human beings, exploitation by prostitution and obscenity which affect the reputation of women shall be prohibited.
Article 48
The State shall protect the rights of children as stipulated in the Convention on Children, in particular, the right to life, education protection during wartime, and from economic and sexual exploitation.
The State shall protect children from acts that are injurious to their educational opportunities, health and welfare.
Article 72
The health of the people shall be guaranteed. The State shall give full consideration to disease prevention and medical treatment. Poor citizens shall receive free medical consultation in public hospitals, infirmaries and maternities.
Article 73
The State shall give full consideration to children and mothers. The State shall establish nurseries to help support children and women who have inadequate support.

(4) The Definition of the Child and Birth Registration
The Marriage age for girls is 18 years, 20 for boys (A,18);
- The Definition of the Child in relation to work states that 16 years is the minimum age, but there are plans to reduce that age to 14 so that children can help their families;
- There is no law on registration of births, although some efforts have been made to institute such as law;
- The Law on the Marriage and Family (1989) states that the age of marriage is eighteen for girls and 20 for boys (as above), then
Article 5
In a special case where a man does not reach the age of 20 years and where a woman does not reach the age of 18 years, a marriage may be legitimized, upon the consent by the parents or guardians, if the woman becomes pregnant.

(5) Child and Maternal Health

Law on Marriage and Family (Decree No. 04 Kr. Feb. 10, 1982, passes July 18 1989).

Article 68

If a wife is pregnant, a husband is not allowed to request divorce until one year after she has delivered the child.

Article 119

Parental power shall be revoked and transferred to any organization or relative by blood, from parent who is at fault as follows:

- The parents treat badly their children.
- All women working in both private and public sectors are entitled to three months maternity leave on full pay; they have the right to nurse their babies at work, and receive social assistance for confinement (D.91);
- The Ministry of Health (MOH) has drawn up a family planning program in order to lower the maternal and infant mortality rates, and to raise the standard of living of families; the program could lower the birth rate by 2.8% (D.94);
- A Ministers' Decision (No. 79, June 23, 1987) lays down the 'political line' (undefined) to be followed for placing orphans and vagrants in State reception centres (D.107);
- The implementation of health care of children and mothers is as follows: 26 units at provincial level for mothers and infants; at district level, 164 maternity and baby care units, at the commune level, there are 1267 infirmaries for the health needs of mothers and children (D.13)

Parental power shall be revoked and transferred to any organization or relative by blood, from parent who is at fault as follows:

- The parents treat badly their children.
- All women working in both private and public sectors are entitled to three months maternity leave on full pay; they have the right to nurse their babies at work, and receive social assistance for confinement (D.91);
- The Ministry of Health (MOH) has drawn up a family planning program in order to lower the maternal and infant mortality rates, and to raise the standard of living of families; the program could lower the birth rate by 2.8% (D.94);
- A Ministers' Decision (No. 79, June 23, 1987) lays down the 'political line' (undefined) to be followed for placing orphans and vagrants in State reception centres (D.107);
- The implementation of health care of children and mothers is as follows: 26 units at provincial level for mothers and infants; at district level, 164 maternity and baby care units, at the commune level, there are 1267 infirmaries for the health needs of mothers and children (D.135);
- All of these units also educate in matters of hygiene and proper nutrition, and medical services for children under 5, including preventive vaccinations (D.135).

(6) Public Health Law

- Many barriers to implementation exist:
- Public health plans cannot be implemented most of the time, as they are very costly and 38% of the population lives below the poverty line (B.3);
- Alternative care facilities for children are not regularly inspected and they need to be monitored by the Royal Government (B.7);
- An extensive vaccination program targeting 6 diseases (not specified was implemented for 70 of the country's children, but the government must import the vaccines as they are in short supply (B.19);
- Many people still resort to traditional medicine and perhaps the government should communicate with these healers to ensure their cooperation (B.24);
- A grave situation is present in regard to environmental health, as only 19% of the population has access to proper sanitation (B.24);
- The National Health Policy should take measures to improve primary and preventive health services (provincial and local) (C.13);
- Infant mortality remains high, despite the efforts of the Royal Government to promote 'preventive vaccination days': according to UNICEF infant mortality rate is 115 for 1,000 and for under fives it is 181 per 1,000 (D.34);

(7) Social Security Issues

- The Royal Government helps with the staff and funding of child-care institutions, helping NGOs with about $10.00 per month (per child?) but many institutions are entirely funded and run by NGOs (b.14);
- Foster care is not regulated and NGOs report to the Ministry of Social and Child Welfare every three months;
- The Bureau of Child Welfare is responsible for monitoring all institutions (B.15).

(8) Anti-Discrimination Law

- The Cambodian National Council for Children (CNCC) was set up in 1995 to verse the implementation of the Convention: it drafted a five-year plan to combat the sexual exploitation of children (A.5);
- The Committee on the Elimination of Racial discrimination reports serious discrimination against Vietnamese children living in Cambodia: for instance there are not facilities for them to learn khmer (A.13);
- Article 31 of the Constitution: Citizens shall be equal before the law without distinction on grounds of race, colour, sex, language, religion, political opinion, national origin and social, property or other status.

(9) Customary and Traditional Law

No specific information is available.

(10) Other Relevant Legislation

- A new civil code of procedure is planned to cover present lacks such as the registration of births and the placement of children in institutions (A.4);
- Questions have been raised about the possibility of creating a Children's Ombudsman t coordinate the functions of the CNCC at the provincial and local levels (A.14);
- The Cambodian National Council for children (CNCE) and UNICEF are working together with the Ministry of the Interior to establish a Bureau for the protection of children's rights due to operate in 2000 (B.12) (no information on present status).

References

A =   Summary Record of the 629th meeting: Cambodia.12/07/2000.CRC/C/SR.629.
B =   Summary Record of the 630th meeting: Cambodia.30/05/2000.CC/C/SR.630.
C =   List of Issues: Cambodia. 01/03/2000.CRC/C/Q/CAM/1.
D =   Initial Reports of State Parties due in 1994: Cambodia.24/06/98.CRC/C/11/Add.16.

GHANA

GENERAL REMARKS
Ghana has been the first State to ratify the *Convention on the Rights of the Child* (Feb. 5, 1990) (C.3). But implementation was thought would be problematic because the general human rights were not adequately protected (c.17). Some of the major problems include:

- the need for a structural adjustment program for Ghana's infrastructure;
- the prevalence of traditional practices and customs, especially in the rural areas;
- specifically regarding children, a serious concern in the institutional use of corporal punishment in schools;
- the absence of laws forbidding cruel, inhuman and degrading treatment against children;
- the problems created by the number of children living and working in the streets in the cities;
- the fact that not enough has been done to implement the principle of 'the best interest of the child' (A. 16, 18, 33);
- 45% of the population is under 15 years (1984 statistics); according to the most recent survey of the Living standards Survey Report, 54% of the population is under 18 years of age (B.5).

(1) International Legal Instruments

International Covenant on Economic, Social and Cultural Rights　　　　Ratified December 7, 2000
(ICESCR (1966) U.N.T.S.3)

A.10.2. Special protection should be accorded to mothers during a reasonable period before and after childbirth. During such period working mothers should be accorded paid leave or leave with adequate social security benefits.

A.12.2 The steps to be taken by the State Parties to the present Covenant to achieve the full realization of this right shall include those necessary for:

(a)　The provisions for the reduction of the stillbirth rate and of infant mortality and for the healthy development of the child;

(b)　The improvement of all aspects of environmental and industrial hygiene;

(c)　The prevention, treatment and control of epidemic, endemic, occupational and other diseases;

(d)　The creation of conditions which would assure to all medical service and medical attention in the event of sickness.

The International Covenant on Civil and Political Rights　　　　Ratified December 7, 2000
(ICCPR (1966) 999U.N.T.S.171)

A.6.1. Every human being has the inherent right to life. This right shall be protected by law. No one shall be arbitrarily deprived of his life.

A.6.4. Sentence of death shall not be imposed for crimes committed by persons below 18 years of age and shall not be carried out on pregnant women.

Optional Protocol to the *International Covenant on Civil and*　　　　Into force Mar. 23, 1976
Political Rights (CCPR-OP1), (G.A. res. 2200A (XXI) 21 U.N.GAOR Supp.　　Ratified December 7, 2000
(No.16), U.N.Doc.A/6316 (1966) 999 U.N.T.S. 302), (a) 28 Nov., 2002

The International Convention on the Elimination of all Forms of　　　　Ratified January 4, 1969
Racial Discrimination (CERD) (U.N.Doc.A/6014 (1966), 660 U.N.T.S. 195)

The Convention of all Forms of Discrimination Against Women　　　　Ratified February 1, 1986
(CEDAW) (U.N.Doc.A/48/49(1993); 14 January 1996

A.5.(b) To ensure that family education includes a proper understanding of maternity as a social function and the recognition of the common responsibility of men and women in the upbringing and development of their children, it being understood that the interest of the children is the primordial consideration in all cases.

A.12.1. State Parties shall take all appropriate measures to eliminate discrimination against women in the field of health care in order to ensure, on a basis of equality of men and women, access to health care services, including those related to family planning.

A.12.2. Notwithstanding the provisions of paragraph 1 of this Article, State Parties shall ensure to women appropriate services in connection with pregnancy, confinement and the post-natal period, granting free services where necessary, as well as adequate nutrition during pregnancy lactation.

The Optional Protocol to the *Convention on the Elimination of All Forms of Discrimination Against Women* (CEDAW-OP)	Signed February 24 – Not ratified

Convention Against Torture and Other Cruel, Inhuman or Degrading Treatment or Punishment (U.N.Doc.A/39/51(1984))	Ratified October 7, 2000

Convention on the Rights of the Child (CRC) (U.N.Doc.A/ RES/44/25/25,	Ratified April 18, 2001

20 November, 1989), 16 July 1995

A.3.1. In all actions concerning children, whether undertaken by public or private social welfare institutions, courts of law, administrative authorities or legislative bodies, the best interests of the child should be the primary consideration.

A.6.1. State Parties recognize that every child has the inherent right to life.

A.6.2. State Parties shall ensure to the maximum extent possible the survival and development of the child.

A.24.1. State Parties recognize the right of the child to the enjoyment of the highest attainable standard of health and to facilities for the treatment of illness and rehabilitation of health. State Parties shall strive to ensure that no child is deprived of his or her right to access to health care services.

A.24.3. State Parties shall take all effective and appropriate measures with a view to abolishing traditional practices prejudicial to the health of children.

Optional Protocol to the *Convention on the Rights of the Child on the Involvement of Children in Armed Conflicts* (CRCOPAC) (U.N.Doc.A/54/49/Vol.III (2000))	Signed September 2, 1990

Optional Protocol to the *Convention on the Rights of the Child on the Sale of Children, Child Prostitution and Child Pornography* (CRCOPSC) (U.N.Doc.A/54/49, Vol. III (2000))	Signed September 8, 2000

(2) Regional Instruments

The African [Banjul] Charter of Human and Peoples Rights (OAU Doc.CAB/LEG/67/3, Rev.5; 21 I.L.M.58 (1982))	No Information on Ratification

The African Charter on the Rights and Welfare of the Child (OAU Doc. CAB/LEG/24.9/49 (1990))	Signed August 8, 1997 Not Ratified

A.5. Survival and Development

1. Every child has an inherent right to life. This right should be protected by law.
2. State Parties to the present Charter shall ensure that, to the maximum extent possible, the survival, protection and development of the child.

A.13. Handicapped Children

1. Every child who is mentally or physically disabled shall have the right to special measures of protection in keeping with his physical and moral needs and under conditions which ensure his dignity, promote his self-reliance and active participation in the community.

A.14. Health and Health Services

1. Every child shall have the right to enjoy the best attainable state of physical, mental and spiritual health.
2. State parties to the present charter shall undertake to pursue the full implementation of this right and in particular shall take measures:
    (a)   to reduce infant and child mortality rate;
    (b)   to ensure the provision of necessary medical assistance and health care to all children with emphasis on the development of primary health care;
    (c)   to ensure the provision of adequate nutrition and safe drinking water;
    (d)   to combat disease and malnutrition within the framework of primary health care through the application of appropriate technology;
    (e)   to ensure appropriate health care for expectant and nursing mothers;
    (f)   to develop preventive health care and family life education and provision of service;
    (g)   to integrate basic health service programmes in national development plans;

(h)   to ensure that all sectors of the society, in particular, parents, children, community leaders and community workers are informed and supported in the use of basic knowledge of child health and nutrition, the advantages of breastfeeding, hygiene and environmental sanitation and the prevention of domestic and other accidents;

(i)   to ensure the meaningful participation of non-governmental organizations, local communities and the beneficiary population in the planning and management of a basic service programme for children;

(j)   to support through technical and financial means, the mobilization of local community resources in the development of primary health care for children.

(3) National Legal Instruments

The 1996 Constitution of the Republic of Ghana

Chapter Five Fundamental Rights and Freedoms

Article 12(2)

Every person in Ghana, whatever his race, place of origin, Political option, creed or gender shall be entitled to the fundamental rights and freedoms for the individual contained in this Chapter, but subject to respect for the rights and freedom of others and the public interest.

Article 27

(1)   Special care shall be accorded to mothers during a reasonable period before and after childbirth;, and during those periods working mothers shall be accorded paid leave.

(2)   Facilities shall be provided for the care of children below school-going age to enable women who have the traditional care of children, realize their full potential;

Article 28

(1)   Parliament shall enact such laws as are necessary to ensure that

   a)   every child has the right to the same measures of special care, assistance and maintenance as necessary for its development from its natural parents, except where those parents have effectively surrendered their rights and responsibilities in respect to the child in accordance with the law;

   b)   every child, whether or not born in wedlock shall be entitled to reasonable provisions out of the estate of its parents;

   c)   parents undertake their natural rights and obligations of care, maintenance and upbringing of their children in cooperation with such institutions as Parliament may, by law, prescribe in such manner that ain all cases the interests of the children are paramount;

   d)   children in young persons receive special protection against exposure to physical and moral hazards; and

(3)   A child shall not be subjected to torture or other cruel, inhuman or degrading treatment or punishment.

(5)   For the purposes of this articles, 'child' means a person below the age of eighteen years.

Birth and Death Registration Act, 1965 (Act 301)

Act (484 of 1994) to Amend the Criminal Code, 1960 (Act 29)

[This Act amends Chana's Criminal Code to insert Section 69A (female circumcision), which reads as follows:]

Section 69A

(1)   Whoever excises, infibulates, or otherwise mutilates the whole or any part of the labia minora, labia majora and the clitoris of another person commits an offence and shall be guilty of a second degree felony and liable on conviction to imprisonment of not less than three years.

(2)   For the purposes of this section, 'excise' means to remove the prepuce, the clitoris and all or part of the labia minora; 'infibulate' includes excision and additional removal of the labia majora.

(4) The Definition of the Child and Birth Registration

Birth and Death Registration Act, 1965 (Act 301)

- In rural areas regulations on birth registration of children is not enforced and those who are not registered will be disadvantaged regarding their rights (A, 15);
- Parliament appointed a Commission to enact laws for child survival and protection (A.26): it established a single definition of the child until age 18 (b.9);
- Children between 14–18 have no legal or social protection (A.26);

- Many children below the minimum age (of 15 when they are allowed to do some light work in domestic or agricultural sectors), are working to survive or to supplement family income;
- No statistics are available on numbers of street/working children;
- Article 6(2) of the Constitution states that any child found in Ghana, if under 7 years of age, will be presumed to be a national of Ghana;

(5) Child and Maternal Health

*Breastfeeding Promotion Regulations, 2000.*L.I. 1667, dated Jan. 19, 2000; into force May 9, 2000.
- Some food distribution is available for under-fives, and mothers are requested to feed their children directly to ensure the supplement goes were it is intended (D.37–38);
- The Government needs to strengthen its programmes of prevention of HIV/AIDS maternal to child transmission, as well as discriminatory attitudes towards affected children (A.41);
- The MOH (with NGO/UNICEF assistance has been training traditional birth attendants to improve child delivery in rural areas (B.86);
- Authorities are encountering problems promoting AIDS prevention because of superstitions;
- Prenatal care has become the government's responsibility since 1997 (E.12);
- Another problem is that if a child of 14 is married, she may be considered mature and therefore no longer protected by legislation;
- The Marriage Ordinance Act (cap. 127), makes the legal age for marriage 18 for girls and 21 for boys, but customary practices still lead to earlier betrothal and marriage for girls, although in principle they have the right to refuse;
- Girls may be forced to live with a man because of poverty.

(6) Public Health Law

- *The Criminal Code*, 1960 (sections 31, 32, 34) protects the child against the use of 'unjustifiable force', but Article 41(a) still authorizes parents and guardians to use reasonable physical force against children;
- The Ministry of Health (MOH) has child Welfare Clinics, and public health nurses visit creches and day-care centres to ensure the welfare of children 0–5 years of age;
- Other services include oral re-hydration therapy, immunization, growth monitoring and anti-malaria therapy;
- There is a major concern about the persistence of malnutrition, a trend that has not yet been reversed, and the increasing spread of HIV/AIDS (A.41);
- To ensure the child's right to life and survival there is a health regulation that stipulates that all babies must be immunized 'against six killer diseases before the age of one' and breast feeding for the first four months of life is actively promoted (B.46);
- Water and sanitation figures vary: 93% of urban centres have access to safe drinking water, but people from smaller communities (500–5,000) have good drinking water from pipes or bore-holes with pumps;
- 46% of people live in rural communities and only 15% have access to safe water;
- 88 our of 136 households have to walk over 20 minutes to reach water (B.104);
- Living space is often unavailable: demand for housing is 70,000 per year, but only 30,000 are available, and 52% of all households in Ghana occupy only one room (B.103);

(7) Social Security Issues

- *The Maintenance of Children Decree 1977* (SMC 133) deals with the 'best interest of the child' in issues regarding paternity, custody and maintenance (B.43);
- Social Services deals with child labour, street children and abandoned and orphaned children (b.3(c));
- The Department of Social Welfare (DSW) operates some children homes for about 400 children, and welfare services are provided in case of child neglect, child abandonment, and short-term care for very young children shoes mother died at childbirth (B.62);
- There are four other NGO run homes but more oversight is needed (B.62)

(8) Anti-Discrimination Law

- Under the *Children's Act* (1998), a Bill to reform the Criminal Code Act prohibits the Tro Kosi system, where girls were given to a priest to atone for family misdeeds (see Section 13(1)).

Children's Act (1998) – Part I. The Rights of the Child

Section 1. Definition of the child. For purposes of this Act, a child is a person below the age of eighteen years.

Section 2. Welfare Principle.

(1) The best interest of the child shall be paramount in any matter concerning a child.

(2) The best interest of the child shall be the primary consideration by any court or person, institution or other body in any matter concerned with a child

Section 6. Parental duty and Responsibility.

1. No parent shall deprive a child of his welfare, whether (a) the parents of the child are married or not at the time of the child's birth; (b) the parents of the child continue to live together or not.

2. Every child has the right to life, dignity, respect, leisure liberty, health, education and shelter from his parents.

3. Every parent has the rights and responsibilities whether imposed by law or otherwise towards his child which include the duty to:

    (a) protect the child from neglect, discrimination, violence, and use, exposure to physical and moral hazards and oppression;

    (b) provide good guidance, care, assistance and maintenance for the child and assurance of the child's survival and development;

    (c) ensure that in the temporary absence of a parent, the child shall be cared for by a competent person and that a child under eighteen months of age shall only be cared for by a person fifteen years and above.

4. Each parent shall be responsible for the registration of the birth of their child and the names of both parents shall appear on the birth certificate except if the father of the child is unknown t the mother.

Section 10. Treatment of the disabled child.

1) No person shall treat a disabled child in an undignified manner.

2) A disabled child has a right to special care, education and training whenever possible to develop his maximum potential and be self-reliant.

(9) Customary and Traditional Law

No specific mention is made of such laws, beyond what emerged in the previous sections.

(10) Other Relevant Legislation with Indirect Impact on Child

● The Ghana National Commission on Children with assistance from NGOs recommends that appropriately disaggregated indicators regarding all children in society should be implemented, as important to monitoring activities (A.30).

References

A = Concluding Observations of the committee on the Rights of the Child: Ghana 18/06/97. CRC/C/15/Add.73.

B = Initial Report of the State Parties due in 1992: Ghana 19/12/85. CRC/C/3/Add.39.

C = Summary Record of the 377th meeting: Ghana.10/06/97.CRC/C/SR.377.

D = Summary Record of the 379th meeting: Ghana.04/09/97.CRC/C/SR.379.

E = Summary Record of the 378th meeting: Ghana.29/05/97.CRC/C/SR.378.

NIGERIA

GENERAL REMARKS

- Only some Nigerian States have adopted the CRC, hence it could not be binding on all of Nigeria;
- In some cases Shariah courts have overturned decisions reached by other courts in children's cases;
- Some states have passed relevant legislation: Edo and Delta States have laws prohibiting circumcision;
- *The Female Circumcision and Genital Mutilations Prohibition law* (1999) in Edo State provides for hefty fines for practitioners, or 6 months imprisonment;
- Cross-River State has the *Girl-Child Marriage and Female Circumcision Prohibition Law* of 2000;
- Cross-River State and Kebbi State have passed a law banning street hawking by girls of school age in the state;
- Sokoto State has banned begging during school hours;
- Several bills relevant to young children are presently to be passed by Lower House of the National Assembly.

(1) International Legal Instruments

International Covenant on Economic, Social and Cultural Rights　　　　　Ratified October 29, 1993
(ICESCR (1966) U.N.T.S.3)

A.10.2. Special protection should be accorded to mothers during a reasonable period before and after childbirth. During such period working mothers should be accorded paid leave or leave with adequate social security benefits.

A.12.2 The steps to be taken by the State Parties to the present Covenant to achieve the full realization of this right shall include those necessary for:

(a)　The provisions for the reduction of the stillbirth rate and of infant mortality and for the healthy development of the child;

(b)　The improvement of all aspects of environmental and industrial hygiene;

(c)　The prevention, treatment and control of epidemic, endemic, occupational and other diseases;

(d)　The creation of conditions which would assure to all medical service and medical attention in the event of sickness.

The International Covenant on Civil and Political Rights (ICCPR (1966)　　　Ratified October 29, 1993
999U.N.T.S.171)

A.6.1. Every human being has the inherent right to life. This right shall be protected by law. No one shall be arbitrarily deprived of his life.

A.6.4. Sentence of death shall not be imposed for crimes committed by persons below 18 years of age and shall not be carried out on pregnant women.

The International Convention on the Elimination of all Forms of Racial　　　Ratified January 4, 1969
Discrimination (CERD) (U.N.Doc.A/6014 (1966), 660 U.N.T.S. 195)

The Convention of all Forms of Discrimination Against Women (CEDAW)　　　Ratified January 14, 1996
(U.N.Doc.A/48/49(1993))

A.5.(b) To ensure that family education includes a proper understanding of maternity as a social function and the recognition of the common responsibility of men and women in the upbringing and development of their children, it being understood that the interest of the children is the primordial consideration in all cases.

A.12.1. State Parties shall take all appropriate measures to eliminate discrimination against women in the field of health care in order to ensure, on a basis of equality of men and women, access to health care services, including those related to family planning.

A.12.2. Notwithstanding the provisions of paragraph 1 of this Article, State Parties shall ensure to women appropriate services in connection with pregnancy, confinement and the post-natal period, granting free services where necessary, as well as adequate nutrition during pregnancy lactation.

The Optional Protocol to the Convention on the Elimination of All Forms　　　Ratified February 22, 2004
of Discrimination Against Women (CEDAW-OP)

Convention Against Torture and Other Cruel, Inhuman or Degrading   Ratified July 28, 2001
Treatment or Punishment (U.N.Doc.A/39/51(1984))

Convention on the Rights of the Child (CRC)   Ratified April 18, 2001
(U.N.Doc.A/RES/44/25/25, 20 November, 1989), 16 July 1995

A.3.1. In all actions concerning children, whether undertaken by public or private social welfare institutions, courts of law, administrative authorities or legislative bodies, the best interests of the child should be the primary consideration.

A.6.1. State Parties recognize that every child has the inherent right to life.

A.6.2. State Parties shall ensure to the maximum extent possible the survival and development of the child.

A.24.1. State Parties recognize the right of the child to the enjoyment of the highest attainable standard of health and to facilities for the treatment of illness and rehabilitation of health. State Parties shall strive to ensure that no child is deprived of his or her right to access to health care services.

A.24.3. State Parties shall take all effective and appropriate measures with a view to abolishing traditional practices prejudicial to the health of children.

Optional Protocol to the *Convention on the Rights of the Child on the*   Signed September 8, 2000
Involvement of Children in Armed Conflicts (CRCOPAC)
(U.N.Doc.A/54/49/Vol.III (2000))

Optional Protocol to the Convention on the Rights of the Child on the   Signed September 8, 2000
Sale of Children, Child Prostitution and Child Pornography (CRCOPSC)
(U.N.Doc.A/54/49, Vol. III (2000))

(2) Regional Instruments

The African Charter on the Rights and Welfare of the Child   Into force Nov. 29, 1999
(OAU Doc.CAB/LEG/24.9/49 (1990))   Ratified January 7, 2000

A.5. Survival and Development

1. Every child has an inherent right to life. This right should be protected by law.
2. State Parties to the present Charter shall ensure that, to the maximum extent possible, the survival, protection and development of the child.

A.13. Handicapped Children

1. Every child who is mentally or physically disabled shall have the right to special measures of protection in keeping with his physical and moral needs and under conditions which ensure his dignity, promote his self-reliance and active participation in the community.

A.14. Health and Health Services

1. Every child shall have the right to enjoy the best attainable state of physical, mental and spiritual health.
2. State parties to the present charter shall undertake to pursue the full implementation of this right and in particular shall take measures:
   (a) to reduce infant and child mortality rate;
   (b) to ensure the provision of necessary medical assistance and health care to all children with emphasis on the development of primary health care;
   (c) to ensure the provision of adequate nutrition and safe drinking water;
   (d) to combat disease and malnutrition within the framework of primary health care through the application of appropriate technology;
   (e) to ensure appropriate health care for expectant and nursing mothers;
   (f) to develop preventive health care and family life education and provision of service;
   (g) to integrate basic health service programmes in national development plans;
   (h) to ensure that all sectors of the society, in particular, parents, children, community leaders and community workers are informed and supported in the use of basic knowledge of child health and nutrition, the advantages of breastfeeding, hygiene and environmental sanitation and the prevention of domestic and other accidents;
   (i) to ensure the meaningful participation of non-governmental organizations, local communities and the beneficiary population in the planning and management of a basic service programme for children;
   (j) to support through technical and financial means, the mobilization of local community resources in the development of primary health care for children.

(3) National Legal Instruments
The Children and Young Persons Act

The Age of Customary Marriage Act (Chapter 218, 1990)

- Consent to Marriage in certain cases necessary
  18. If either party to an intended marriage, not being a Consent widower or widow, is under twenty-one years of age, the written consent of the father, or if he be dead or of unsound mind or absent from Nigeria, of the mother, or if both be dead or of unsound mind or absent from Nigeria, of the guardian of such party, must be produced annexed to such affidavit as aforesaid before a licence can be granted or a certificate issued.
- Various infants laws of the States (B.22);

The Constitution of the Federal Republic of Nigeria, 1999 Chapter IV – Fundamental Rights
- 33 (1) Every person has a right to life, and no one shall be deprived intentionally of his life, save in the execution of the sentence of the court in respect of a criminal offence of which he has been found guilty in Nigeria.
- 35 (1) Every person shall be entitled to his personal liberty and no person shall be deprived of such liberty save in the cases and in accordance with a procedure permitted by law – (d) in the case of a person who has not attained the age of eighteen years for the purpose of education or welfare;

(4) The Definition of the Child and Birth Registration
- No uniform definition of the child: examples include voting age of 18, but Immigration Act stipulates that everyone under 16 is a minor;
- Compulsory education ends at age 15
- Employment is allowed as 'apprenticeship and regular employment at 18'
- The age of sexual consent is 18 in most states; two states have that age as 13; in the west the age of marriage varies between 16–19;
- In the North-East Islamic religion does not allow sexual consent;

(5) Child and Maternal Health
- Institutional programmes exist to protect Maternal and Child Health;

(6) Public Health Law
- National Policy on Health (1989) intended to protect mothers and children;
- By 1990 'it was estimated that only 17% of Nigerians had access to health facilities;
- National Primary Health Care Development Agency (1992) was developed (B.103-104);
- The Bamako Initiative provides basic drugs, helps with financial arrangements and implements its principle: 'children from disadvantaged families, particularly poor families, are guaranteed access to health care' (1999) (B.106);

(7) Social Security Issues
No specific information.

(8) Anti-Discrimination Laws
No specific information.

(9) Customary and Traditional Laws
- Shariah laws are sometimes in conflict with other court decisions (A.28)
- Different States and regions handle situations dealing with children and women's rights in different ways;

(10) Other Relevant Legislation
No specific information.

References
A = Summary Record of the 1022nd Meeting: Nigeria 03/02/2005.CRC/c/SR.1033;
B = Committee on the Rights of the Child—Consideration of Reports Submitted by State Parties under Article 44 of the Convention. Second Periodic Reports of State Parties due in 1998, Nigeria, 30 January 2003.

SOUTH AFRICA

GENERAL REMARKS

South Africa is constitutionally committed to be responsible for child health, at least in principle, although some of the obstacles and other difficulties that lie in the path of their commitment will emerge below.

The first thing to note is that 'morbidity and mortality indicators...provide a crude albeit incomplete measure of the extent to which children's rights are being met...' (A.29). Hence, before looking in detail at what has been accomplished, and what needs to be done, we need to keep in mind the obstacles to implementation (of the CRC): (1) the need to overcome the legacy of apartheid; (2) 'the relatively high levels of unemployment and poverty' that persist (Summary Record of the 611th Meeting, S. Africa 02/02/2000. CRC/C/SR.611. p.3); and (3) the existence of 'vast economic and social disparities'. It is important to note that the South African Human Rights Commission has appointed a Director with specific responsibilities for children's rights (A.2); Equally important, the Principle of the Best Interest of the Child is now accepted and commonly used (A.3; F.3). Family Courts have been developed while there are continuing efforts to ensure that legal reforms conform to the CRC. Although S. Africa is a Signatory to the ICESCR (1966, U.N.T.S.3), it now needs to proceed to ratification (F.5).

Aside from direct constitutional measures and legislative responses, there are a number of government policies to address children's needs, such as the African National Congress's National Health Plan for South Africa (ANC 1994), the Reconstruction and Development Plan (1994), and the White Paper for the Transformation of the Health System in South Africa (Department of Health, 1997). These documents include the following:

- Free health care for children under six and for pregnant women;
- Immunization;
- Reduction in morbidity and mortality from common conditions;
- Improved nutrition

Most of these documents recognize the health rights of children and cite 'this as a basis for the development of the policy and/or programme' (B, 139–140).

However, several serious problems remain. First, the data collection mechanisms in existence are insufficient (C.4); second, there is no specific budget for children and in that regard, it would be useful to know exactly how much money is spent on grants, as income provided specifically for children under 7 years of age (A.3); the state budget itself should be a means of transferring funds to vulnerable groups including children (D.1–2).

On the question of the relation between mortality and childhood disease, there is an urgent need for combined statistics about tuberculosis and HIV/AIDS mortality, as the latter appear to affect the gravity and extent of the former (A.6). Environmental degradation, especially around waste disposal sites, seriously affect the health of children, and no action has been taken or is presently being considered on this issue (A.5). Finally, there are serious implementation difficulties for any kind of health care: maternal, child and infant mortality require greater access to services as well as safe drinking water and sanitation (C.8). A great number of illegal abortions are still taking place and one of the most grave issues is the mother-to-child-transmission of HIV/AIDS, but programmes are being put in place to combat that threat (B.145, ff.).

(1) International Legal Instruments

International Covenant on Economic, Social and Cultural Rights   Signed but not ratified
(ICESCR (1966) U.N.T.S.3)

A.10.2. Special protection should be accorded to mothers during a reasonable period before and after childbirth. During such period working mothers should be accorded paid leave or leave with adequate social security benefits.

A.12.2 The steps to be taken by the State Parties to the present Covenant to achieve the full realization of this right shall include those necessary for:

(a) The provisions for the reduction of the stillbirth rate and of infant mortality and for the healthy development of the child;
(b) The improvement of all aspects of environmental and industrial hygiene;
(c) The prevention, treatment and control of epidemic, endemic, occupational and other diseases;
(d) The creation of conditions which would assure to all medical service and medical attention in the event of sickness.

The International Covenant on Civil and Political Rights (ICCPR (1966) 999U.N.T.S.171)   Ratified

A.6.1. Every human being has the inherent right to life. This right shall be protected by law. No one shall be arbitrarily deprived of his life.

A.6.4. Sentence of death shall not be imposed for crimes committed by persons below 18 years of age and shall not be carried out on pregnant women.

Optional Protocol to the *International Covenant on Civil and Political Rights*   Into force Mar. 23, 1976
(CCPR-OP1), (G.A. res. 2200A (XXI) 21 U.N.GAOR Supp. (No.16),   Ratified
U.N.Doc.A/6316 (1966) 999 U.N.T.S. 302), (a) 28 Nov., 2002

Optional Protocol to the *International Covenant on Civil and Political Rights*   Into force July 11, 1991
(U.N.Doc.A/A/44/49 (1989)), (a) Nov.28, 02   Ratified

The International Convention on the Elimination   Into force Jan. 4, 1969
of all Forms of Racial Discrimination (CERD)   State party has recognized the
(U.N.Doc.A/6014 (1966), 660 U.N.T.S. 195)   instrument (9 January 1999)

The Convention of all Forms of Discrimination Against Women (CEDAW)   Ratified
(U.N.Doc.A/48/49(1993); 14 January 1996

A.5.(b) To ensure that family education includes a proper understanding of maternity as a social function and the recognition of the common responsibility of men and women in the upbringing and development of their children, it being understood that the interest of the children is the primordial consideration in all cases.

A.12.1. State Parties shall take all appropriate measures to eliminate discrimination against women in the field of health care in order to ensure, on a basis of equality of men and women, access to health care services, including those related to family planning.

A.12.2. Notwithstanding the provisions of paragraph 1 of this Article, State Parties shall ensure to women appropriate services in connection with pregnancy, confinement and the post-natal period, granting free services where necessary, as well as adequate nutrition during pregnancy lactation.

Convention Against Torture and Other Cruel,   Into force June 26, 1987
Inhuman or Degrading Treatment or Punishment   State party has recognized the
(U.N.Doc.A/39/51(1984))   instrument (9 January 1999)

Convention on the Rights of the Child (CRC)   Ratified 16 July 1995
(U.N.Doc.A/RES/44/25/25, 20 November, 1989)

A.3.1. In all actions concerning children, whether undertaken by public or private social welfare institutions, courts of law, administrative authorities or legislative bodies, the best interests of the child should be the primary consideration.

A.6.1. State Parties recognize that every child has the inherent right to life.

A.6.2. State Parties shall ensure to the maximum extent possible the survival and development of the child.

A.24.1. State Parties recognize the right of the child to the enjoyment of the highest attainable standard of health and to facilities for the treatment of illness and rehabilitation of health. State Parties shall strive to ensure that no child is deprived of his or her right to access to health care services.

A.24.3. State Parties shall take all effective and appropriate measures with a view to abolishing traditional practices prejudicial to the health of children.

Optional Protocol to the *Convention on the Rights of the Child*   Into force 12 February, 2002
on the Involvement of Children in Armed Conflicts (CRCOPAC) (U.N.Doc.A/   Ratified
54/49/Vol.III (2000)) s.08 February 2002

Optional Protocol to the *Convention on the Rights of the Child on the*   Into force Jan. 18, 2002
Sale of Children, Child Prostitution and Child Pornography (CRCOPSC)   Ratified
(U.N.Doc.A/54/49, Vol. III (2000)), a-30 July 2003.

(2) Regional Instruments

The African [Banjul] Charter of Human and Peoples Rights (OAU Doc.   Into force October 1, 1986
CAB/LEG/67/3 Rev.5;21 I.L.M.58 (1982))   Ratified July 9, 1996

A.4. Human beings are inviolable. Every human being shall be entitled to respect for his life and the integrity of his person. No one may be arbitrarily deprived of this right.

A.16.1. Every individual shall have the right to enjoy the best attainable state of physical and mental health.
A.16.2. State Parties to the present Charter shall take all necessary measures to protect the health of their people and to ensure that they receive medical attention when they are sick.

The African Charter on the Rights and Welfare of the Child (OAU Doc.   Into force Nov. 29, 1999
CAB/LEG/24.9/49 (1990))   Ratified January 7, 2000
A.5. Survival and Development
1. Every child has an inherent right to life. This right should be protected by law.
2. State Parties to the present Charter shall ensure that, to the maximum extent possible, the survival, protection and development of the child.
A.13. Handicapped Children
1. Every child who is mentally or physically disabled shall have the right to special measures of protection in keeping with his physical and moral needs and under conditions which ensure his dignity, promote his self-reliance and active participation in the community.
A.14. Health and Health Services
1. Every child shall have the right to enjoy the best attainable state of physical, mental and spiritual health.
2. State parties to the present charter shall undertake to pursue the full implementation of this right and in particular shall take measures:
    (a) to reduce infant and child mortality rate;
    (b) to ensure the provision of necessary medical assistance and health care to all children with emphasis on the development of primary health care;
    (c) to ensure the provision of adequate nutrition and safe drinking water;
    (d) to combat disease and malnutrition within the framework of primary health care through the application of appropriate technology;
    (e) to ensure appropriate health care for expectant and nursing mothers;
    (f) to develop preventive health care and family life education and provision of service;
    (g) to integrate basic health service programmes in national development plans;
    (h) to ensure that all sectors of the society, in particular, parents, children, community leaders and community workers are informed and supported in the use of basic knowledge of child health and nutrition, the advantages of breastfeeding, hygiene and environmental sanitation and the prevention of domestic and other accidents;
    (i) to ensure the meaningful participation of non-governmental organizations, local communities and the beneficiary population in the planning and management of a basic service programme for children;
    (j) to support through technical and financial means, the mobilization of local community resources in the development of primary health care for children.

(3) National Legal Instruments
The Constitution of South Africa
Article 27. (1) Everyone has the right to have access to
a. health care services, including reproductive health care;
b. sufficient food and water, and
c. social security, including, if they are unable to support themselves and their dependents, appropriate social assistance.
(2) The state must take reasonable legislative and other measures, within its available resources, to achieve the progressive realization of each of these rights.
(3) No one may be refused emergency medical treatment.
Article 28. (1) Every child has the right
a. To a name and nationality from birth;
b. To family or parental care, or to appropriate alternative care when removed from the family environment;
c. To basic nutrition, shelter, basic health care services and social services;
d. To be protected from maltreatment, neglect, abuse or degradation;
(2) A child's best interests are of paramount importance in every matter concerning the child;
(3) In this section 'child' means a person under the age of 18 years.

(4) The Definition of the Child and Birth Registration
The Birth and Deaths Act (Act. No.51, 1992)
Provides for the registration of all children at birth. Many children are not registered, so that it becomes necessary to put in place new initiatives to facilitate registration such as mobile clinics and hospitals to ensure accessibility.(C.5); efforts should be made to encourage birth registration.(D.1).
- How are children born outside of marriage to be registered? No specific provision presently exists for them at this time(F.9);
- On the question of the Definition of the child, there is a discrepancy between the age of sexual consent to intercourse: 12 for girls and 14 for boys.

(5) Public Health Law
The National Health Act (Act. No.61 of 2003) recognizes children as a group deserving special attention, but offers no clear legislative framework to ensure that children's rights are met (B.139).
Chapter 1
Objects of Act
2. The objects of this Act are to regulate national health and to provide uniformity in respect of health services across the nation by-
    (a) establishing a national health system which-
        (i) encompasses public and private providers of health services; and
        (ii) provides in an equitable manner the population of the Republic with the best possible health services that available resources can afford;
    (b) setting out the rights and duties of health care providers, health workers, health establishments and users; and
    (c) protecting, respecting, promoting and fulfilling the rights of-
        (i) the people of South Africa to the progressive realisation of the constitutional right of access to health care services, including reproductive health care;
        (ii) the people of South Africa to an environment that is not harmful to their health or well-being;
        (iii) children to basic nutrition and basic health care services contemplated in section 28(1)(c) of the Constitution; and
        (iv) vulnerable groups such as women, children, older persons and persons with disabilities.
Eligibility for free health services in public health establishments
4 (1) The Minister, after consultation with the Minister of Finance, may prescribe conditions subject to which categories of persons are eligible for such free health services at public health establishments as may be prescribed.
   (2) In prescribing any condition contemplated in subsection (1), the Minister must have regard to-
        (a) the range of free health services currently available;
        (b) the categories of persons already receiving free health services;
        (c) the impact of any such condition on access to health services; and
        (d) the needs of vulnerable groups such as women, children, older persons and persons with disabilities.
   (3) Subject to any condition prescribed by the Minister, the State and clinics and community health centres funded by the State must provide-
        (a) pregnant and lactating women and children below the age of six years, who are not members or beneficiaries of medical aid schemes, with free health services;
        (b) all persons, except members of medical aid schemes and their dependants and persons receiving compensation for compensable occupational diseases, with free primary health care services; and
        (c) women, subject to the Choice on Termination of Pregnancy Act, 1996 (Act No. 92 of 1996), free termination of pregnancy services.

(6) Child and Maternal Health
- A great number of illegal abortions are still taking place;
- One of the most grave issues is the Mother-to-Child Transmission of HIV/AIDS and programs are being put in place to combat that threat (B.145 ff).

(7) Social Security Issues
Social Assistance Act (No.13 of 2004, No.26446)
Chapter 2
Provision of social grants
4. The Minister must, with the concurrence of the Minister of Finance, out of moneys appropriated by
    Parliament for that purpose, make available-
    (a)   a child support grant;
    (b)   a care dependency grant;
    (c)   a foster child grant;
    (d)   a disability grant;

Child Care Act (Act No. 74,1983)

(8) Anti-Discrimination Law
No specific information.

(9) Customary and Traditional Law
●   There is yet to be a well-organized campaign to eradicate female genital mutilation (FGM) (C.9);
●   There are concerns about non-sterile conditions for male circumcision;
●   Traditional laws are important in South Africa, but legislation has been enacted to allow courts to take
    judicial notice of customary laws, 'provided that it was not in conflict with principles of public policy or
    of natural justice' (F.7);
●   Some of the traditional laws and practices are deleterious to children health and should be proscribed
    (F.5).

(10) Other Relevant Legislation
●   Article 18 of the CRC requires 'parental guidance' so policies should be enacted to ensure that child
    health can be pursued even in child-headed households, in single parent and polygamous families;
●   The *Prevention of Family Violence Act* suggests studies of domestic violence, ill-treatment and abuse including
    sexual abuse are needed;
●   The *Standard Rules on the Equalization of Opportunities for Persons with Disabilities* (Gen Assembly res. 48/96),
    and the Children with Disabilities Act (A/53/41, Chapter IV, sect. C), both need technical assistance and
    cooperation from UNICEF and WHO (C.9);
●   The Refugee and Asylum Seeking children should be better protected: S. Africa should finalize the
    adoption of the 1951 Convention on the Status of Refugees, and the 1967 Protocol (C.9).

References
A = Concluding Observations of the Committee on the Rights of the Child: South Africa. 23/02/2000.
    CRC/C/15/Add.122.
B = Chapter Four, 'Children's Right to Health', M. Shing-King, Lori Michels, Thokozani Kaime, Pasula
    Proudlock, Alexandra Vennekens-Poane and Nhlanhla Ndlovu.
C = Summary Record of the 611th meeting: South Africa. 02/02/2000.
D = Summary Record of the 610th meeting: South Africa. 19/05/2000.
E = Implementation of the Convention of the Rights of the Child, List of Issues: South Africa. 17/09/99.
    CRC/C/Q/SAFR/1.
F = Summary record of the 609th meeting: South Africa. 01/02/2000. CRC/C/SR.609.

List of Abbreviations and Acronyms

ASEAN	Association of Southeast Asian Nations
ATCA	Alien Torts Claims Act
BGH	Bovine Growth Hormone
CAH	Department of Child and Adolescent Health and Development
CEDAW	Convention on the Elimination of all Forms of Discrimination Against Women
CELA	Canadian Environmental Law Association
CEPA	Canadian Environmental Protection Act
CHM	Common Heritage of Mankind
CITES	Convention on International Trade in Endangered Species of Wild Flora and Fauna
CRC	Convention on the Rights of the Child
DALY	disability-adjusted life year
DMF	dimethylformamide
ECHR	European Convention on Human Rights
ECJ	European Court of Justice
EEOC	Equal Employment Opportunity Commission
EMEA	European Medicines Agency
EPA	Environmental Protection Agency (US)
FAO	Food and Agriculture Organization
FDA	Food and Drug Administration (US)
GATT	General Agency for Tariffs and Trade
GLWQA	Great Lakes Water Quality Agreement
IBI	Index of Biotic Integrity
ICC	International Criminal Court
ICCPR	International Convention on Civil and Political Rights
ICESCR	International Convention on Economic, Social and Cultural Rights
ICJ	International Court of Justice
ILC	International Law Commission
IMF	International Monetary Fund
IPCC	International Panel on Climate Change
IUCN	International Union for the Conservation of Nature
MDG	Millennium Development Goals
MNR	Ministry of Natural Resources
MOE	Ministry of the Environment
MOSOP	Movement for Survival of the Ogoni People
NAFTA	North American Free Trade Association
NGO	non-governmental organization
NIEO	New International Economic Order
OEPA	Ontario Environmental Protection Act
OMAFRA	Ontario Ministry of Agriculture and Farming

OSHA	Occupational Safety and Health Act
PAH	polycyclic aromatic hydrocarbon
PCB	polychlorinated biphenyl
PTP	presently threatened populations
SSHRC	Social Sciences and Humanities Research Council
TNC	transnational corporation
TVPA	Torture Victim Protection Act
UDHR	Universal Declaration of Human Rights
UN	United Nations
UNCLOS	United Nations Convention on the Law of the Sea
UNEP	United Nations Environment Programme
UNICEF	United Nations International Child and Environment Fund
WCED	World Commission on Environment and Development
WHA	World Health Assembly
WHO	World Health Organization
WTO	World Trade Organization

CANADA

A.G. Canada v. Mossop (1993) 1 S.C.R. 554

Allaire v. St. Luke Hospital et al, 184 I11.359; 56 N.E. 638, Feb. 19, 1990

Cherry (Guardian ad litem of) v. Borsman [1990] B.C.J. No.2576, Vancouver Registry No.C845601; Judgment Dec.3, 1990

Customs and Excise v. Samex [1983], 1 All E.R. 1042, 1056

Dobson (Litigation Guardian of) v. Dobson, [1999] 2 S.C.R. 753

Droit de la Famine, 323, [1988] R.J.Q. 1542 (C.A.)

E. (Mrs.) v. Eve, [1986] 2 S.C.R. 388, [1986] S.C.J. No.60 (S.C.C.)

Egan v. Canada (1993) 3 S.C.R. 513

Evans v. UK [2006] E.C.H.R. 6339/05, 7 March 2006

Forliti (Guardian ad litem of) v. Woolley, [2003] B.C.J. No.1627, 2003 BCSC 1082; Judgment: July 10, 2003

Hepton v. Maat [1957], S.C.R. 606

In Re X [1975] 1 All E.R. 697

Joyce v. Director of Public Prosecution [1946] A.C. 347 (H.L.)

Keys v. Mistashia Regional Health Authority, [2001] A.J. No.461, Action No.9703 14590, Judgment April 10, 2001

M.V.R. 2231R. v. Muise (1990)

Moge v. Moge (1992) 3 R.F.L. 3d 345

Montreal Tramways v. Leveille, 4 D.L.R. 337 [1933]

Northwest Area v. D.F.G. [1997] 3 S.C.R. 926

Pappajohn v. the Queen (1980), 2 S.C.R. 120.

R.B. v. Children's Aid Society of Metro Toronto [1995] 1 S.C.R. 315

Snell v. Farrell (1990) 72 D.L.R. (4th) 289 SCC

Trinity Western (1996) 2 O.R. 3d 132, D.L.R. 4th.

Vriend v. Alberta Alta. (1994) 1 S.C.R. 493

Ward v. Canada (Attorney General) (2002) 1 S.C.R. 569

Winnipeg Child and Family Services (Northwest Area) v. D.G.F. [1997] S.C.J. No.96 (S.C.C.)

Winnipeg Child and Family Services v. K.L.W. [2000] 2 S.C.R. 519

EUROPE

Brüggemann and Scheuten v. Federal Republic of Germany, ECHR Appl. No. 6959;3 E.H.R.R. 244/245

Calvelli and another v. Italy [2001] ECHR 3296/96

Comm. Rep. No 6959/75, 12.7.77, DR 10

Donaghue v. Stevenson [1932] A.C. 562

ECJ Celex Lexis 1991 6962; p.2

Gabcikovo-Nagymaros (1997) ICJ, Rep.7, Judge C. Weeramantry, separate opinion

Guerra v. Italy (1998) Rep. 1998-I, no.64, p.21026 EHRR 357

Hatton and Others v. United Kingdom, 37 EHRR 28(2003) Grand Chamber Judgment; see also 34 EHRR 1 (2002)

In re Urios, France's court of Cassation (criminal Chamber), 15 January, 192, (1919–1922), I Annual Digest 107

Lender v. Sweden, A/116 (1987) 9 E.HR.R. 433

Lopez-Ostra v. Spain (1994) Series A, no 303, 20 EHRR 330

Officier van Justitie v. Sandoz, 174/82, BV [1983] ECR 2445

Olsson v. Sweden, Judgment of 24 March 1988, Series A no.130, (1988)

Paton v. UK, No 8416/78 Dec.13.5.80, DR 19,p.244, 3 EHRR 408

Portugal v. Council, Case C-149/96, (1999) ECR I-8395

Preussen–Elektra AG v. Schleswag AG, [2001] Case c–379/98, ECR 1-2099

Rewe-Zentrale AG v. Bundesmonopolverwaltung fur Brantwein Case 120/78

Rieme v. Sweden, Judgment of 22 April 1992, Series A no.226 B, (1992)

Rutili [1975] Case 36/75, ECR 1219

Simmenthal SpA v. Commission (Case 92/78) [1979] ECR 777, [1980] 1 CMLR

Skinner v. Warner, Dickens 799, 21 E.R. 473 (Ch. 1792)

Society for the Protection of Unborn Children (Ireland) Limited v. Stephen Grogan and Others (no. 5), The Supreme Court, 1998 4 IR 343, 6 March 1997

Tank Haulage Ltd., Case no. 1381/80, March 26,1980; [1981] 1 RLR 13 (EAT)

Vo v. France (Application No. 53924/00, July 8, 2004)

W. v. United Kingdom, Judgment of 8 July 1987, Series A no.121, (1987)

X v. U.K. (1970) App. no. 3868/68, 34 C.D. 10,18)

X v. U.K. (1974) App. no. 5877/7 45 C.D. 90.93

Z. v. Finland, 1997-I 323; 25 EHRR 371 (1998) Judge Meyer in his 'partly dissenting opinion'

INTERNATIONAL

Corfu Channel Case, U.K. v. Albania 1949 I.C.J., Rep. 4

Farooque v. Government of Bangladesh 1997 I.L.R. (AD) 1

Le Louis, 2 Dodson Rep., 238

Maritime Delimitation in the Area Between Greenland and Jan Meyer, (Denmark v. Norway) 1993 I.C.J. 38

Minors Oposa v. Secretary of the Department of the Environment and Rural Resources, 33 I.L.M. 173 (1994)

Rex v. Nuemann (Special Criminal Court, Transvaal), 1949 (3) S.A. 1238

UK v. Iceland, 1973 I.C.J. Rep.3

Watt v. Rama, Supreme Full Court of Victoria; 1971 Vic Lexis 143; Y1972U VR 3531 Dec. 14, 1971

UNITED STATES

United States v. Canada, 31 A. A 1911 (1941)

United States v. Carolene Prod. Co., 304 US 144, 152-53, n.4 (1938) (dictum)

United States v. Iran (1980) I.C.J. 3 69

United States District Court S.D. Florida, Sinaltral the Estate of Isidro Segundo Gil, Plaintiffs v. Coca-Cola Company et al, 256 F. Supp. 2d 1345

Webster v. Reproductive Health Services, 492 US 490 (1989)

White Motor Corporation v. Stewart, 465 F.2d 1085, 1088-1089 (10th Cir.)

Whitner v. South Carolina, 523 U.S. 1145 (1998)

Wiwa v. Royal Dutch Petroleum Co. et al, Feb. 8, 2002, 226 H.3d 88 (2d Cir., 2000)

WTO

Appellate Body Hormones Decision, EC Measures Concerning Meat and Meat Products (Hormones), AB-1997-4, WT/DS26/AB/R, WT/DS48/AB/R

Measures Affecting Agricultural Products, report of the Panel, adopted March 19, 1999, WTO Doc. WTDS76/R; Report of the Appellate Body, adopted March 19, 1999, WTO Doc. DT/DS76/AB/R

Measures Affecting the Importation of Salmon, report of the Panel, adopted November 6, 1998, WTO Doc. WT/DS18/R; Report of the Appellate Body, adopted November 6, 1998, WTO Doc. WT/DS18/AB/R; Abitration under Article 21.3(c) of the Understanding on Rules and Procedures Governing the Settlement of Disputes, February 23, 1999, WTO Doc. WT/DS18/9

List of Documents

African Charter on Human and Peoples Rights (1981) A.16

African Convention on the Conservation of Nature and Natural Resources (1968), in force 16 June 1969

Agreement Establishing the World Trade Organization (1994) Marrakesh Agreement Establishing The World Trade Organization, WTO Legal Texts, 3, 'Chapeau,' and (b) and (g)

Agreement Governing the Activities of States on the Moon and Other Celestial Bodies, 18 ILM (1979), 1434; in force 11 July 1984

Agreement on the Application of Sanitary and Phytosanitary Measures, 15 April 1994, final act embodying the results of the Uruguay Round of Multilateral Trade Negotiations, MTN/FA II-A1A-4

Alien Torts Claims Act (1789) 28 USC §1350

American Convention on Human Rights (1969) OAS Tr. Ser./No.36; 1144 U.N.T.S. 123

Antarctic Treaty on Environmental Protection, 1991

Arkansas Code Ann. (Michie 1991 Supp.) §5-14-123(b)

ASEAN Agreement on the Conservation of Nature and Natural Resources, Kuala Lumpur, 9 July 1985

The Ashbrook proposal, H.R.J. Res. 13, 97th Cong., 1st Sess. (1981)

Bamako Convention on the Ban of the Import into Africa and the Control of Transboundary Movement and Management of Hazardous Waste within Africa, 29 January1991, 30 I.L.M. 775 (1991)

Basel Protocol on Liability and Compensation for Damage Resulting from Transboundary Movements of Hazardous Wastes and their Disposal (2000)

Biodiversity Convention (Convention on Biological Diversity or CBD), adopted at the Earth Summit in Rio de Janeiro, Brazil, June 1992, in force December 1993

Biosecurity Act (1993) no. 95

Cal.Penal Code (1986) §187 (a), West Supp.

Canadian Environmental Protection Act (1985) R.S.C. 1985 Ch.16, amended 1999, in force 1999

Child, Family and Community Services Act, R.S.B.C. 1996, c.46, s.2(a) and 4(1)

Child and Family Services Act (1990) R.S.O.; s.1(a), amended, R.S.) c.11, s.37(3)

Code Napoleon (cited in Ross, Alf, 1958, *On Law and Justice,* Steven and Sons Ltd., p246)

Concluding Observations of CEDAW Committee on Third and Fourth Periodic Reports of China, (1999) CEDAW/C/1999/1/L.1/Add.7

Constitution of Pennsylvania, September 1776

Constitution of the Republic of S. Africa (1996) S.11

Constitution of the United States of America, (1787)

Constitution of the World Health Organization, as adopted by the International Health conference, New York, 19 June–20 July, 1946; signed on July 22, 1946 by the representatives of 51 states; Official Records of the World Health Organization, no. 2, p. 100 and entered into force on 7 April 1948

Convention against Torture and Other Cruel, Inhuman or Degrading Treatment or Punishment, U.N.Doc. A/39/51 (1984)

Convention for the Protection of the Ozone Layer (Vienna) UKTS 1 (1990), 26 ILM (187), 1529; in force 22 September 1988

Convention for the Protection of Human Rights and Dignity of the Human Being with Regard to the Application of Biology and Medicine, and the Additional Protocol on the Prohibition of Cloning Human Beings, Oviedo, April 4 (1997) in force December 1, 1999

Convention for the Protection of World Cultural and Natural Heritage, 1972

Convention on the Elimination of All Forms of Discrimination Against Women (CEDAW), effective 1981, 165 State Parties in March 2000

Convention on International Trade in Endangered Species of Wild Flora and Fauna, 993 UNTS 243, 3 March 1973

Convention on the Law of the Sea (Montego Bay) 21 ILM (1982), 1261; in force 16 November 1994

Convention on the Prevention and Punishment of the Crime of Genocide (1951) 78 U.N.T.S. 277

Convention on the Protection of the Rhine Against Chemical Pollution (Bonn) (1977) 1124 U.N.T.S. 375; I.L.M., 243. In force February 1, 1973

Convention on the Protection of the Rhine from Pollution by Chlorides (Bonn) (1997) 16 I.L.M. 265. In force 5 July 1985; Amended by the 1991 Protocol

Convention on the Rights of the Child (1990) U.N.Doc E/CN.4/1989/29; in force Nov. 20, 1990 (henceforth CRC)

Council Directive 83/129, 1983 O.J. (L.91) 30, *Marine Mammals Regulations*

Council of Europe Communities Directive on Major-Accident Hazards of Certain Industrial Activities (Seveso Directive) (82/501/EEC, 24 June 1982; as amended by 87/2161 ECC, 19 March 1987 and 88/8610/EEC, 24 November 1988)

Decision no. 74054 of January 15, 1975

Declaration of the Environmental Leader of the Eight on Children's Environmental Health (1997) (Miami, FL, 5–6 May 1997; www.g7.utoronto.ca/g7/environment/1997 Miami/children.html)

Declaration of the Rights of the Child, drafted by Eglantyne Jebb, adopted by the International Save the Children Union, Geneva, 23 February 1923; endorsed by the League of Nations General Assembly, 26 November 1924

Declaration of the UN Conference on Environment and Development, UN Doc. A/CONF.151/26/Rev.1

Delaney Clause (1994) USC 348 (C) (3) (A), 1994

Doc. Parl. Ch.S.O. 1989-1990, No.1033/1p.11.

EEOC Interpretive Guidelines on Employment Discrimination and Reproductive Hazards, 45 Fed. Reg. 7514 (Feb.1, 1980) (corrected in 45 Fed. Reg.16, 501 (1980))

European Convention for the Protection of Human Rights and Fundamental Freedoms, Nov. 4, 1950, 213 U.N.T.S. 221

European Group on Ethics in Science and New Technologies at the European Commission, 5th Framework Program, 23 November, 1998

European Social Charter, 529 U.N.T.S. 89, in force 26 February 1965

*G.A.Res.2200,*U.N. GADR,21st Sess., Supp.No.16, U.N.Doc.A/6316(1966)

The Garn-Rhodes proposal, S.J. Res. 17, 97th Cong., 1st Sess. (1981)

Great Lakes Water Quality Agreement (GLWQA) (1978), ratified 1987

H.R.Rep. No.948, 95th Cong., 2d Sess. 5, reprinted in US Code Cong.Ad.News 4749, 4753

Hazardous Substances and New Organisms Act (1996) no. 30

Health Protection and Promotion Act; R.S.O. 1990, see especially Chapter H.7, Part III, 'Community Health Protection'; and Part IV Communicable Diseases

The Helles-Dorman proposal, S.J. Res. 19, 97th Cong., 1st Sess (1981)

The Helms-Hyde human life bill, S. 158, 97th Cong., 1st Sess. (1981)

Idaho Code §39-608 (1992 Supp.)

ILC Rep. 242

Ill. Rev. Stat., Ch. 38, 9-1.2, 12-3.1 (1986 Supp.)

Illinois Criminal Code, ch. 38, secs. 4–6 and 12–5 (in 'Reckless Conduct')

Implications of the Industrial Disaster in Bhopal, India: Hearing before the Subcomm. on Asia and Pacific Affairs of the House Comm. on Foreign Affairs, 98th Con.. 2d Sess. 3, 6, 28 (1984) (statements of Robert A. Peck, Deputy Assistant Secretary for Near Eastern and South Asian Affairs, Department of State, and Ronald Wishart, Vice President for Government Relations, Union Carbide Corporation)

Indiana Statute, Ind. Code Ann. §35-42-1-7, Burns 1992, Supp.

International Commission on Intervention in State Sovereignty (ICISS), December 2001; www.iciss.gc.ca report – e.asp

International Convention on the Elimination of all Forms of Racial Discrimination, A.5 (e)(iv)(1965)

International Covenant on Civil and Political Rights (ICCPR), G.A. res. 2200A (XXI), 21 U.N. GAOR Supp. No. 16 at 52, U.N. Doc. A/6316, (1966) 999 U.N.T.S.171, in force March 23, 1986

International Covenant on Economic, Social and Cultural Rights (ICESCR), G.A. Res. 2200A, 21 GAOR Supp. 16 at 49, UN Doc. A/6316 (1966), 993 U.N.T.S. 3, in force January 3, 1976

International Criminal Court, Rome Statute, in force, July 12, 2002

International Law Commission (ILC) Fifty-fifth Session, Geneva 5 May–6 June and 7 July–8 August, 2003

International Law Commission (ILC) Report of the Working Group on International Liability for Injurious Consequences Arising Out of Acts not Prohibited by International Law, in Rpt. Of the ILC (1996) GAOR A/51/10, Annex 1

International Law Commission Rpt. of the ILC (2001) GAOR A/56/10

International Law Commission; Special Rapporteur Srenivasa Rao, 1 X.B. I.L.C. 61 (1998)

International Law Convention on Transboundary Harm, Special Rapporteur Rao's 1st Report (1988) UN Doc.A/CN 487/Add. 1; *2nd Report* (1999) UN Doc.A/Cn.4/501; *3rd Report* (2000) UN Doc. A/CN 4/510

The Irish Constitution, 1937 (but see *McGee v. Attorney General* [1974] I.R. 284)

Legality of the Use by a State of Nuclear Weapons in Armed Conflict, [1996] I.C.J. Rep. 66; Dissenting Opinion of Judge Weeramantry (1996) I.C.J. Rep. 429, at 433

Martin's Criminal Code, 1996 (Canada)

Minn.Stat. Ann. § 609.266 (1987 Supp.)

Missouri Ann. Stat. §1.205.2 (Vernon's 1992 Supp.)

New York City Health Code (3-31-93), Ch. 11.47 (RCNY: 103039-10312)

New York Penal Law 120.25

New Zealand Bill of Rights Act 1990, no. 109

New Zealand Children, Young Persons and Their Families Act (1989 s.2(1))

New Zealand Contraception, Sterilization and Abortion Act, 1977, ss.182, 187

New Zealand Crimes Act (1961) no. 63

New Zealand Guardianship Act, 1968, s.7

New Zealand Resource Management Act, 1991, s.5(2)

Nuremberg Charter (1945) Charter of the Military Tribunal, 82 U.N.T.S. 279

Occupational Safety and Health Act, 29 USC § 651–678 (1976)

Ocean Dumping Act (1971), 33 USC §1411 (a)

Patient's Rights and Quality of Health Services Act (Law No. 2002-203)

Pregnancy Amendment to Title VII; Supreme Court Decision, 429 US 125 (1976) 42 USC§ 2000e–(k) (Supp.1980)

Protocol on Substances that Deplete the Ozone Layer (Montreal), 26 ILM (1987), 1550, in force 1 January 1989

Protocol to the Framework Convention on Climate Change (Kyoto), 37 I.L.M. (1998), 22

Report by the Majority Staff on EEOC, Title VII and Workplace Fetal Protection Policies in the 1980s, House Education and Labor Committee, 101st Cong., 2d sess., April 1990: 16

Reproductive Health Hazards in the Workplace, Office of Technology Assessment's document, US Congress, US Government Printing Office, Washington, DC, 1985

Respect for the Human Body, Law no. 94-653 of 29 July 1994 (Article 16 of the Civil Code)

Restatement (Third) of the Foreign Relations Law of the United States (1987)

Rio Declaration on Environment and Development, Annex 1 of the *Report of the United Nations Conference on Environment and Development*, 1992, A/CONF.151/26 (Vol. I)

Rome Declaration on World Food Security, www.fao.org/wts/policy/english/96-eng.html

The State of the World's Children, UNICEF, 1994, Oxford University Press, New York

Stockholm Convention on Persistent Organic Pollutants (see A.1, 'Objectives')

Stockholm Declaration of the United Nations Conference on the Human Environment, June 16 1972, 11 ILM 1416

Title VII of the Civil Rights, 42 USC §§ 20000e to 2000e-17 (1976 and Supp.1980)

UNECE Environment and Human Settlement Division, 'Convention on access to information, public participating in decision-making and access to justice in environmental matters', Aarhus, Denmark, June 1998)

United Nations Charter of the Rights of the Child, GA Res. 1386 XIV

United Nations Conference on Trade and Development Draft International Code of Conduct on the Transfer of Technology, May 6 1980, rep. 19 I.L.M. 773 (1980)

United Nations Convention on the Rights of the Child (UNCROC), 20 November 1989, GA44/25

United Nations Declaration of Human Rights, (1948) Res. 217A(III) U.N.Doc.A/810)

United Nations Declaration on the Establishment of a New Economic International Order, May 9, 1974, G.A. Res. 3201, 29 U.N. GAOR Supp. (No.31), C 50, U.N. Doc.A/9631 (1975)

Universal Declaration of Human Rights, G.A.Res.217, U.N.GAOR 3d. Sess., at 71, U.N.Doc.A/810 (1948)

Vienna Convention on the Law of Treaties (1969) 1155 U.N.T.S. 331, in force 1980, 8ILM

Voluntary Termination of Pregnancy Act of 17 January 1975 (Law no. 75-17)

Whaling Convention (*International Convention for the Regulation of Whaling*), signed by 42 nations in Washington, DC on 2 December 1946, in force 10 November 1948

WHO Framework Convention on Tobacco Control, WHA 56.1, 21 May, 2003; A56/INF.Doc./7

World Heritage Convention (*The Convention Concerning the Protection of the World Cultural and Natural Heritage*), adopted by the UNESCO General Conference at its 17th session, Paris, 16 November 1972; in force 1975

Abbassi, K. (1999) 'Changing sides', *British Medical Journal*, vol 318

Abraham, C. (2005) 'No faith in science', *The Globe and Mail*, Canada, April 9

Adams, H. M. (1995) 'Somalia environmental degradation and environmental racism' in L. Westra and P. Wenz (eds) *Faces of Environmental Racism*, Rowman and Littlefield, Lanham, MD

Agius, Emmanuel (1998) 'Obligations of justice towards future generations: A revolution in social and legal thought', in E. Agius and Salvino Busuttil (eds) *Future Generations and International Law*, Earthscan, London, UK

Ago, R. (1988) 'The concept of the international community as a whole', in J. Weiler, A. Cassese and M. Spinedi (eds) *International Crime of State: A Critical Analysis of the ILC Draft Article 19 on State Responsibility*, Walter de Gruyter, Berlin

Albritton, R. (2004) 'Eating the future', unpublished manuscript, on file with the author

Ament, M. (1974) 'The right to be well-born', *Journal of Legal Medicine*, November–December

Amnesty International (1995) 'Nigeria historical fact sheet: June 1993, February 1995', Amnesty International, Washington, DC

Arendt, H. (1964) *Eichmann in Jerusalem: A Report on the Banality of Evil*, Viking Press, New York

Aristotle *De Generatione Animalium II*

Aristotle *De Anima II*

Aristotle (1992) *Nicomachean Ethics*, edited by R. McKeon, Random House, New York

Aron, J. L. and Patz, J. A. (2001) *Ecosystem Change and Public Health: A Global Perspective*, Johns Hopkins University Press, Baltimore, MD

Ashford, N. (1999) 'A conceptual framework for the use of the precautionary principle in law' in *Protecting Public Health and the Environment*, Island Press, Washington, DC, pp189–206

Atias, C. (1985) 'Les personnes – les incapacités', Droit Civil, PUF, Paris, France, p14

Baker, J. H. (1979) *An Introduction to English Legal History*, 2nd edn, Butterworths, London, p273

Bala, N. C., Hornick, J. P. and Vogel, R. (2004) *Canadian Child Welfare Law*, 2nd edn, Thompson Educational Publications, Toronto, Canada

Baram, M. J. (1989) 'Corporate risk management and risk communication in the European Community and the United States', *Harvard Journal of Law and Technology*, no 2

Barash, D. D. (2000) 'International law' in D. Barash (ed) *Approaches to Peace*, Oxford University Press, Oxford

Barlow, M. (1999) *Blue Gold*, special report issued by the International Forum of Globalization (IFG), Ottawa, Canada

Barlow, M. and Clarke, T. (2002) *Global Showdown*, Stoddard Publishing House, Don Mills, Ontario

Barlow, S. M. and Sullivan, F. M. (1982) *Reproductive Hazards of Industrial Chemicals*, Academic Press, London

Barresi, P. A. (1997) 'Beyond fairness to future generations: An intergenerational alternative to intergenerational equity in the intergenerational environmental arena', *Tulaine Environmental Law Journal*, vol 11, no 1

Barry, B. M. (1966) 'The use and abuse of the public interest', in C.-J. Friedrich (ed) *The Public Interest*, Atherton Press, NY, pp191–204

Baxi, Upendra, (1999) 'Voices of suffering and the future of human rights', *Transnational and Contemporary Problems*, vol 8, p125

Beaglehole, R. and Bonita, R. (2004) *Public Health at the Crossroads*, Cambridge University Press, Cambridge, UK, p270

Beal, R. (1984) 'Can I sue Mommy? An analysis of a women's tort liability for prenatal injuries to her child born alive', *San Diego Law Review*, vol 21, no 325

Bearer, C. F. (1995) 'How are children different from adults?', *Environmental Health Perspectives*, vol 102, pp7–12

Beck, J. (1860) *Elements of Medical Jurisprudence*, 11th edn, Lippincott, Philadelphia, PA, p253

Bederman, D. (2001) *International Law Frameworks*, Foundation Press, New York

Beetham, D. (1995) 'What future for economic and social rights?' *Political Studies*, vol 43, p47

Bennett, C. (1965) 'The liability of the manufacturers of thalidomide to the affected children', *American Law Journal*, vol 39, p256

Berlin, I. (1969) 'Two concepts of liberty' in *Four Essays on Liberty*, Oxford University Press, Oxford, p130

Bernstein, A. (1997) 'Formed by thalidomide: Mass torts as a false cure for toxic exposure', *Columbia Law Review*, p2153

Bertin, J. E. (1989) 'Reproductive hazards in the workplace' in S. Cohen and N. Taub (eds) *Reproductive Laws for the 1990s*, Humana Press, Clifton, NJ

Beyleveld, D. and Brownsword, R. (2001) *Human Dignity in Bioethics and Biolaw*, Oxford University Press, Oxford

Birnie, P. and Boyle, A. E. (1992) *International Law and the Environment*, Clarendon Press, New York

Birnie, P. and Boyle, A. E. (2002) *International Law and the Environment*, 2nd edn, Oxford University Press, Oxford

Black, R. E., Morris, S. S. and Bryce, J. (2003) 'Where and why are 10 million children dying every year?', *The Lancet*, vol 361, pp2226–2234

Black's Law Dictionary (1979) *Black's Law Dictionary*, 5th edn, West Publishing Co., St Paul, MN

Blackstock, C. and Trocme, N. (2004) 'Pathways to the overrepresentation of aboriginal children in Canada's child welfare system', *Social Service Review*, vol 10, August

Boos-Hersberger, A. (1997) 'Transboundary water pollution and state responsibility: The Sandoz spill', *Annual Survey International and Comparative Law*, vol 4

Bosselmann, K. (1999) 'Justice and the environment: A theory on ecological justice', in K. Bosselmann and B. Richardson (eds) *Environmental Justice and Market Mechanisms*, Kluwer Law International, London

Bourette, S. (2000) 'Editorial', *The Globe and Mail*, Canada, June 7

Bradshaw, J. S., (1982) 'The medical dimension', in D. M. Clarke (ed) *Morality and the Law*, Mercier Press, Dublin

Braybrook, D. (1966) 'The public interest: The present and future of the concept', in C. J. Frierich (ed) *The Public Interest*, Atherton Press, New York, pp129–154

Breen, C. (2002) *The Standard of the Best Interests of the Child*, Kluwer Law International, the Hague, The Netherlands

Brennan, T. A. (1988) 'Causal chains and statistical links: The role of scientific uncertainty in hazardous substance litigation', *Cornell Legal Review*, vol 73, pp469, 491

Brook, C. G. D. (1978) 'Influence of nutrition in childhood on the origins of coronary heart disease', *Postgraduate Medical Journal*, vol 54, pp171–175

Brooks, G. (1994) 'Slick alliance', 'Shell's Nigerian fields produce few benefits for region's villagers', 'How troops handle protests', *The Wall Street Journal*, May 6, ppA1, A4

Brown, D. (1995) 'The role of law in sustainable development and environmental protection decision-making', in *Sustainable Development: Science, Ethics and Public Policy*, Kluwer Academic Press, Dordrecht, The Netherlands, pp64–76

Brown, D. (2000) *American Heat*, Rowman and Littlefield, Lanham, MD

Brown-Weiss, E. (1988) 'The planetary trust: Conservation and intergenerational equity', *Ecology Law Journal*, vol 11

Brown-Weiss, E. (1990) 'Our Rights and Obligations to Future Generations for the Environment', *American Journal of International Law*, vol 84

Brown-Weiss, E. (ed) (1992) *Environmental Change and International Law*, United Nations University Press, Tokyo

Brown-Weiss, E. (1993) 'Intergenerational equity: Toward an international legal framework', in Nazli Chourcri (ed) *Global Accord*, MIT Press, Cambridge, MA

Bruckmann, E. (2000) 'Rural Ontario: Industrial hog barns, industrial waste', *Intervenor*, vol 25, no 1, January–March

Brunnee, J. and Toope, S. J. (1997) 'Environmental security and freshwater resources: Ecosystem regime building', *American Journal of International Law*, vol 91, p26

Bullard, R. (1994) *Dumping in Dixie*, Westview Press, Boulder, CO

Bullard, R. (2001) 'Decision making' in L. Westra and B. Lawson (eds) *Faces of Environmental Racism*, Rowman and Littlefield, Lanham, MD, pp3–28

Burkitt, D., MD (1991) 'Are our commonest diseases preventable?', *The Pharos of Alpha Omega*, vol 54, no 1, Winter, 19-22

Burley, D. M., Clarke, J. M. and Lasagna, L. (1993) *Pharmaceutical Medicine*, 2nd edn, Edward Arnold, London

Business India (1985) 'Bhopal: What really happened', *Business India*, February 25–March 10, p102

Callicott, J. B. (1999) *The Land Ethic Revisted*, Suny Press, New York

Callicott, J. B. (2000) 'Animal liberation: A triangular affair', in L. Pojman (ed) *Environmental Ethics*, Wadsworth Publishing, Belmont, CA

Carlson, J. and Tamburlini, G. (2002) 'Policy developments', in Tamburlini et al (2002)

Cassese, A. (1996) *International Law in a Divided World*, Clarendon Press, Oxford

Caulfield, L. E., de Onis, M., Blossner, M. and Black, R. E. (2004) 'Undernutrition as an underlying cause of child deaths associated with diarrhea, pneumonia, malaria, and measles', *American Journal of Clinical Nutrition*, vol 80, pp193–198

Center for Disease Control (1992) 'The second 100,000 cases of A.I.D. syndrome US June 1981–December 1991', *Morbidity and Mortality Weekly*, no 41, report no 2, January 17

Charnovitz, S. (1994) 'Free trade, fair trade, green trade: Defogging the debate', *Cornell International Law Journal*, vol 27, pp459–525

Chaskalson, Justice A. (2002) Address at the Summit for the Johannesburg Principles on the Role of Law and Sustainable Development, August 27

Cheng, B. (1980) 'The legal regime of airspace and outer space in the boundary problem, functionalism versus spatialism: The major promises', *Annals of Air Space Law*, vol 5, pp323–337

Chomsky, N. (2004) *Hegemony or Survival: American Quest for Global Dominance*, Owl Books (imprint of Henry Holt and Company), New York

Chopra, S. (1994) 'Increased radiation levels were found in Scandinavia, Poland, France, United Kingdom, Finland, Ireland and West Germany', in W. P. Weiner, D. S. Favre and S. Chopra (eds), Sudhir *International Environmental Law*, Lupus Publications, Detroit, MI

Clark, K. and Yacoumidis, A. (2001) *CELN 5 Year Report on The Common Sense Revolution*, Canadian Environmental Law Association, Toronto, Canada

Clarkson, T. (1993) *International Organization*, no 50, p3

Cohen, J. (1962) 'A lawman's view of the public interest', in C. J. Friedrich (ed) *Nomos V: The Public Interest*, Atherton Press, New York, p156

Cohen, R. (1998) *Milk, The Deadly Poison*, Argus Publishing, New York

Colborn, T., Dumanski, D. and Myers, J. P (1996) *Our Stolen Future*, Dutton, imprint of Penguin Books USA, New York

Cooney, J. F., Starr, J. W., Block, J. G., Kelly, T. J., Herrup, A. R., Mann, V. K. and Braker, G. S. (1996) *Environmental Crimes Deskbook*, Environmental Law Institute, Washington, DC

Courage, C. M. (2002) 'Environmental tobacco smoke', in Tamburlini et al (2002), p142

Crawford, J. (2002) *The International Law Commission's Articles on State Responsibility*, Cambridge University Press, Cambridge, UK

Daily Labor Report (1987) 'British EEO Agency warns employers that discharge for pregnancy is illegal', *Daily Labor Report*, vol 175, September 11, pA5

Daily, G. (1997) *Nature's Services: Societal Dependence on Natural Ecosystems*, Island Press, Washington, DC, pp3–4

Daly, H. (1996) *Beyond Growth*, Beacon Press, Boston, MA

D'Amato, A. (1990) 'Agora: What obligation do our generation owe to the next? An approach to global environmental responsibility', *American Journal of International Law*, vol 84, p190

Davis, K. (1996) *Prisoned Chickens, Poisoned Eggs: An Inside Look at the Poultry Industry*, The Book Publishing Co., Summertown, TN

Davis, M. (1995) 'Arresting the white death: Preventive detention, confinement for treatment, and medical ethics', *APA Newsletter*, vol 94, no 2, Association Central Meeting, April

De Burca, G. and Craig, P. (2003) *EU Law: Text, Cases and Materials*, Oxford University Press, Oxford

De George, R. (1981) 'The environment, rights and future generations', in E. Partirdge (ed) *Responsibilities to Future Generations*, Prometheus Books, Buffalo, NY

De Grazia, D. (1995) *Taking Animals Seriously*, Cambridge Univeristy Press, New York

de Sousa Santos, B. (2002) *Towards a New Legal Common Sense: Law, Globalization and Emancipation*, Butterworth, London

Detricks, S. (1999) *A Commentary on the United Nations Convention on the Rights of the Child*, Kluwer Law International, the Hague, The Netherlands

Dhoge, L. J. (2003) 'The Alien Torts Claims Act and the modern transnational enterprise: Deconstructing the mythology of judicial activism', *Georgetown Journal of International Law*, vol 35, no 1

Diamond, S. (1985) 'The Bhopal disaster: How it happened', *The New York Times*, January 28, pA1

Dinstein, Y. (1981) 'The right to life, physical integrity and liberty', in L. Henki (ed) *The International Bill of Rights: The Covenant on Civil and Political Rights*, Columbia University Press, New York, pp114–137

Donald T. W. (2003) *Child Health and the Environment*, Oxford University Press, New York

Donnelly, J. (1995) 'States sovereignty and international intervention: The case of human rights' G. M. Lyons and M. Mastanduno (eds) *Beyond Westphalia? State Sovereignty and International Intervention*, Johns Hopkins University Press, Baltimore, MD, pp115–146

Dooley-Clark, D. (1982) 'Abortion and the law', in D. Clarke (ed) *Morality and the Law*, Mercier Press, Dublin, pp31–46

Dorland's Illustrated Medical Dictionary (1985) *Dorland's Illustrated Medical Dictionary*, 26th edn, W. B. Saunders, Philadelphia, PA

Downs, J. (1993) 'A healthy and ecologically balanced environment: An argument for a third generation right', *Duke Journal of Comparative and International Law*, no 3, p351

Draper, E. (1991) *Risky Business*, Cambridge University Press, Cambridge, MA

Durning, A. T. (1992) *How Much is Enough?*, W.W. Norton and Co., New York, p71

Dworkin, G. (1971) 'Paternalism', in R. A. Wasserstrom (ed) *Morality and the Law*, Wadsworth Publishing, Belmont, CA

Dworkin, R. M. (1977) 'What rights do we have?', in *Taking Rights Seriously*, Harvard University Press, Cambridge, MA

Dyson, R. (2000) *Mind Abuse: Media Violence in an Information Age*, Black Rose Books, Montreal, Canada

Ebi, K. L. (2002) 'Electromagnetic fields', in Tamburlini et al (2002), p172

Edgerton, H. W. (1928) 'Negligence, inadvertence and indifference', *Harvard Law Review*, vol 39, p849

Eisnitz, G. (1997) *Slaughterhouse: The Shocking Story of Greed, Neglect and Inhumane Treatment Inside the US Meat Industry*, Prometheus Books, New York

Epstein, F. H. (1979) 'Predicting, explaining and preventing coronary heart disease', *Modern Concepts in Cardiovascular Disease*, vol 48

Epstein, R. A. (1989) 'Justice across the generations', *Texas Law Review*, vol 67, p1465

Falk, R. (1998) *Law in an Emerging Global Village*, Transnational Publishers, Ardsley, NY

Farber, D. A. (2003) 'From here to eternity: Environmental law and future generations', *University of Illinois Law* Review, vol 2, p289

Feinberg, J. (1973) *Social Psychology*, Prentice Hall, Englewood Cliffs, NJ, p94

Feinberg, J. (1980) *Rights, Justice and the Bounds of Liberty*, Princeton University Press, Princeton, NJ

Fidler, D. (1998) 'The future of the World Health Organization: What role for international law?', *Vanderbilt Journal of Transnational Law*, vol 31, pp1079–1126

Fidler, D. (2000) *International Law and Public Health*, Trans National Publishers, Ardsley, NY

Fionda, J. (2001) *Legal Concepts of Childhood*, Hart Publishing, Oxford

Fletcher, A. C. (1985) *Reproductive Hazards of Work*, Equal Opportunity Commission, Manchester, UK

Fletcher, G. P. (1971) 'The theory of criminal negligence: A comparative analysis', *Universitym of Pennsylvania Law Review*, vol 119, no 3, pp401–437

Fluss, S. S. (1998) 'The Role of the WHO in health legislation: Some historical perspectives', *International Digest of Health Legislation*, vol 49, p111

Forsythe, C. D. (1987) 'Homicide of the unborn child: The born alive rule and other legal anachronisms', *Valparaiso University Law Review*, vol 21

Freedman, L. P., Waldman, R. J., de Pinho, H., Wirth, M. E., Mushtaque, A., Chowdury, R. (coordinator) and Rosenfield, A. (coordinator) (2005) *Who's Got the Power? Transforming Health Systems for Women and Children*, UN Millennium Project Task Force on Child and Maternal Health, Earthscan, London, p31

French, Howard, W. (1995) 'Nigeria executes activist playwright', in *New York Times*, reprinted in *San Francisco Chronicle* 11 Nov., ppA1 and A13.

Friedman, M. (1993) 'The social responsibility of business is to increase its profits', in T. Donaldson and P. Werhane (eds) *Ethical Issues in Business*, Prentice Hall, Englewood Cliffs, NJ, pp249–254

Fuchs, F. and Galba-Araujo, J. (1980) 'Perinatal diseases and injuries', in F. Falkner (ed) *Prevention in Childhood of Health, Problems in Adult Life*, WHO, Geneva

Gallagher, J. (1989) 'Fetus as a patient', in S. Cohen and N. Taub (eds) *Reproductive Laws for the 1990s*, Humana Press, Clifton, NJ, pp185–236

Gaylord, C. and Bell, E. (1995) 'Environmental justice: A national priority', in Westra and Wenz (1995), pp29–40

Gbadegesin, S. (2001) 'Multinational corporations, developed nations and environmental racism: Toxic waste, oil exploration and ecocatastrophy', in Westra and Lawson (2001), pp187–202

Gelbspan, Ross (2005) 'Katrina's Real Name', *The Boston Globe*, Boston, MA, August 30

George, S. (2003) 'Globalizing rights?', in Matthew Gibney (ed) *Globalizing Rights: Oxford Amnesty Lectures 1999*, Oxford University Press, Oxford, pp15–33

Gewirth, A. (1982) *Starvation and Human Rights: Essays in Justification and Application*, University of Chicago Press, Chicago, IL

Gilbert, P. (1994) *Terrorism, Security and Nationality*, Routledge, London

Glasbeek H. and Rowland, S. (1986) 'Are injuring and killing in the workplace crimes?', in N. Boyd (ed) *The Social Dimensions of Law*, Prentice-Hall, Scarborough, Ontario

The Globe and Mail (1995) *The Globe and Mail*, Canada, November 21, 1995, pA17

The Globe and Mail (1997) *The Globe and Mail*, Canada, January 3, 1997, pA3

The Globe and Mail (2000) *The Globe and Mail*, Canada, July 3, 2000, A11

Goedhuis, D. (1981) 'Some recent trends in the interpretation and the implementation of international space law', *Columbia Journal of Transnational Law*, no 19

Goerner, S. J. (1994) *Chaos and Evolving Ecological Universe*, Gordon and Breach Science Publishers, Amsterdam, The Netherlands

Goldstein, J., Freud, A., Solnit, A. and Beynel, A. (1980) *The Best Interests of the Child*, Burnett Books, London/The Free Press, New York, pp51–2

Gonzales, C. (2001), 'Beyond eco-imperialism: An environmental justice critique of free trade', *Denver University Law Review*, no 78, p979

Goodland, R. and Daly, H. (1995) 'Universal environmental sustainability and the principle of integrity', in Westra and J. Lemons (1995), pp102–124

Goodwin, N. R. (2000) 'Consumption?', in A. R. Chapman, R. L. Peterson and B. Smith-Moran (eds) *Population and Sustainability*, Island Press, Washington, DC, p248

Gordenker, L. (1994) 'The World Health Organization: Sectoral leader or occasional benefactor?', in R. Coate (ed) *US Policy and The Future of The United Nations*, Twentieth Century Fund Press, New York, pp167–191

Gordon, B. (1965) 'The unborn plaintiff', *Michigan Law Review*, vol 63, p579

Gordon, B., Mackay, R. and Rehfuess, E. (2004) *Inheriting the World: The Atlas of Children's Health and the Environment*, Myriad Editions, Brighton

Gostin, L. O. (2000) *Public Health Law (Power, Duty and Restraint)*, University of California Press, Berkeley, CA

Grandjean, P. (2005) 'Only to develop a brain: Consequence of developmental neurotoxicity', paper presented at the meeting of the Collegium Ramazzini, Bologna, Italy, September 20

Grandjean, P. and White, R. (2002) 'Neurodevelopmental disorders', in Tamburlini et al (2002), p66

Grotius, H. (1625) *De Jure belli ac Pacis, libri tres*, Buon, Paris

Gruskin, S. (2001) 'A world fit for children: Are the world's leaders being passed on the fast lane?', *Health and Human Rights*, Harvard School of Public Health, vol 5, no 2, pp1–7

Guha, R. (1989) 'Radical environmentalism and wilderness preservation: A third world critique' in L. Pojman (ed) *Environmental Ethics*, 4th edn, Wadsworth Publishing, Belmont, CA, pp312–319

Hanson, J. W., Streissguth, A. P. and Smith, D. W. (1978) 'The effects of moderate alcohol consumption during pregnancy on fetal growth and morphogenesis', *Journal of Pediatrics*, vol 92, pp457–460

Harjuila, H. (2005) 'Hazardous waste: Recognition of the problem and response', paper presented at the meeting of the Collegium Ramazzini, Bologna, Italy, September 19

Harold, C. (2004) 'Ethics of seeing: Consuming environments', *Ethics and the Environment*, vol 9, no 2, p1

Hart , H. L. A. (1961) *The Concept of Law*, Clarendon Press, Oxford

Harvard Law Review (1985) 'The Supreme Court, 1984 Term – Foreword: The Civil Rights Chronicles', *Harvard Law Review*, vol 99, no 4, pp4–7

Harvard Law Review (1995) 'FDA reforms and the European Medicines Evaluation Agency', *Harvard Law Review*, vol 108, p2009

Hauskeller, M. (2002) unpublished paper, presented in July 2005 at the meeting of the Global Ecological Integrity Group (GEIG) in Venice

Hazarika, S. (1984) 'Gas leak in India kills at least 410 in City of Bhopal', *The New York Times*, December 4, pAl

Health and Safety Information Bulletin (1981) 'Ban on woman transporting DMF NOT unlawful discrimination', *Health and Safety Information Bulletin*, vol 62, February, pp18–19

Healy, P. (1993) 'The Creighton Quartet: Enigma variations in the lower key', 23 Criminal Reports (4th), Carswell Publishers, Toronto, p265

Heath, J. (2001) *The Efficient Society*, Penguin Books, Toronto

Held, D. and McGrew, A. (2002) *Globalization and Anti-Globalization*, Polity Press, Cambridge, UK

Hermann, D. H. (1990) 'Criminalizing conduct related to HIV transmission', *St Louis University Public Law Review*, vol 9

Hertsgaard, M. (1996) 'Benefit of the doubts', *Nation*, July 8, p10

Higgins, R. (1994) *Problems and Process: International Law and How We Use It*, Clarendon Press, Oxford

Hirsch Ballin, E. (1999) 'Children as world citizens', in S. Detrick and P. Vlaardingerbroek (eds) *Globalization of Child Law*, Martinus Nijhoff Publishers, Dordrecht, The Netherlands, p7

Hiskes, R. P. (1998) *Democracy, Risk and Community*, Oxford University Press, New York

Hoffman, E. (2003) 'The balm of recognition: Rectifying wrong through the generations', in N. Owen (ed) *Human Rights, Human Wrongs: Amnesty International Lectures*, Oxford University Press, Oxford, p280

Hogerzeil, H. (2003) 'Access to essential medicines as a human right', *Essential Drugs Monitor*, no 33

Holmes, O. W. (1881) *The Common Law*, Little Brown, Boston, MA

Holmes, O. W. (1897) 'The path of law', *Harvard Law Review*, vol 10, p547

Homer-Dixon, T. F. (1999) *Environmental Scarcity and Violence*, Princeton University Press, Princeton, NJ

Homer-Dixon, T. F. and Gizewski, P. (1996) *Environmental Scarcity and Violent Conflict: The Case of Pakistan*, Project on Environment, Population and Security, University of Toronto Press, Toronto

Houlihan, J., Kropp, T., Wiles, R., Gray, S. and Campbell, C. (2005) 'Body burden in the pollution in newborns', report, July 14, Environmental Working Group, Washington, DC, available at www.ewg.org/report_content/bodyburden2/pdf/bodyburden2_final.pdf

Howe of Aberavon, Lord (1996) *E.L. Rev.*, June, 187, pp190–193

Howse, R. (2000) 'Democracy, science, and free trade: Risk regulation on trial at the World Trade Organization', *Michigan Law Review*, vol 98, pp2329–2357

Human Resources Development (2000) *Child Welfare in Canada*, Human Resources Development, Canada

Hummel, M. (1989) *Endangered Spaces: The Future of Canada's Wilderness*, Key Porter Books, Toronto

Hutt, P. B. (1993) 'The regulation of pharmaceutical products in the USA', *Pharmaceutical Medicine*, pp216–17

Ibbitson, J. (2000) 'Harris's denials are floundering', *The Globe and Mail*, Canada, June 8, pA7

ICISS (2001) *The Responsibility to Protect: Report of the International Commission on Intervention and State Sovereignty*, available at www.iciss.ca/report-en.asp

Ikenberry, J. (2002) 'National security strategy of the United States of America', *Foreign Affairs*, September–October

India Today (1984) 'Bhopal: City of death', *India Today*, December 31, p6

IPCC (2005) *IPCC Second Assessment Synthesis of Scientific-Technical Information relevant to interpreting Article 2 of the UN Framework Convention on Climate Change*, available at www.ipcc.ch/pub/sarsyn. htm

Jacobson, J. L. and Jacobson, S. W. (1996) 'Intellectual impairment in children exposed to polychlorinated biphenyls in utero', *New England Journal of Medicine*, vol 335, pp783–789

Jansen, M. (2000) 'Children and the right to grow up in an environment provided for and encapsulated in the convention on the rights of the child', in A. Fijalkowski and M. Fitzmaurice (eds) *The Rights of the Child to a Clean Environment*, Ashgate Publishing, Aldershot, pp209–236

Jenkins, M. and Houbé, J. (2004) 'Review of the best practices in Canada and internationally for healthy child development', working paper, Healthy Child Forum, Vancouver, BC

Jensen T. K. (2002) 'Birth defects', in Tamburlini et al (2002), p99

Ji, B., Shu, X. and Linet, S. M. (1997) 'Paternal cigarette smoking and the risk of childhood cancer among offspring of non-smoking mothers', *Journal of National Cancer Institute*, vol 89

Johnsen, D. (1986) 'The creation of fetal rights: Conflicts with women's constitutional rights to liberty, privacy and equal protection', *Yale Law Journal*, vol 95, no 3, January

Jonas, H. (1984) *The Imperative of Responsibility*, University of Chicago Press, Chicago, IL

Jones, C (2000) *Cosmopolitanism*, Oxford University Press, Oxford, pp51–64

Kafka, S. (1984) 'The European chemical industry's view of major hazards legislation', paper presented to the 1984 European Major Hazards Conference, organized by the Oyes Scientific and Technical Service, London, May

Kamm, T. and Greenberger, R. (1995) 'Nigeria executions raise sanction "threat"', *The Wall Street Journal*, November 13, p10

Karr, J. (2000) 'Defining and measuring river health', in Pimentel et al (2000)

Karr, J. and Chu, E. (1995) 'Ecological integrity: Reclaiming lost connections', in Westra and J. Lemons (1995), pp34-48

Karr, J. and Chu, E. (1999) *Restoring Life in Running Waters*, Island Press, Washington, DC

Katz, E. M. (1993) 'Europe's centralized new drug procedures: Is the United States prepared to keep pace?', *Food Drug Law Journal*, no 48, p577

Kay, J. J. and Schneider, E. (1994) 'Embracing complexity: The challenge of the ecosystem approach', *Alternatives*, vol 20, no 3, pp1-6, reprinted in L. Westra and J. Lemons (1995), pp49–59

Kendall, H. W. and D. Pimentel (1994) 'Constraints on the expansion of the global food supply', *AMBIO*, vol 23, no 3, pp1998-2005

Kenney, S. J. (1992) *For Whose Protection? Reproductive Hazards and Exclusionary Policies in the United States and Britain*, University of Michigan Press, Ann Arbor, MI

Kilkenny, U. (1999) *The Child and the European Convention on Human Rights*, Ashgate Publishing, Aldershot, UK, pp18–21

Kindred, H. M., Mickelson, K., Provost, R., McDonald, T. L., de Mistral, A. and Williams, S. A. (2000) *International Law*, 6th edn, Edmond Montgomery Publications, Ottawa

Kingham, R. F., Bogaert, P. W. L. and Eddy, P. S. (1994) 'The new European medicines agency', *Food and Drug Law Journal*, vol 49

Kingsbury, B. (2005) 'The international legal order', New York University School of Law, The Berkeley Electronic Press, http://lsr.mellco.org/nyu/plltwp/papers/6

Kiralfy, A. and Routledge, R. A. (1980) 'An historical perspective of the child without family ties', *Journal of Legal History*, vol 1, p165

Kiss, A. (1989) *Droit International de l'environment*, Pedone, Paris, pp719–727

Kiss, A. and Shelton, D. (1997) *Manual of European Environmental Law*, 2nd edn, Cambridge University Press, Cambridge

Kohn, D. (2004) 'Solvents are linked to drop in kids' IQ', *The Toronto Star*, Friday October 29, pF2

Korten, D. (1995) *When Corporations Rule the World*, Kumarian Press, Hartford, CT

Koskenniemi, M. (1992) 'Breach of treaty or non-compliance? Reflections on the enforcement of the Montreal Protocol', *Yearbook of International Environmental Law*, vol 3, pp123–128

Labbée, X. (1984) 'L'insémination artificielle pratiquée après la mort du donneur', *La Gazette du Palais*, September, pp401–404

Lagrega, M. D., Buckingham, P. L. and Evans, C. J. (1994) *Hazardous Waste Management*, McGraw-Hill, New York

Larschan, B. and Brennan, B. C. (1983) 'The common heritage of mankind principle in international law', *Columbia Journal of Transnational Law*, vol 21, pp305–337

Last, J. M. (1997) *Public Health and Human Ecology*, 2nd edn, Appleton and Lange, Hartford, CT

Last, J. M. (2001) *A Dictionary of Epidemiology*, 4th edn, Oxford University Press, Oxford

Lauterpacht, Sir H. (1968) *International Law and Human Rights*, Archon Books, New York

Laxer, J. (1991) *Inventing Europe: The Rise of a New World Power*, Lester Publications, Toronto

Lazarus, R. (1995) 'A new fault line – mens rea', *Environmental Law*, May/June

Leff, A. (1997) 'The Leff Dictionary of Law: A fragment', *Yale Law Journal*, vol 94, p1855

Leopold, A. (1949) *A Sand County Almanac and Sketches Here and There*, Oxford University Press, New York

Licari, L., Nemer, L. and Tamburlini, G. (2005) *Children's Health and the Environment*, World Health Organization Regional Office for Europe, Copenhagen, Denmark

Linn, S. (2004) *Consuming Kids: The Hostile Takeover of Childhood*, The New Press, New York

Lisi, G. (2003) 'Major accidents involving dangerous substances', 18 June, available at www.europarl.org.uk/news/infocus/seveso2003.htm (accessed March 2005)

Lopen, L. (1987) *Health Promotion: A Discussion Document*, WHO, Geneva, pp5–28

Lutz, R., Nanda, V., Wirth, D., Magraw, D., and Handl, G. (1985) 'International transfer of hazardous technology and substances: Caveat emptor or state responsibility?', *American Society of International Law – Proceedings*, vol 79, pp303–322

Machine, R. (2000) 'Water sewage not a priority for superbuild', *The Globe and Mail*, Canada, June 8, pA7

Majupuria, S. (1993) 'A new theory oil Bhopal leak', *India Abroad*, March 5, p30.

Malhotra, A. (1988) 'A commentary on the status of future generations as a subject of international law', in E. Agius and S. Busuttil (eds) *Future Generations and International Law*, Earthscan, London, pp41–42

Malone, L. A. (1987) 'The Chernobyl accident: A case study in international law regulating state responsibility for transboundary nuclear pollution', *Columbia Journal of Environmental Law*, vol 12, p203

Manson, J. M. (1978) 'Human and laboratory animal test systems available for detection of reproductive failure', *Preventive Medicine*

Marquis, D. (1989) 'Why abortion is immoral', *The Journal of Philosophy*, vol 89, pp183–202

Massager, N. (1996) *Les Droits de l'Enfant à Naître*, Université Libre de Bruxelle, Brussels

Mathiew, D. (1996) *Preventing Prenatal Harm: Should the State Intervene?*, Georgetown University Press, Washington, DC

McBride, S. and Shields, J. (1993) 'Embracing free trade: Embedding neo-liberalism', in *Dismantling a Nation: Canada and the New World Order*, Fernwood, Halifax, NS, pp161–187

McCalman, I., Penny, B. and Cook, M. (1998) *Mad Cows and Modernity*, Humanities Research Centre, Australian National University, Canberra, Australia

McMichael, A. J. (1995a) *Planetary Overload*, Cambridge University Press, Cambridge, UK

McMichael A. J. (1995b) 'The health of persons, populations and planets: Epidemiology comes full circle', *Epidemiology and Society*, Epidemiology Resources, London

McMichael, A. J. (2000) 'Global environment change in the coming century: How sustainable are recent health gains?' in Pimentel et al (2000)

McMichael A. J., Haines, A., Slooff, R., and Kovats, S. (eds) (1996) *Climate Change and Human Health*, WHO Publications, Geneva

Mellon, M. and Fondriest, S. (2001) 'Hogging it: Estimates of animal abuse in livestock', *Nucleus*, vol 23, no 1, Spring

Mémenteau, G. (1983) 'Le prélevement a fins therapeutique sur le fetus *de lege ferenda*', *La Gazette du Palais*, p332

Meulders-Klein, M-T. (1975) 'Le corps humain, personalité jurisique famille en droit belge', *Travaux de l'Association Henry Capitant*, vol 26, p20

Meyer, F. (1987) 'La protection juridique de la vie anténatale', *Revue de Droit, Sanitaire et Sociale*, October–December, p578

Michales, D. (2005) 'Doubt is their product', *Scientific American*, vol 292, no 6, June, pp96–101

Mill, J. S. (1910) *On Liberty*, Everyman Edition, London

Mnookin, R. H. (1985) *In the Interest of Children*, W. Freeman Company, New York

Moffatt, A. (no date) 'Fetal alcohol syndrome, fetal alcohol effects and the impact of alcohol exposure during pregnancy on school performance and behavior in school age children in a First Nation community', unpublished paper on file with author

Morin, M. (1990) 'La competence parens patriae et le droit privé', *Revue de Barreau*, vol 50, no 5

Mowbray, A. (2004) 'European Convention on Human Rights: The issuing of practice directions and recent cases', *Human Rights Law Review*, vol 4, no 1

Murray, T. M. (1996) 'Moral obligations to the not-yet-born: The fetus as a patient', in T. A. Mappes and D. De Grazia (eds) *Biomedical Ethics*, 4th edn, McGraw-Hill, New York, pp464–473

Nanda, V. P. and Bailey, B. C. (1988) 'Export of hazardous waste and hazardous technology: Challenge for international environmental law', *Denver Journal of International law and Policy*, vol 17, pp165–170

Nichter, S. (1973) 'The children of drug users', *Journal of American Academy of Child Psychiatry*, vol 12, no 24

Norton, B. (1995) 'Why I am not a Nonanthropocentrist: Calicott and the failure of monistic inherentism', *Environmental Ethics*, vol 17, Winter

Noss, R. F. (1992) 'The Wildlands Project: Land conservation strategy', *Wild Earth*, Special Issue, pp10–25

Noss, R. F. and Cooperrider, A. Y. (1994) *Saving Nature's Legacy*, Island Press, Washington, DC

Oke, Y. (2005) 'Intergenerational sustainability and traditional knowledge in Africa', paper presented at the Ecological Integrity Conference, Venice, Italy, July 2

O'Neill, J. (1994) *The Missing Child in Liberal Theory*, University of Toronto Press, Toronto, p4

O'Neill, J. S. (1976) *Fetus-in-Law*, Independent Publishing Co., Dunedin, New Zealand

O'Neill, O. (1996) *Towards Justice and Virtue*, Cambridge University Press, Cambridge, UK

Ottawa (2002) www.hrdc.gc.ca/sp-ps/socialp-psociale/cfs/rpt2000/rpt 2000e_toc.shmtl

Palaia, N. (1974) *L'Ordine Pubblico Internazionale*, CEDAM, Padova, Italy, p115

Parfit, D. (1984) *Reasons and Persons*, Oxford University Press, Oxford

Parnet, W. E. (1996) 'From slaughter-house to Lochner: The rise and fall of the constitutionalization of public health', *American Journal of Legal History*, vol 40, p502

Parsons, J. (2000) 'Banality on our dinner plates', unpublished paper presented at Sarah Lawrence College, May

Partridge, E. (1990) 'On the rights of future generations', in D. Scherer (ed) *Upstream/Downstream*, Temple University Press, Philadelphia, PA, pp40–66

Pauly, D. (2000) 'Global change, fisheries, and the integrity of marine ecosystems: The future has already begun', in Pimentel et al (2000)

Pelletier, D. L., Frongillo E. A. and Habicht, J. P. (1993) 'Epidemiologic evidence for a potentiating effect of malnutrition on child mortality', *American Journal of Public Health*, vol 83, no 8, pp1130–1133

Petros-Barzavian, A., 1980, 'Foreword' in F. Falkner (ed) *Prevention in Childhood of Health Problems in Adult Life*, WHO 1960, pvii

Pimentel, D. and Goodland, R. (2000) 'Environmental sustainability and integrity in the agriculture sector', in Pimentel et al (2000), pp121–137

Pimentel D., Tor, M., D'Anna, L. and Krawic, A. (1998) 'Ecology of increasing disease', *Bioscience*, vol 48, no 10, pp817–816

Pimentel, D., Westra, L. and Noss, R. (eds) (2000) *Ecological Integrity: Integrating Environment, Conservation and Health*, Island Press, Washington, DC

Plant, R. (1991) *Modern Political Thought*, Blackwell, Oxford, p290

Plunkett, L. M., Turnbull, D. and Rodricks, J. V. (1992) ' Differences between adults and children affecting exposure assessment', in P. S. Guzelian, C. J. Henry and S. S. Olin (eds) *Similarities and Differences between Children and Adults: Implications for Risk Assessment*, ILSI Press, Washington, DC, pp79–94

Plutarch *Lycurgus*

Pogge, T. W. (2001a) *Global Justice*, Blackwell Publishers, Oxford

Pogge, T. W. (2001b) 'Priorities in global justice', in T. Pogge (ed) *Global Justice*, Blackwell Publishers, Oxford

Pond, K. (2002) 'Waterborne gastrointestinal diseases', in Tamburlini et al (2002), p113

Post, H. (2000) 'The right of the child to a clean environment in European Union law', in A. Fijalkowski and M. Fitzmaurice (eds) *The Right of the Child to a Clean Environment*, Ashgate Publishing, Aldershot, pp61–102

Postiglione, A. (2001) *Giustizia e Ambiente Globale*, Giuffré, Milan, Italy

Postman, N. (1994) *The Disappearance of Childhood*, Vintage, London, pxi

Pritchard, J. and MacDonald, P. (1980) *Williams Obstetrics*, 16th edn, Appleton-Century-Crofts, New York, pvii

Pritchard, J., MacDonald, P. and Gant, N. (1985) *Williams Obstetrics*, 17th edn, Appleton-Century-Crofts, Norwalk, CT

Prosser, W. L. (1964) *Handbook on the Law of Torts*, 3rd edn, West Publishing Co., St Paul, MN

Rachels, J. (1997) 'Vegetarianism and the other weight problem', in L. Pojman (ed.) *Environmental Ethics*, Wadsworth, Belmont, CA, pp367–373

Raffensperger, C. and Tickner, J. (1999) *Protecting Public Health and the Environment (Implementing the Precautionary Principle)*, Island Press, Washington, DC

Ragazzi, M. (1997) *The Concept of International Obligations Erga Omnes*, Clarendon Press, Oxford

Rapport, D. (1995) 'Ecosystem health: More than a metaphor?', *Environmental Values*, vol 4, no 4, pp287–309

Rawls, J. (1971) *A Theory of Justice*, Harvard University Press, Cambridge, MA

Raz, J. (1986) *The Morality of Freedom*, Clarendon Press, Oxford

Rees, W. (2000) 'Patch disturbance, ecofootprints, and biological integrity: Revisiting the limits to growth or why industrial society is inherently unsustainable', in Pimentel et al (2000)

Rees, W. and Westra, L. (2003) 'When consumption does violence: Can there be sustainability and environmental justice in a resource limited world?', in J. Agyeman, R. Evans and R. D. Bullarad (eds) *Just Sustainabilities*, Earthscan, London, pp99–124

Regan, T. (1983) *The Case for Animal Rights*, University of California Press, Berkeley, CA

Rehfuss, E. A. and von Ehrenstein, O. S. (2002) 'Ultraviolet radiation', in Tamburlini et al (2002), p161

Reinisch, A. (2001) 'Governance without accountability', *German Yearbook of International Law*, pp270–306

Remington, J. S. and Klein, J. O. (1976) *Infectious Diseases of the Fetus and Newborn Infant*, Saunders, Philadelphia, PA, pp1–32

Report of the Aboriginal Justice Inquiry of Manitoba (1991) *Report of the Aboriginal Justice Inquiry of Manitoba: The Justice System and Aboriginal People*, Province of Manitoba, Winnipeg

Report of the Presidential Commission (1987) *Report of the Presidential Commission on the Human Immunodeficiency Virus Epidemic*, pXVII

Rice, D. and Barone, S. (2002) 'Critical periods of vulnerability for the developing nervous system: Evidence from human and animal models', *Environmental Health Perspectives*, vol 108, supp 3, pp511–533

Rifkin, J. (1992) *Beyond Beef: The Rise and Fall of the Cattle Culture*, Plume Books, New York

Rifkin, J. (2004) *The European Dream*, Penguin, New York

Rockefeller, S. (2002) 'Foreword' in P. Miller and L. Westra (eds) *Just Ecological Integrity*, Rowman and Littlefield, Lanham, MD, ppx–xiv

Rodriguez-Pineau, E. (1994) 'European Union international *ordre public*', *Spanish Yearbook of International Law*, vol 3, pp43–85

Rossetti, L. (2002) 'The oldest known ecological law in context', in L. Westra and T. Robinson (eds) *Thinking about the Environment: Our Debt to the Ancient and Medieval Past*, Lexington Books, Lanham, MD

Ross, A. (1958) *On Law and Justice*, Stevens and Sons, London

Ruskin, G. (1999) 'Commercial alert, psychologists, psychiatrists call for limits on the use of psychology to influence and exploit children for commercial purposes', press release, September 30

Sachs, J. (2005) *The End of Poverty*, Penguin, New York

Sagoff, M. (1988) *The Economy of the Earth: Philosophy, Law and the Environment*, Cambridge University Press, Cambridge, UK

Sandoz (1996) 'Safety and environmental protection at Sandoz, ten years after Schweizerhalle', report, October

Sands, P. (2005) *Lawless World*, Penguin, New York

Saro-Wiwa, K. (1994a) 'Right Livelihood Award acceptance speech', Right Livelihood Award Foundation, Stockholm, Sweden, December 9

Saro-Wiwa, K. (1994b) 'Human rights, democracy and an African gulag', unpublished talk, New York, March 2

Savitz, D. A. (1989) 'Effects of parents occupational exposures on risk of stillbirth, preterm delivery, and small for gestational age infants', *American Journal of Epidemiology*, vol 129, pp1201–1210

Schabas, W. (2000) *On Genocide*, Kluwer Law Publishers, Dordrecht, The Netherlands

Schindler, D. (2000) *The Globe and Mail*, Canada, June 7, pA5

Schmidt, C. W. (2004) 'Battle scars: Global conflicts and environmental health', *Environmental Health Perspectives*, vol 11, no 1, December

Schmitz, K. L. (2005) 'The ontology of rights', *Ave Maria Law Review*, vol 3, pp275–281

Schor, J. (1999) 'The new politics of consumption: Why Americans want so much more than they need', *Boston Review*, vol 24, no 3–4, Summer

Schroedel, J. R. and Fiber, P. (2004) 'Punitive versus public health oriented responses to drug use by pregnant women', *Yale Journal of Health Policy, Law and Ethics*, vol 1

Schudson, M. (1984) *Advertising the Uneasy Persuasion: Its Dubious Impact*, Basic Books, New York

Scott, C. (2000) *Torture as Tort*, Hart Publishing, Oxford

Scott, C. (2001) 'Interpreting intervention', *The Canadian Yearbook of International Law*, pp333–369

Seck, S. (1999) 'Environmental harm in developing countries caused by subsidiaries of Canadian mining corporations: The interface of public and private international law', *The Canadian Yearbook of International Law*, vol 37, pp139–221

Seidman, L. M. and Tushnet, M. V. (1996) 'Remnants of belief', *Contemporary Constitutional Issues*, vol 52, p54

Seremba, G. (1995) 'Playwright grieves for Saro-Wiwa and Africa', *The Globe and Mail*, Canada, November 18, pH3

Shiva, V. (1989) *Staying Alive*, Zed Books, London

Shiva, V. (2002) *Water Wars*, Between the Lines, Toronto

Shrader-Frechette, K. (1991) *Risk and Rationality*, University of California Press, Berkeley, CA

Shue, H. (1979) 'Rights in the light of duties', in P. G. Brown and D. MacLean (eds) *Human Rights and US Foreign Policy*, Lexington Books, Lexington, MA, p65–84

Shue, H. (1996a) *Basic Rights: Subsistence, Affluence, and American Foreign Policy*, Princeton Univeristy Press, Princeton, NJ

Shue, H. (1996b) 'Solidarity among strangers and the right to food', in H. La Follette and W. Aiken (eds) *World Hunger and Morality*, Prentice-Hall, Upper Saddle River, NJ, pp114–115

Silverstein, D. (1995) 'Nigeria's Ken Saro-Wiwa on trial for his life', Goldman Environmental Prize Foundation, San Francisco, CA, February 23

Simon, D. (1976) 'Ordre public et libertes publiques dans les Communautées Européennes', *Revue Marché Commun*, p221

Simon, J. G., Powers, C. W. and Gunneman, J. P. (1972) *The Ethics of Investment*, Yale University Press, New Haven, CT

Sinclair, M., Bala, N., Lilles, H. and Blackstock, C. (2004) *Canadian Child Welfare Law*, 2nd edn, Thompson Educational Publishers, Toronto

Singer, P. (1975) *Animal Liberation: A New Ethics for Our Treatment of Animals*, Random House, New York

Singer, P. (1995) *How Are We to Live? Ethics in the Age of Self-Interest*, Prometheus Books, Amherst, NY

Singer, P. (2003) 'How can we prevent crimes against humanity?', *Human Rights, Human Wrongs: Oxford Amnesty Lectures 2001*, Oxford University Press, Oxford

Snodgrass, W. R. (1992) 'Physiological and biochemical differences between children and adults as determinants of toxic exposure to environmental pollutants', in P. S. Guzelian, C. J. Henry and S. S. Olin (eds) *Similarities and Differences between Children and Adults: Implications for Risk Assessment*, ILSI Press, Washington, DC, pp35–42

Soskolne, C. (2001) 'International transport of hazardous waste: Legal and illegal trade in the context of Professional Ethics', *Global Bioethics*, vol 1, March, pp3–9

Soskolne, C and Bertollini, R. (1999) 'Ecological integrity and "sustainable development": Cornerstones of public health', discussion document based on an international workshop at the World Health Organization European Centre for Environment and Health, Rome Division, Rome, Italy, 3–4 December 1998, available at www.euro.who.int/document/gch/ecorep5.pdf

Soyinka, W. (1994) 'Nigeria's long, steep, bloody slide', *The New York Times*, August 22

Stedman's Medical Dictionary (1990) *Stedman's Medical Dictionary*, 25th edn, Lippincott, Williams and Wilkins, Hagerstown, MD, pp1139–1140, 1205

Steinbock, B. (1992) *Life Before Birth* , Oxford University Press, Oxford, p92

Sterba, J. (1998) *Justice Here and Now*, Cambridge University Press, Cambridge

Stokes, J., III, Noren, J. J. and Shindell, S. (1997) 'Definition of terms and concepts applicable to clinical preventive medicine', *Journal of Community Health and Human Ecology*, 2nd edn, Appleton and Lange, Harford, CT

Strasser, T. (1978) 'Rheumatic fever and rheumatic heart disease in the 1970s', *WHO Chronicle*, vol 32, pp18–25

Tamburlini, G. (2002) 'Children's special vulnerability to environmental health hazards: An overview', in Tamburlini et al (2002), p18

Tamburlini, G., von Ehrenstein, O. and Bertollini, R. (2002) *Children's Health and Environment: A Review of the Evidence*, EEA Report No.29, World Health Organization, Geneva

Tanzi, A. (1987) 'Diritto di veto ed esecuzione della sentenza della Corte Internazionale di Giustizia fra Nicaragua e Stati Uniti', *Rivista di Diritto Internazionale*, vol 70, no 12, pp293–308

Taylor, A. S. (1861) *Medical Jurisprudence*, 7th edn, London

Taylor, A. L. (1998) 'Globalization and public health: Regulations, norms and standards at the global level', background paper for the Conference on World Health Cooperation, Mexico City, Mexico, March 29–April 1

Taylor, D. (2004) 'Is environmental health a basic human right?', *Environmental Health Perspectives*, vol 112, no 17, December, pA1007

Taylor, P. (1998) 'From environmental to ecological human rights: A new dynamic in international law?', *The Georgetown International Environmental Law Review*, vol 10

Taylor, P. (2004) 'Child neurodevelopmental outcome and maternal occupational exposure to solvents', *Archives of Pediatric and Adolescent Medicine*, vol 158

Terracini, B. (2002) 'Cancer' in Tamburlini et al (2002), p79

Thompson, J., Baird, P. and Downie, J. (2001) *The Olivieri Report*, James Lorimer and Company, Toronto

Thomson, J. J. (1990) *The Realm of Rights*, Harvard University Press, Cambridge, MA

Tickner, J. (1999) 'A map toward precautionary decision making', in J. Tickner and C. Raffensperger (eds) *Protecting Public Health and the Environment*, Island Press, Washington, DC, pp162–186

Timoshenko, A. S. (1994) 'Intergenerational equity: Legal and international implications', in E. Agius, and S. Busuttil (eds) *What Future for Future Generations?*, Union Print, Malta, pp209–215

Tirado, C. (2002) 'Pesticides', in Tamburlini et al (2002), p152

Tobey, J. A. (1926) *Public Health: A Manual of Law for Sanitarians*, Commonwealth Press, New York

Tomuschat, C. (1991) 'International liability for injurious consequences arising out of acts not prohibited by international law: The work of the International Law Commission', in F. Francioni and T. Scovazzi (eds) *International Responsibility for Environmental Harm*, Graham Trottman, UK, pp37–72, 58

Tooley, M. (1983) *Abortion and Infanticide*, Clarendon Press, Oxford

Tridimas, T. (1996) 'The course of justice and judicial activism', *Environmental Law Review*, June, pp199–210

Turman, T., Trocdsson, H. and Stahlhofer, M. (2001) 'A human rights approach to public health: WHO capacity building in the area of children's rights', *Health and Human Rights*, Harvard School of Public Health, vol 5, no 2, pp147–154

Ugelow, J. L. (1982) 'A survey of recent studies on costs of pollution control and the effects on trade', in S. Rubin and T. R. Graham (eds) *Environment and Trade*, Allanheld, Osmun, Totowa, NJ, p167

Ulanowicz, R. (1995) 'Ecosystem integrity: A causal necessity', in L. Westra and J. Lemons (eds) *Perspectives on Ecological Integrity*, Kluwer Academic Press, Dordrecht, The Netherlands, pp 77–87

Ulanowicz, R. (2000) 'Towards the measurement of ecological integrity', in Pimentel et al (2000)

Van Bueren, G. (1995) *The International Law on the Rights of the Child*, Martinus Nijhoff, Leiden, The Netherlands

Velasquez, M. (2000) *Business Ethics: Concepts and Cases*, Prentice Hall, Belmont, CA

Vincent, R. J. (1996) *Human Rights and International Relations*, Cambridge University Press, Cambridge, p90

Visser 't Hooft, H. P. (1999) *Justice to Future Generations and the Environment*, Kluwer Academic Publishers, Dordrecht, The Netherlands

von Ehrenstein, O. S. (2002) 'Asthma, allergies and respiratory health', in Tamburlini et al (2002), p44

Wackernagel, M. and Rees, W. (1996) *Our Ecological Footprint*, New Society Publishers, Gabriola Island, BC, Canada

Wallach, L. and Sforza, M. (1999) *Whose Trade Organization? Corporate Globalization and the Erosion of Democracy: An Assessment of the World Trade Organization*, Public Citizen, Washington, DC

Wanamaker, D. A. (1993) 'From mother to child . . . a criminal pregnancy: Should criminalization of the prenatal transfer of AIDS/HIV be the next step in the battle against the deadly epidemic?', *Dickinson Law Review*, vol 97, Winter

Warren, M-A. (1991) 'On the moral and legal status of abortion', *The Monist*, vol 57, no 1, reprinted in T. Mappes and J. Zembaty (eds), *Biomedical Ethics*, McGraw-Hill, New York, pp438–444

Westfall, D. (1982) 'Beyond abortion: The potential reach of the Human Life Amendment', *American Journal of Law and Medicine*, vol 8, no 2, pp97–135

Westra, L. (1994) *An Environmental Proposal for Ethics*, Rowman and Littlefield, Lanham, MD

Westra, L. (1998) *Living in Integrity*, Rowman and Littlefield, Lanham, MD

Westra, L. (2000a) 'The disvalue of "contingent valuation" and the problem of the "expectation gap"', *Environmental Values*, vol 9, no 2, White Horse Press, Lancaster, UK, pp153–171

Westra, L. (2000b) 'Conclusions', in P. Crabbé, A. Holland, L. Ryszkpwski and L. Westra (eds) *Implementing Ecological Integrity*, NATO Science Series, Kluwer Academic Publishers, Dordrecht, The Netherlands, pp465–476

Westra, L. (2003) 'The ethics of integrity and the law in global governance', *Environs, Environmental Law and Policy Journal*, Fall, vol 27, no 1, p136

Westra, L. (2004a) *Ecoviolence and the Law (Supranational Normative Foundations of Ecocrime)*, Transnational Publishers, Ardsley, New York

Westra, L. (2004b) 'Environmental rights and human rights: The final enclosure movement', in Roger Brownsword (ed) *Global Governance and the Quest for Justice, Vol4: Human Rights*, Hart Publishing, Oxford

Westra, R. (2006) 'Socio-material communication community, and eco-sustainability in the global era', in C. A. Maida (ed) *Sustainability and Communities of Place*, Environmental Anthropology Series (Roy Ellen, ed), Berghahn Books, Oxford and New York

Westra, L. and Lawson, B. (2001) *Faces of Environmental Racism*, 2nd edn, Rowman and Littlefield, Lanham, MD

Westra, L. and Lemons, J. (eds) (1995) *Perspectives on Ecological Integrity*, Kluwer Academic Press, Dordrecht, The Netherlands

Westra, L. and Wenz, P. (1995) *The Faces of Environmental Racism: The Global Equity Issues*, Rowman and Littlefield, Lanham, MD

Wigle, D. T. (2003) *Child Health and the Environment*, Oxford University Press, New York

Williams Obstetrics (1985) *Williams Obstetrics*, 17th edn, J. A. Pritchard, P. C. MacDonald and N. F. Gant (eds) Appleton-Century-Crofts, New York

Williams, G. L. (1948) 'The correlation of allegiance and protection', *Cambridge Law Journal*, vol 10, pp54–76

Wilson, G. H., Murdina, D. and Verniaud, W. M. (1973) 'Early development of infants of heroin-addicted mothers', *American Journal of Diseases of Children*, vol 126, p457

Wolf, L. E., Lo, B. and Gostin, L. (2004) 'Legal barriers to implementing recommendations for universal, routine prenatal HIV testing', *Journal of Law, Medicine and Ethics*, vol 32, pp137–147

Wood, P. (1996) 'Intergenerational equity and climate change', *Georgetown International Environmental Law Review*, vol 8, pp293–307

World Bank (1993) *World Development Report 1993: Investing in Health*, Oxford University Press, New York

World Bank (1999) *Entering the 21st Century: World Development Report 1999/2000*, Oxford University Press, New York

World Health Organization (1980) *Sixth Report on The World Health Situation, 1973-1977*, WHO, Geneva

Zeeman, M. (1996) 'Our fate is connected with the animals', *Bioscience*, vol 46, p542